ECGs MADE EASY

Barbara Aehlert, RN, BSPA
Southwest EMS Education, Inc.

ELSEVIER

Fifth Edition

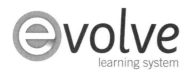
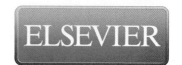
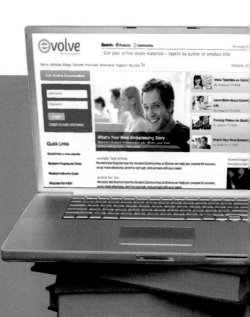

Preface To The Fifth Edition

This book is designed for use by paramedic, nursing, and medical students; ECG monitor technicians; nurses; and other allied health personnel working in emergency departments, critical care units, postanesthesia care units, operating rooms, and telemetry units who wish to master the skill of basic ECG recognition. This book may be used alone or as part of a formal course of instruction in basic dysrhythmia recognition.

The information presented in this book focuses on the essential information you need to know to interpret ECGs and understand their significance. Each ECG rhythm is described and accompanied by a sample rhythm strip. Possible patient signs and symptoms related to the rhythm and, where appropriate, current recommended treatment for the rhythm are discussed. Additional rhythm strips, and their answers, are provided for practice at the end of each chapter. All rhythm strips shown in this text were recorded in lead II unless otherwise noted. The Stop and Review exercises at the end of each chapter are self-assessment exercises that allow the reader to check his or her learning. Green button icons ▶ appearing throughout the text indicate additional content pertaining to the subject that can be found on the Evolve website.

Every attempt has been made to provide information that is consistent with current literature, including current resuscitation guidelines. However, medicine is a dynamic field. Resuscitation guidelines change, new medications and technology are being developed, and medical research is ongoing. As a result, be sure to learn and follow local protocols as defined by your medical advisors.

Best regards,
Barbara Aehlert

3251 Riverport Lane
St. Louis, Missouri 63043

ECGs MADE EASY, FIFTH EDITION   978-0-323-17057-4

Notices

Knowledge and best practice in this field are constantly changing. As new research and experience broaden our understanding, changes in research methods, professional practices, or medical treatment may become necessary.

Practitioners and researchers must always rely on their own experience and knowledge in evaluating and using any information, methods, compounds, or experiments described herein. In using such information or methods they should be mindful of their own safety and the safety of others, including parties for whom they have a professional responsibility.

With respect to any drug or pharmaceutical products identified, readers are advised to check the most current information provided (i) on procedures featured or (ii) by the manufacturer of each product to be administered, to verify the recommended dose or formula, the method and duration of administration, and contraindications. It is the responsibility of practitioners, relying on their own experience and knowledge of their patients, to make diagnoses, to determine dosages and the best treatment for each individual patient, and to take all appropriate safety precautions.

To the fullest extent of the law, neither the Publisher nor the authors, contributors, or editors, assume any liability for any injury and/or damage to persons or property as a matter of products liability, negligence or otherwise, or from any use or operation of any methods, products, instructions, or ideas contained in the material herein.

978-0-323-17057-4

Executive Content Strategist: Jennifer Janson
Associate Content Development Specialist: Andrea Hunolt
Publishing Services Manager: Julie Eddy
Senior Project Manager: Andrea Campbell
Design Direction: Maggie Reid

Printed in the United States of America

Last digit is the print number: 9 8 7 6 5 4 3 2

Acknowledgments

I would like to thank the manuscript reviewers for their comments and suggestions, which helped to improve the clarity of the information presented in this text, and the following healthcare professionals who provided many of the rhythm strips used in this book: Andrew Baird, CEP; James Bratcher; Joanna Burgan, CEP; Holly Button, CEP; Gretchen Chalmers, CEP; Thomas Cole, CEP; Brent Haines, CEP; Paul Honeywell, CEP; Timothy Klatt, RN; Bill Loughran, RN; Andrea Lowrey, RN; Joe Martinez, CEP; Stephanos Orphanidis, CEP; Jason Payne, CEP; Steve Ruehs, CEP; Patty Seneski, RN; David Stockton, CEP; Jason Stodghill, CEP; Dionne Socie, CEP; Kristina Tellez, CEP; and Fran Wojculewicz, RN.

I would also like to thank the editorial and production teams at Elsevier, who continue to provide helpful guidance, humor, and support throughout the development and production of this book and its ancillary materials.

Publisher Acknowledgments

Timothy Scott Brisbin, BSN, RN, NCEE, NREMT-P
Nurse Manager/Team Leader
MedCenter Air
Carolinas Medical Center
Charlotte, North Carolina

Kristen D. Borchelt, RN, CPN, NREMTP
Cincinnati Children's Hospital
Cincinnati, Ohio

John S. Cole, MD, EMT-P
EMS Fellowship Director
Allegheny General Hospital
Pittsburgh, Pennsylvania

Joshua J. Neumiller, PharmD, CDE, CGP, FASCP
Assistant Professor of Pharmacotheraphy
Washington State University
Spokane, Washington

Larry Richmond, AS, NREMT-P, CCEMT-P
Aberdeen Area IHS EMS Program
Rapid City, South Dakota

John N. Schupra, BS, EMT-P I/C, CCEMTP
LIFE EMS Ambulance
Grand Rapids, Michigan

Everett Stephens, MD, FAAEM
University of Louisville, Department of Emergency Medicine
Louisville, Kentucky

About the Author

Barbara Aehlert, RN, BSPA, is the President of Southwest EMS Education, Inc. She has been a registered nurse for more than 35 years with clinical experience in medical/surgical and critical care nursing and prehospital education. Barbara is an active CPR, First Aid, Paramedic, ACLS, and PALS instructor and takes a special interest in teaching basic dysrhythmia recognition and ACLS to nurses and paramedics.

Contents

Anatomy and Physiology

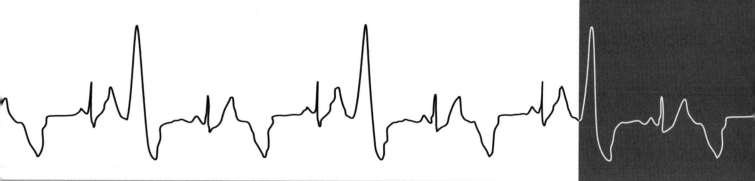

LEARNING OBJECTIVES

After reading this chapter, you should be able to:

1. Describe the location of the heart.
2. Identify the surfaces of the heart.
3. Describe the structure and function of the coverings of the heart.
4. Identify the three cardiac muscle layers.
5. Identify and describe the chambers of the heart and the vessels that enter or leave each.
6. Identify and describe the location of the atrioventricular (AV) and semilunar (SL) valves.
7. Explain atrial kick.
8. Name the primary branches and areas of the heart supplied by the right and left coronary arteries.
9. Define and explain acute coronary syndromes.
10. Discuss myocardial ischemia, injury, and infarction, indicating which conditions are reversible and which are not.
11. Compare and contrast the effects of sympathetic and parasympathetic stimulation of the heart.
12. Identify and discuss each phase of the cardiac cycle.
13. Beginning with the right atrium, describe blood flow through the normal heart and lungs to the systemic circulation.
14. Identify and explain the components of blood pressure and cardiac output.

KEY TERMS

Acute coronary syndrome (ACS): A term used to refer to distinct conditions caused by a similar sequence of pathologic events—a temporary or permanent blockage of a coronary artery; these conditions are characterized by an excessive demand or inadequate supply of oxygen and nutrients to the heart muscle associated with plaque disruption, thrombus formation, and vasoconstriction. ACSs consist of three major syndromes: unstable angina (UA), non–ST-segment elevation myocardial infarction (NSTEMI), and ST-segment elevation myocardial infarction (STEMI)

Adrenergic: Having the characteristics of the sympathetic division of the autonomic nervous system

Afterload: The pressure or resistance against which the ventricles must pump to eject blood

Angina pectoris: Chest discomfort or other related symptoms of sudden onset that may occur because the increased oxygen demand of the heart temporarily exceeds the blood supply

Aortic valve: SL valve on the left of the heart; separates the left ventricle from the aorta

Apex of the heart: Lower portion of the heart that is formed by the tip of the left ventricle

Arteriosclerosis: A chronic disease of the arterial system characterized by abnormal thickening and hardening of the vessel walls

Atherosclerosis: A form of arteriosclerosis in which the thickening and hardening of the vessel walls are caused by a buildup of fatty deposits in the inner lining of large and middle-sized muscular arteries (from *athero*, meaning gruel or paste, and *sclerosis*, meaning hardness)

Atria: Two upper chambers of the heart (singular, atrium)

Atrial kick: Blood pushed into the ventricles because of atrial contraction

Atrioventricular valve: valve located between each atrium and ventricle; the tricuspid separates the right atrium from the right ventricle, and the mitral (bicuspid) separates the left atrium from the left ventricle

Atypical presentation: Uncharacteristic signs and symptoms perceived by some patients experiencing a medical condition, such as an ACS

Base of the heart: Posterior surface of the heart

Blood pressure: Force exerted by the blood against the walls of the arteries as the ventricles of the heart contract and relax

Cardiac output: The amount of blood pumped into the aorta each minute by the heart; defined as the stroke volume multiplied by the heart rate

Catecholamines: Natural chemicals produced by the body that have sympathetic actions; epinephrine, norepinephrine, dopamine

Cholinergic: Having the characteristics of the parasympathetic division of the autonomic nervous system

Chordae tendineae (tendinous cords): Thin strands of fibrous connective tissue that extend from the AV valves to the papillary muscles that prevent the AV valves from bulging back into the atria during ventricular systole (contraction)

Chronotropy: A change in (heart) rate

Circumflex artery: Division of the left coronary artery

Coronary sinus: Outlet that drains five coronary veins into the right atrium

Diastole: Phase of the cardiac cycle in which the atria and ventricles relax between contractions and blood enters these chambers; when the term is used without reference to a specific chamber of the heart, the term implies ventricular diastole

Dromotropy: Refers to the speed of conduction through the AV junction

Dysrhythmia: Any disturbance or abnormality in a normal rhythmic pattern; any cardiac rhythm other than a sinus rhythm

Ejection fraction: The percentage of blood pumped out of a heart chamber with each contraction

Endocardium: Innermost layer of the heart that lines the inside of the myocardium and covers the heart valves

Epicardium: Also known as the visceral pericardium; the external layer of the heart wall that covers the heart muscle

Great vessels: Large vessels that carry blood to and from the heart: superior and inferior venae cavae, pulmonary veins, aorta, and pulmonary trunk

Heart failure: A condition in which the heart is unable to pump enough blood to meet the metabolic needs of the body; it may result from any condition that impairs preload, afterload, cardiac contractility, or heart rate

Hypercapnea: A condition in which there is an elevated concentration of carbon dioxide in the blood

Hypovolemia: Inadequate tissue perfusion caused by inadequate vascular volume

Infarction: Death of tissue because of an inadequate blood supply

Inotropy: Refers to a change in myocardial contractility

Ischemia: Decreased supply of oxygenated blood to a body part or organ

Left anterior descending artery: Division of the left coronary artery

Mediastinum: Middle area of the thoracic cavity; contains the heart, great vessels, trachea, and esophagus, among other structures; extends from the sternum to the vertebral column

Mitochondria: The energy-producing parts of a cell

Myocardium: Middle and thickest layer of the heart; contains the cardiac muscle fibers that cause contraction of the heart and contains the conduction system and blood supply

Myofibril: Slender striated strand of muscle tissue

Neurotransmitter: A chemical released from one nerve that crosses the synaptic cleft to reach a receptor

Pericardium: A double-walled sac that encloses the heart and helps protect it from trauma and infection

Peripheral resistance: Resistance to the flow of blood determined by blood vessel diameter and the tone of the vascular musculature

Preload: Force exerted by the blood on the walls of the ventricles at the end of diastole

Proximal: Location nearer to the midline of the body or the point of attachment than something else is

Pulmonary circulation: Flow of unoxygenated (venous) blood from the right ventricle to the lungs and oxygenated blood from the lungs to the left atrium

Sarcolemma: Membrane that covers smooth, striated, and cardiac muscle fibers

Sarcomere: Smallest functional unit of a myofibril

Sarcoplasm: Semifluid cytoplasm of muscle cells

Sarcoplasmic reticulum: Network of tubules and sacs that plays an important role in muscle contraction and relaxation by releasing and storing calcium ions

Semilunar valves: Valves shaped like half moons that separate the ventricles from the aorta and pulmonary artery

Septum: An internal wall of connective tissue

Shock: Inadequate tissue perfusion that results from the failure of the cardiovascular system to deliver sufficient oxygen and nutrients to sustain vital organ function

Stroke volume: The amount of blood ejected from a ventricle with each heartbeat

Sulcus: Groove

Syncytium: Unit of combined cells

Systole: Contraction of the heart (usually referring to ventricular contraction) during which blood is propelled into the pulmonary artery and aorta; when the term is used without reference to a specific chamber of the heart, the term implies ventricular systole

Tone: A term that may be used when referring to the normal state of balanced tension in body tissues

Venous return: Amount of blood flowing into the right atrium each minute from the systemic circulation

Ventricle: Either of the two lower chambers of the heart

LOCATION, SIZE, AND SHAPE OF THE HEART

[Objective 1]

The heart is a hollow muscular organ that lies in the space between the lungs (i.e., the **mediastinum**) in the middle of the chest (Figure 1-1). It sits behind the sternum and just above the diaphragm. Approximately two thirds of the heart lies to the left of the midline of the sternum. The remaining third lies to the right of the sternum.

The adult heart is approximately 5 inches (12 cm) long, 3.5 inches (9 cm) wide, and 2.5 inches (6 cm) thick (Figure 1-2). It typically weighs between 250 and 350 g (about 11 oz) and is about the size of its owner's fist. The weight of the heart is about 0.45% of a man's body weight and about 0.40% of a woman's. A person's heart size and weight are influenced by their age, body weight and build, frequency of physical exercise, and heart disease. ▶

SURFACES OF THE HEART

[Objective 2]

The **base**, or posterior surface of the heart, is formed by the left atrium, a small portion of the right atrium, and **proximal** portions of the superior and inferior venae cavae and the pulmonary veins (Figure 1-3). The front (anterior) surface of the heart lies behind the sternum and costal cartilages. It is formed by portions of the right atrium and the left and right ventricles (Figure 1-4). However, because the heart is tilted slightly toward the left in the chest, the right ventricle is the area of the heart that lies most directly behind the sternum.

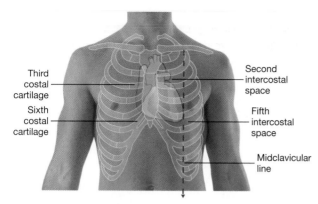

Figure 1-1   Anterior view of the chest wall of a man showing skeletal structures and the surface projection of the heart.

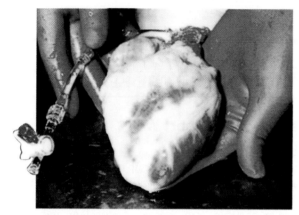

Figure 1-2   Appearance of the heart. This photograph shows a living human heart prepared for transplantation into a patient. Note its size relative to the hands that are holding it.

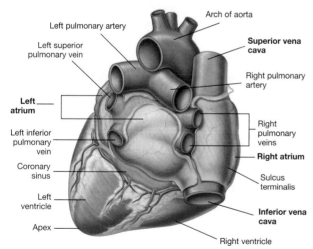

Figure 1-3   The base of the heart.

The heart's **apex**, or lower portion, is formed by the tip of the left ventricle. The apex lies just above the diaphragm at approximately the level of the fifth intercostal space, in the midclavicular line.

The heart's left side (i.e., left lateral surface) faces the left lung and is made up mostly of the left ventricle and a portion

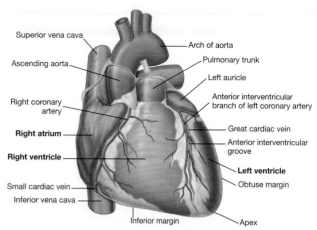

Figure 1-4   The anterior surface of the heart.

of the left atrium. The right lateral surface faces the right lung and consists of the right atrium. The heart's bottom (i.e., inferior) surface is formed primarily by the left ventricle with small portions of the right ventricle and right atrium. The right and left ventricles are separated by a groove containing the posterior interventricular vessels. Because the inferior surface of the heart rests on the diaphragm, it is also called the *diaphragmatic surface* (Figure 1-5).

COVERINGS OF THE HEART

[Objective 3]

The **pericardium** is a double-walled sac that encloses the heart and helps protect it from trauma and infection. The tough outer layer of the pericardial sac is called the *fibrous parietal pericardium* (Figure 1-6). It anchors the heart to some of the structures around it, such as the sternum and diaphragm, by means of ligaments. This helps prevent excessive movement of the heart in the chest with changes in body position.

CLINICAL CORRELATION

The right and left phrenic nerves, which innervate the diaphragm, pass through the fibrous pericardium as they descend to the diaphragm. Because these nerves supply sensory fibers to the fibrous pericardium, the parietal serous pericardium, and the mediastinal pleura, discomfort related to conditions affecting the pericardium may be felt in the areas above the shoulders or lateral neck.

The inner layer of the pericardium, the *serous pericardium*, consists of two layers: parietal and visceral (Figure 1-7). The parietal layer lines the inside of the fibrous pericardium. The visceral layer attaches to the large vessels that enter and exit the heart and covers the outer surface of the heart muscle (i.e., the epicardium).

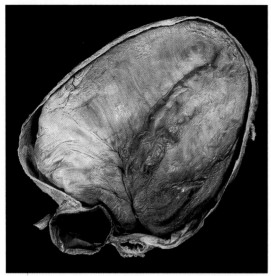 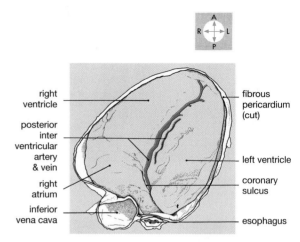

Figure 1-5   The inferior surface of the heart. The inferior part of the fibrous pericardium has been removed with the diaphragm.

Between the visceral and parietal layers is a space (the pericardial space) that normally contains about 20 mL of serous (pale yellow and transparent) fluid. This fluid acts as a lubricant, preventing friction as the heart beats.

CLINICAL CORRELATION

If the pericardium becomes inflamed (pericarditis), excess pericardial fluid can be quickly generated in response to the inflammation. Pericarditis can be caused by a bacterial or viral infection, rheumatoid arthritis, tumors, destruction of the heart muscle in a heart attack, and other causes.

Heart surgery or trauma to the heart, such as a stab wound, can cause a rapid buildup of blood in the pericardial space. The buildup of excess blood or fluid in the pericardial space compresses the heart. This can affect the heart's ability to relax and fill with blood between heartbeats. If the heart cannot adequately fill with blood, the amount of blood the ventricles can pump out to the body (cardiac output) will be decreased. As a result, the amount of blood returning to the heart is also decreased. These changes can result in a life-threatening condition called *cardiac tamponade*. The amount of blood or fluid in the pericardial space needed to impair the heart's ability to fill depends on the rate at which the buildup of blood or fluid occurs and the ability of the pericardium to stretch and accommodate the increased volume of fluid.

The rapid buildup of as little as 100 to 150 mL of fluid or blood can be enough to result in signs and symptoms of shock. Conversely, 1000 mL of fluid may build up over a longer period without any significant effect on the heart's ability to fill. This is because the pericardium accommodates the increased fluid by stretching over time.

The symptoms of cardiac tamponade can be relieved by removing the excess fluid from the pericardial sac. *Pericardiocentesis* is a procedure in which a needle is inserted into the pericardial space and the excess fluid is sucked out (aspirated) through the needle. If scarring is the cause of the tamponade, surgery may be necessary to remove the affected area of the pericardium.

STRUCTURE OF THE HEART

Layers of the Heart Wall

[Objective 4]

The walls of the heart are made up of three tissue layers: the endocardium, myocardium, and epicardium (Figure 1-8, Table 1-1). The heart's innermost layer, the **endocardium**, is made up of a thin, smooth layer of epithelium and connective tissue and lines the heart's inner chambers, valves, chordae tendineae (tendinous cords), and papillary muscles. The endocardium is continuous with the innermost layer of the arteries, veins, and capillaries of the body, thereby creating a continuous, closed circulatory system.

The **myocardium** (middle layer) is a thick, muscular layer that consists of cardiac muscle fibers (cells) responsible for the pumping action of the heart. The myocardium is subdivided into two areas. The innermost half of the myocardium is called the *subendocardial area*. The outermost half is called the *subepicardial area*. The muscle fibers of the myocardium are separated by connective tissues that have a rich supply of capillaries and nerve fibers.

Did You Know?

The thickness of a heart chamber is related to the amount of pressure or resistance that the muscle of the chamber must overcome to eject blood.

The heart's outermost layer is called the **epicardium**. The epicardium is continuous with the inner lining of the pericardium at the heart's apex. The epicardium contains blood capillaries, lymph capillaries, nerve fibers, and fat. The main coronary arteries lie on the epicardial surface of the heart. They feed this area first before entering the myocardium and supplying the heart's inner layers with oxygenated blood. **Ischemia** is a decreased supply of oxygenated blood to a

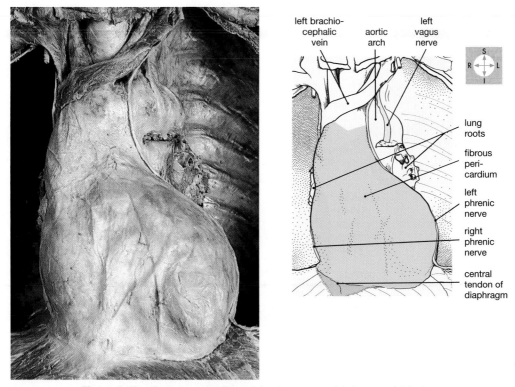

Figure 1-6   The fibrous pericardium and phrenic nerves revealed after removal of the lungs.

Labels for Figure 1-6:
- left brachio-cephalic vein
- aortic arch
- left vagus nerve
- lung roots
- fibrous peri-cardium
- left phrenic nerve
- right phrenic nerve
- central tendon of diaphragm

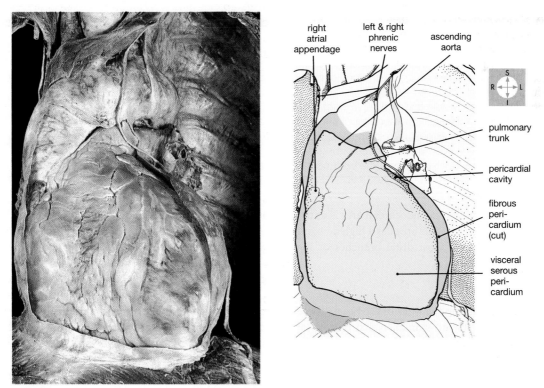

Figure 1-7   The fibrous pericardium has been opened to expose the visceral pericardium covering the anterior surface of the heart.

Labels for Figure 1-7:
- right atrial appendage
- left & right phrenic nerves
- ascending aorta
- pulmonary trunk
- pericardial cavity
- fibrous peri-cardium (cut)
- visceral serous peri-cardium

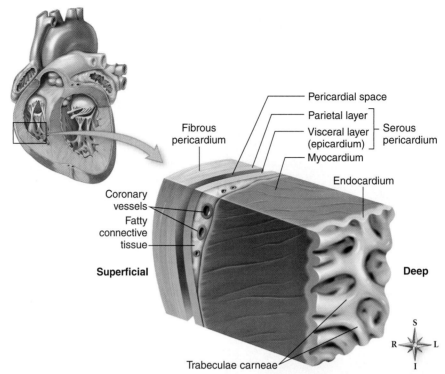

Figure 1-8   Wall of the heart. The cutout section of the heart wall shows the outer fibrous pericardium and the parietal and visceral layers of the serous pericardium (with the pericardial space between them). Note that a layer of fatty connective tissue is located between the visceral layer of the serous pericardium (epicardium) and the myocardium. Note also that the endocardium covers beamlike projections of myocardial muscle tissue, called *trabeculae carneae* (meaning "fleshy beams") that help to add force to the inward contraction of the heart wall.

Table 1-1	Layers of the Heart Wall
Heart Layer	**Description**
Epicardium	• External layer of the heart • Coronary arteries, blood capillaries, lymph capillaries, nerve fibers nerves, and fat are found in this layer
Myocardium	• Middle and thickest layer of the heart • Muscular component of the heart; responsible for the heart's pumping action
Endocardium	• Innermost layer of the heart • Lines heart's inner chambers, valves, chordae tendineae, and papillary muscles • Continuous with the innermost layer of arteries, veins, and capillaries of the body

body part or organ. The heart's subendocardial area is at the greatest risk of ischemia because this area has a high demand for oxygen and is fed by the most distal branches of the coronary arteries.

Cardiac Muscle

Cardiac muscle fibers make up the walls of the heart. These fibers have striations, or stripes, similar to that of skeletal muscle. Each muscle fiber is made up of many muscle cells (Figure 1-9, A). Each muscle cell is enclosed in a membrane called a **sarcolemma**. Within each cell (as with all cells) are **mitochondria**, the energy-producing parts of a cell, and hundreds of long, tube-like structures called **myofibrils**. Myofibrils are made up of many **sarcomeres**, the basic protein units responsible for contraction. The process

of contraction requires adenosine triphosphate (ATP) for energy. The mitochondria that are interspersed between the myofibrils are important sites of ATP production.

The sarcolemma has holes in it that lead into tubes called *T (transverse) tubules*. T tubules are extensions of the cell membrane. Another system of tubules, the **sarcoplasmic reticulum** (SR), stores calcium. Muscle cells need calcium in order to contract. Calcium is moved from the sarcoplasm of the muscle cell into the SR by means of "pumps" in the SR.

There are certain places in the cell membrane where sodium (Na^+), potassium (K^+), and calcium (Ca^{++}) can pass. These openings are called *pores* or *channels*. There are specific channels for sodium (sodium channels), potassium (potassium channels), and calcium (calcium channels).

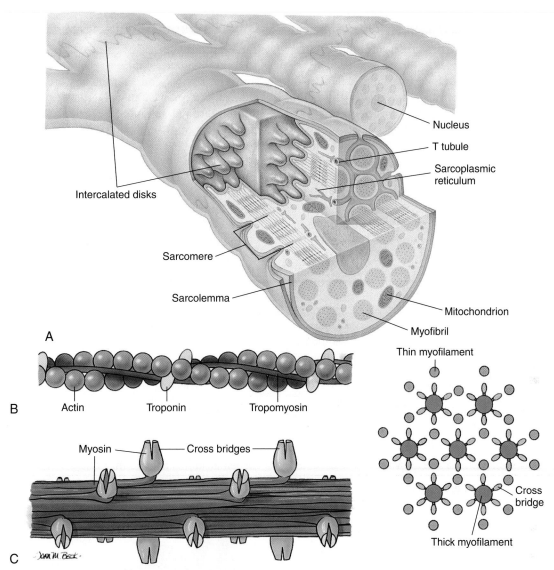

Nucleus

T tubule

Sarcoplasmic reticulum

Intercalated disks

Sarcomere

Sarcolemma

Mitochondrion

Myofibril

A

Thin myofilament

Actin Troponin Tropomyosin

B

Myosin Cross bridges

Cross bridge

Thick myofilament

C

Figure 1-9 **A,** Cardiac muscle fiber. Unlike other types of muscle fibers, the cardiac muscle fiber is typically branched and forms junctions, called *intercalated disks*, with adjacent cardiac muscle fibers. **B,** Thin myofilament. **C,** Thick myofilament.

When the muscle is relaxed, the calcium channels are closed. As a result, calcium cannot pass through the membrane of the SR. This results in a high concentration of calcium in the SR and a low concentration in the sarcoplasm, where the muscle cells (sarcomeres) are found. If the muscle cells do not have calcium available to them, contraction is inhibited (the muscle stays relaxed).

T tubules pass completely through the sarcolemma and go around the muscle cells. The job of the T tubules is to conduct impulses from the cell's surface (sarcolemma) down into the cell to the SR. When an impulse travels along the membrane of the SR, the calcium channels open. Calcium rapidly leaves the SR and enters the sarcoplasm. The muscle cells are then stimulated to contract.

Much of the calcium that enters the cell's sarcoplasm comes from the interstitial fluid surrounding the cardiac muscle cells through the T tubules. This is important because without the extra calcium from the T tubules, the strength of a cardiac muscle contraction would be considerably reduced. Thus, the force of cardiac muscle contraction depends largely on the concentration of calcium ions in the extracellular fluid.

Each sarcomere is composed of thin filaments and thick filaments. The thin filaments are made up of actin and actin-binding proteins. Actin-binding proteins include tropomyosin and troponin-T, troponin-C, and troponin-I, among others. The thick filaments are made up of hundreds of myosin molecules. Contraction occurs when the muscle is stimulated. Projections on the thin actin filaments (Figure 1-9, B) interact with the thick myosin filaments and form crossbridges (Figure 1-9, C). The crossbridges use energy (ATP) to bend. This allows the actin filaments to slide over the myosin filaments toward the center of the sarcomere and overlap. This overlap causes shortening of the muscle cells, resulting in contraction. Actin-binding proteins hinder the formation of crossbridges with myosin. When crossbridge formation is hindered, the muscle is relaxed.

Cardiac muscle fibers are long branching cells that fit together tightly at junctions called *intercalated disks*. The arrangement of these tight-fitting junctions gives an appearance of a **syncytium**, that is, resembling a network of cells with no separation between the individual cells. The intercalated disks fit together in such a way that they form *gap junctions*. Gap junctions allow cells to communicate with each other. They function as electrical connections and permit the exchange of nutrients, metabolites, ions, and small molecules. As a result, an electrical impulse can be quickly conducted throughout the wall of a heart chamber. This characteristic allows the walls of both atria (likewise, the walls of both ventricles) to contract almost at the same time.

ECG Pearl

The heart consists of two syncytiums: atrial and ventricular. The *atrial syncytium* consists of the walls of the right and left atria. The *ventricular syncytium* consists of the walls of the right and left ventricles. Normally, impulses can be conducted only from the atrial syncytium into the ventricular syncytium by means of the atrioventricular (AV) junction. The AV junction is a part of the heart's electrical system. This allows the atria to contract a short time before ventricular contraction.

Heart Chambers and Valves

The heart has four chambers, two atria and two ventricles. The outside surface of the heart has grooves called *sulci*. The coronary arteries and their major branches lie in these grooves. The coronary **sulcus** (groove) encircles the outside of the heart and separates the atria from the ventricles. It contains the coronary blood vessels and epicardial fat. ▶

Atria
[Objective 5]

The two upper chambers of the heart are the right and left **atria** (singular, *atrium*) (Figure 1-10). An earlike flap called an *auricle* (meaning "little ear") protrudes from each atrium.

The purpose of the atria is to *receive* blood. The right atrium receives blood low in oxygen from the superior vena cava (which carries blood from the head and upper extremities), the inferior vena cava (which carries blood from the lower body), and the coronary sinus, which is the largest vein that drains the heart. The left atrium receives freshly oxygenated blood from the lungs via the right and left pulmonary veins.

The four chambers of the heart vary in muscular wall thickness, reflecting the degree of pressure each chamber must generate to pump blood. For example, the atria encounter little resistance when pumping blood to the ventricles. As a result, the atria have a thin myocardial layer. The wall of the right atrium is about 2 mm thick and the wall of the left atrium is about 3 mm thick. Blood is pumped from

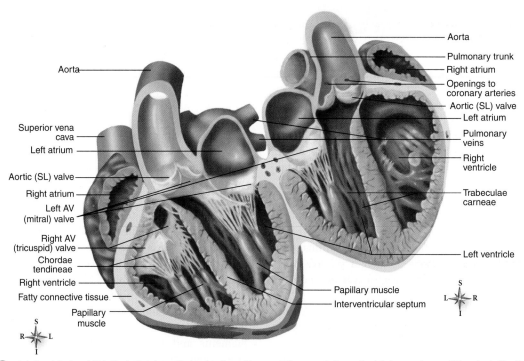

Figure 1-10   Interior of the heart. This illustration shows the heart as it would appear if it were cut along a frontal plane and opened like a book. The front portion of the heart lies to the reader's right; the back portion of the heart lies to the reader's left. (Note each portion has a separate anatomical rosette to facilitate orientation.) The four chambers of the heart—two atria and two ventricles—are easily seen. AV, atrioventricular; SL, semilunar.

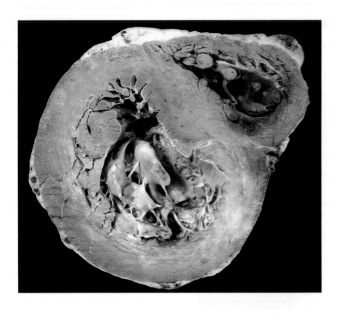
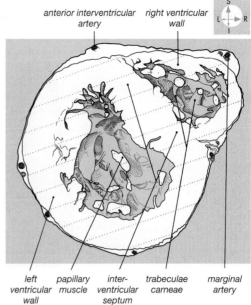

anterior interventricular artery   right ventricular wall

left ventricular wall   papillary muscle   inter-ventricular septum   trabeculae carneae   marginal artery

Figure 1-11 Section through the heart showing the apical portions of the left and right ventricles.

the atria through an AV valve and into the ventricles. The valves of the heart are discussed later in this chapter.

ECG Pearl

Think of the atria as "holding tanks" or "reservoirs" for blood.

Ventricles

[Objective 5]

The heart's two lower chambers are the right and left ventricles. Their purpose is to *pump* blood. The right ventricle pumps blood to the lungs. The left ventricle pumps blood out to the body. Because the ventricles must pump blood to either the lungs (the right ventricle) or to the rest of the body (the left ventricle), the ventricles have a much thicker myocardial layer than the atria. The wall of the left ventricle is three times thicker than that of the right because the left ventricle propels blood to most vessels of the body (Figure 1-11). The right ventricle moves blood only through the blood vessels of the lungs and then into the left atrium.

CLINICAL CORRELATION

When the left ventricle contracts, it normally produces an impulse that can be felt at the apex of the heart (*apical impulse*). This occurs because as the left ventricle contracts, it rotates forward. In a normal heart, this causes the apex of the left ventricle to hit the chest wall. You may be able to see the apical impulse in thin individuals. The apical impulse is also called the *point of maximal impulse* (PMI) because it is the site where the left ventricular contraction is most strongly felt.

Heart Valves

The heart has a skeleton, which is made up of four rings of thick connective tissue. This tissue surrounds the bases of the pulmonary trunk, the aorta, and the heart valves. The inside of the rings provides secure attachments for the heart valves. The outside of the rings provides for the attachment of the cardiac muscle of the myocardium (Figure 1-12). The heart's skeleton also helps form the partitions (septa) that separate the atria from the ventricles.

There are four one-way valves in the heart: two sets of AV valves and two sets of SL valves. The valves open and close in a specific sequence and assist in producing the pressure gradient needed between the chambers to ensure a smooth flow of blood through the heart and prevent the backflow of blood.

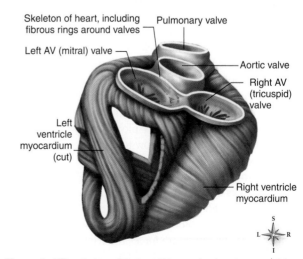

Skeleton of heart, including fibrous rings around valves   Pulmonary valve

Left AV (mitral) valve   Aortic valve

Right AV (tricuspid) valve

Left ventricle myocardium (cut)

Right ventricle myocardium

Figure 1-12 Skeleton of the heart. This posterior view shows part of the ventricular myocardium with the heart valves still attached. The rim of each heart valve is supported by a fibrous structure, called *the skeleton of the heart*, which encircles all four valves. *AV*, Atrioventricular.

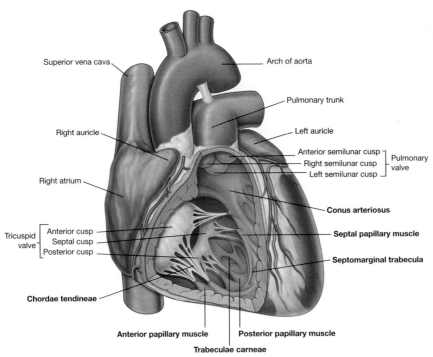

Figure 1-13   Internal view of the right ventricle.

Atrioventricular Valves

[Objectives 6, 7]

Atrioventricular (AV) valves separate the atria from the ventricles. The two AV valves consist of the following:

- Tough, fibrous rings (annuli fibrosi)
- Flaps (leaflets or cusps) of endocardium
- Chordae tendineae
- Papillary muscles

The tricuspid valve is the AV valve that lies between the right atrium and right ventricle. It consists of three separate cusps or flaps (Figure 1-13). It is larger in diameter and thinner than the mitral valve. The mitral valve, which is also called the *bicuspid valve*, has only two cusps and lies between the left atrium and left ventricle (Figure 1-14). The mitral valve is so named because of its resemblance to a miter, which is a double-cusp bishop's hat, when open.

The AV valves open when a forward pressure gradient forces blood in a forward direction. They close when a backward pressure gradient pushes blood backward. The AV valves require almost no backflow to cause closure.[1]

The flow of blood from the superior and inferior venae cavae into the atria is normally continuous. About 70% of this blood flows directly through the atria and into the ventricles before the atria contract; this is called *passive filling*. As the atria fill with blood, the pressure within the atrial chamber rises. This pressure forces the tricuspid and mitral valves open and the ventricles begin to fill, gradually increasing the pressure within the ventricles. When the atria contract, an additional 10% to 30% of the returning blood is added to filling of the ventricles. This additional contribution

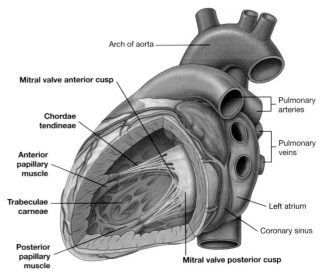

Figure 1-14   Internal view of the left ventricle.

of blood resulting from atrial contraction is called **atrial kick**. On the right side of the heart, blood low in oxygen empties into the right ventricle. On the left side of the heart, freshly oxygenated blood empties into the left ventricle. When the ventricles then contract (i.e., systole), the pressure within the ventricles rises sharply. The tricuspid and mitral valves completely close when the pressure within the ventricles exceeds that of the atria.

Chordae tendineae are thin strands of connective tissue. On one end, they are attached to the underside of the

AV valves. On the other end, they are attached to small mounds of myocardium called **papillary muscles**. Papillary muscles project inward from the lower portion of the ventricular walls. When the ventricles contract and relax, so do the papillary muscles. The papillary muscles adjust their tension on the chordae tendineae, preventing them from bulging too far into the atria. For example, when the right ventricle contracts, the papillary muscles of the right ventricle pull on the chordae tendineae. The chordae tendineae prevent the flaps of the tricuspid valve from bulging too far into the right atrium. Thus, the chordae tendineae and papillary muscles serve as anchors. Because the chordae tendineae are thin and string-like, they are sometimes called *heart strings*.

Semilunar Valves
[Objective 6]
The pulmonic and aortic valves are **SL valves**. The SL valves prevent the backflow of blood from the aorta and pulmonary arteries into the ventricles. The SL valves have three cusps shaped like half-moons. The openings of the SL valves are smaller than the openings of the AV valves and the flaps of the SL valves are smaller and thicker than the AV valves. Unlike the AV valves, the SL valves are not attached to chordae tendineae.

When the ventricles contract, the SL valves open, allowing blood to flow out of the ventricles. When the right ventricle contracts, blood low in oxygen flows through the pulmonic valve into the pulmonary trunk, which divides into the right and left pulmonary arteries. When the left ventricle contracts, freshly oxygenated blood flows through the aortic valve into the aorta and out to the body (Figure 1-15). The SL valves close as ventricular contraction ends and the pressure in the pulmonary artery and aorta exceeds that of the ventricles.

CLINICAL CORRELATION

Blood flow through the heart can be hampered if a valve does not function properly. *Valvular heart disease* is the term used to describe a malfunctioning heart valve. Types of valvular heart disease include the following:

- *Valvular prolapse.* If a valve flap inverts, it is said to *prolapse*. Prolapse can occur if one valve flap is larger than the other is. It can also occur if the chordae tendineae stretch markedly or rupture.
- *Valvular regurgitation.* Blood can flow backward, or regurgitate, if one or more of the heart's valves does not close properly. Valvular regurgitation is also known as *valvular incompetence* or *valvular insufficiency*.
- *Valvular stenosis.* If a valve narrows, stiffens, or thickens, the valve is said to be *stenosed*. The heart must work harder to pump blood through a stenosed valve.

Papillary muscles receive their blood supply from the coronary arteries. If a papillary muscle ruptures because of an inadequate blood supply (as in a **myocardial infarction [MI]**), the attached valve cusps will not completely close and may result in a *murmur*. If a papillary muscle in the left ventricle ruptures, the leaflets of the mitral valve may invert (i.e., prolapse). This may result in blood leaking from the left ventricle into the left atrium (e.g., regurgitation) during ventricular contraction. Blood flow to the body (i.e., cardiac output) could be decreased as a result.

Heart Sounds

Heart sounds occur because of vibrations in the tissues of the heart caused by the closing of the heart's valves. Vibrations are created as blood flow is suddenly increased or slowed with the contraction and relaxation of the heart

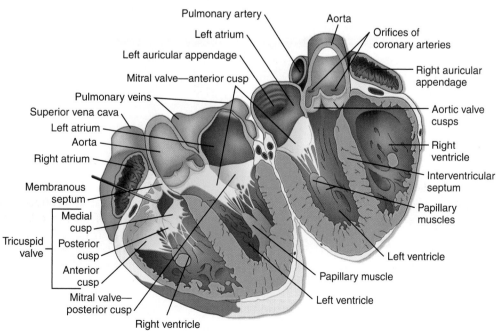

Figure 1-15   Drawing of a heart split perpendicular to the interventricular septum to illustrate the anatomic relationships of the leaflets of the atrioventricular and aortic valves.

chambers and with the opening and closing of the valves. The location of the heart's AV and SL valves for auscultation is shown in Figure 1-16. A summary of the heart's valves and auscultation points for heart sounds appears in Table 1-2. ▶

CLINICAL CORRELATION

Normal heart sounds are called *S1* and *S2*. (S1 = sound one; S2 = sound two). The first heart sound ("lubb") occurs during ventricular contraction when the tricuspid and mitral (atrioventricular [AV]) valves are closing. The second heart sound ("dupp") occurs during ventricular relaxation when the pulmonic and aortic (semilunar [SL]) valves are closing.

A third heart sound is produced by ventricular filling. In persons younger than 40 years of age, the left ventricle normally permits rapid filling. The more rapid the ventricular filling, the greater the likelihood of hearing a third heart sound. A third heart sound (S3) heard in persons older than 40 years of age is considered abnormal. An abnormal third heart sound is frequently associated with heart failure. An S1-S2-S3 sequence is called a *ventricular gallop* or *gallop rhythm.* It sounds like Ken (S1)–tuck (S2)–y (S3).

Turbulent blood flow within the cardiac chambers and vessels can produce *heart murmurs.* An inflamed pericardium can produce a *pericardial friction rub,* which sounds like rough sandpaper.

The Heart's Blood Supply

The coronary circulation consists of coronary arteries and veins. The right and left coronary arteries encircle the myocardium like a crown, or corona.

Coronary Arteries
[Objective 8]

The main coronary arteries lie on the outer (epicardial) surface of the heart. Coronary arteries that run on the surface of the heart are called *epicardial coronary arteries.* They branch into progressively smaller vessels, eventually becoming arterioles, and then capillaries. Thus, the epicardium has a rich blood supply to draw from. Branches of the main coronary arteries penetrate into the heart's muscle mass and supply the subendocardium with blood. The diameter of these "feeder branches" (i.e., collateral circulation) is much narrower. The tissue supplied by these "feeder branches" gets enough blood and oxygen to survive, but they do not have much extra blood flow.

The work of the heart is important. To ensure that it has an adequate blood supply, the heart makes sure to provide itself with a fresh supply of oxygenated blood before supplying the rest of the body. This freshly oxygenated blood is supplied mainly by the branches of two vessels: the right and left coronary arteries.

The right and left coronary arteries are the very first branches off the base of the aorta. The openings to these

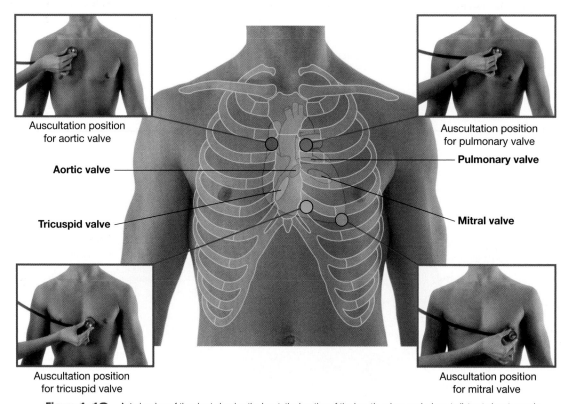

Auscultation position for aortic valve

Auscultation position for pulmonary valve

Aortic valve

Pulmonary valve

Tricuspid valve

Mitral valve

Auscultation position for tricuspid valve

Auscultation position for mitral valve

Figure 1-16   Anterior view of the chest showing the heart, the location of the heart's valves, and where to listen to heart sounds.

Table 1-2 Heart Valves and Auscultation Points

Valve Name	Valve Type	Location	Auscultation Point
Tricuspid	Atrioventricular	Separates right atrium and right ventricle	Just to the left of the lower part of the sternum near fifth intercostal space
Mitral (bicuspid)	Atrioventricular	Separates left atrium and left ventricle	Heart apex in left fifth intercostal space at midclavicular line
Pulmonic (pulmonary)	Semilunar	Between right ventricle and pulmonary artery	Left second intercostal space close to sternum
Aortic	Semilunar	Between left ventricle and aorta	Right second intercostal space close to sternum

vessels lie just beyond the cusps of the aortic SL valve. When the left ventricle contracts (systole) the force of the pressure within the left ventricle pushes blood into the arteries that branch from the aorta. This causes the arteries to fill. However, the heart's blood vessels (i.e., the coronary arteries) are compressed during ventricular contraction, reducing blood flow to the tissues of the heart. Thus, the coronary arteries fill when the aortic valve is closed and the left ventricle is relaxed (i.e., diastole).

The three major coronary arteries include the left anterior descending (LAD) artery, circumflex (CX) artery, and the right coronary artery (RCA). A person is said to have coronary artery disease (CAD) if there is more than 50% diameter narrowing (i.e., stenosis) in one or more of these vessels.

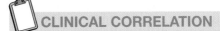

CLINICAL CORRELATION

Because a heart attack, which is also called a *myocardial infarction*, is usually caused by a blocked coronary artery, it is worthwhile to become familiar with the arteries that supply the heart. When myocardial ischemia or infarction is suspected, an understanding of coronary artery anatomy and the areas of the heart that each vessel supplies makes it possible to predict the coronary artery blocked and the problems that can be anticipated related to blockage of that vessel.

Right Coronary Artery

The RCA originates from the right side of the aorta (Figure 1-17. It travels along the groove between the right atrium and

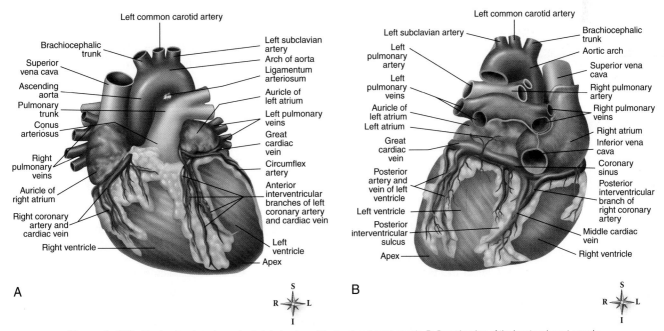

Figure 1-17 The heart and great vessels. **A,** Anterior view of the heart and great vessels. **B,** Posterior view of the heart and great vessels.

right ventricle. A branch of the RCA supplies the following structures:

- Right atrium
- Right ventricle
- Inferior surface of the left ventricle in about 85% of individuals
- Posterior surface of the left ventricle in 85%
- Sinoatrial (SA) node in about 60%
- AV bundle in 85% to 90%

Left Coronary Artery

The left coronary artery (LCA) originates from the left side of the aorta (see Figure 1-17). The first segment of the LCA is called the *left main coronary artery*. It is about the width of a soda straw and less than an inch long. Blockage of the left main coronary artery has been referred to as the *widow maker* because of its association with sudden cardiac arrest when it is blocked.

The left main coronary artery supplies oxygenated blood to its two primary branches: the LAD, which is also called the *anterior interventricular artery*, and the CX. These vessels are slightly smaller than the left main coronary artery.

The LAD can be seen on the outer (i.e., epicardial) surface on the front of the heart. It travels along the groove that lies between the right and left ventricles (i.e., the anterior interventricular sulcus) toward the heart's apex. In most patients, the LAD travels around the apex of the left ventricle and ends along the left ventricle's inferior surface. In the remaining patients, the LAD does not reach the inferior surface. Instead, it stops at or before the heart's apex. The major branches of the LAD are the septal and diagonal arteries. The septal branches of the LAD supply blood to the interventricular septum. The LAD supplies blood to the following:

- The anterior surface of the left ventricle
- Part of the lateral surface of the left ventricle
- The anterior two thirds of the interventricular septum

The CX coronary artery circles around the left side of the heart in a groove on the back of the heart that separates the left atrium from the left ventricle called the *coronary sulcus* (see Figure 1-17). The CX supplies blood to the following:

- The left atrium
- Part of the lateral surface of the left ventricle
- The inferior surface of the left ventricle in about 15% of individuals
- The posterior surface of the left ventricle in 15%
- The SA node in about 40%
- The AV bundle in 10% to 15%

A summary of the areas of the heart supplied by the three major coronary arteries is shown in Table 1-3.

Coronary Artery Dominance

In about 50% of people, the RCA forms the posterior descending artery. In about 20% of people, the circumflex artery forms the posterior descending artery. The coronary artery that forms the posterior descending artery is considered the *dominant* coronary artery. If a branch of the RCA becomes the posterior descending artery, the coronary artery arrangement is described as a *right dominant system*. If the CX branches and ends at the posterior descending artery, the coronary artery arrangement is described as a *left dominant system*. In about 30% of people, neither coronary artery is dominant. If damage to the posterior wall of the left ventricle is suspected, a cardiac catheterization usually is necessary to determine which coronary artery is involved.

Acute Coronary Syndromes

[Objectives 9, 10]

Acute coronary syndrome is a term that is used to refer to distinct conditions caused by a similar sequence of pathologic events and that involve a temporary or permanent blockage of a coronary artery. This sequence of events results in conditions that range from myocardial ischemia or injury

Table **1-3** Coronary Arteries		
Coronary Artery	**Portion of Myocardium Supplied**	**Portion of Conduction System Supplied**
Right	• Right atrium • Right ventricle • Inferior surface of left ventricle (about 85%)* • Posterior surface of left ventricle (85%)*	• Sinoatrial (SA) node (about 60%)* • Atrioventricular (AV) bundle (85% to 90%)*
Left anterior descending	• Anterior surface of left ventricle • Part of lateral surface of left ventricle • Anterior two thirds of interventricular septum	• Most of right bundle branch • Anterior-superior fascicle of left bundle branch • Part of posterior-inferior fascicle of left bundle branch
Circumflex	• Left atrium • Part of lateral surface of left ventricle • Inferior surface of left ventricle (about 15%)* • Posterior surface of left ventricle (15%)*	• SA node (about 40%)* • AV bundle (10% to 15%)*

*Of population.

to death (i.e., necrosis) of the heart muscle. The usual cause of an ACS is the rupture of an atherosclerotic plaque. **Arteriosclerosis** is a chronic disease of the arterial system characterized by abnormal thickening and hardening of the vessel walls. **Atherosclerosis** is a form of arteriosclerosis in which the thickening and hardening of the vessel walls are caused by a buildup of fat-like deposits (e.g., plaque) in the inner lining of large and middle-sized muscular arteries. As the fatty deposits build up, the opening of the artery slowly narrows and blood flow to the muscle decreases (Figure 1-18).

The complete blockage of a coronary artery may cause a myocardial infarction (MI). However, because a plaque usually increases in size over months and years, other vascular pathways may enlarge as portions of a coronary artery become blocked. These vascular pathways (i.e., collateral circulation) serve as an alternative route for blood flow around the blocked artery to the heart muscle; thus the presence of collateral arteries may prevent infarction despite complete blockage of the primary artery.

CLINICAL CORRELATION

Any artery in the body can develop atherosclerosis. If the coronary arteries are involved (i.e., coronary artery disease [CAD]) and if blood flow to the heart is decreased, angina pectoris or more serious signs and symptoms may result. If the arteries in the leg are involved (i.e., peripheral vascular disease), leg pain (i.e., claudication) may result. If the arteries supplying the brain are involved (i.e., carotid artery disease), a stroke or transient ischemic attack (TIA) may result.

Angina pectoris is chest discomfort or other related symptoms of sudden onset that may occur because the increased oxygen demand of the heart temporarily exceeds the blood supply. Angina is not a disease. Rather, it is a symptom of myocardial ischemia. Angina most often occurs in patients with CAD that involves at least one coronary artery. However, it can be present in patients with normal coronary arteries. Angina also occurs in persons with uncontrolled high blood pressure or valvular heart disease. Possible causes of myocardial ischemia are shown in Box 1-1.

The term *angina* refers to squeezing or tightening rather than pain. The discomfort that is associated with angina occurs because of the stimulation of nerve endings by lactic acid and carbon dioxide that builds up in ischemic tissue. Examples of common words and phrases used by patients experiencing angina to describe the sensation they are feeling include "heaviness," "squeezing," "a band across my chest," "a weight in the center of my chest," and "a vise tightening around my chest."

Chest discomfort associated with myocardial ischemia usually begins in the central or left chest and then radiates to the arm (especially the little finger [ulnar] side of the left arm), the wrist, the jaw, the epigastrium, the left shoulder, or between the shoulder blades. Ischemic chest discomfort is usually not sharp; it is not worsened by deep inspiration, it is not affected by moving muscles in the area where the discomfort is localized, nor is it positional in nature. Other symptoms associated with ACSs include shortness of breath, sweating, nausea, vomiting, dizziness, and discomfort in other areas of the upper body.[2]

Not all patients experiencing an ACS present similarly. **Atypical presentation** refers to the uncharacteristic signs and symptoms that are experienced by some patients. Atypical chest discomfort is localized to the chest area but may have musculoskeletal, positional, or pleuritic features.

Patients who are experiencing an ACS who are most likely to present atypically include older adults, diabetic individuals, women, patients with prior cardiac surgery, and patients during the immediate postoperative period after noncardiac surgery.[3] Older adults may have atypical symptoms such

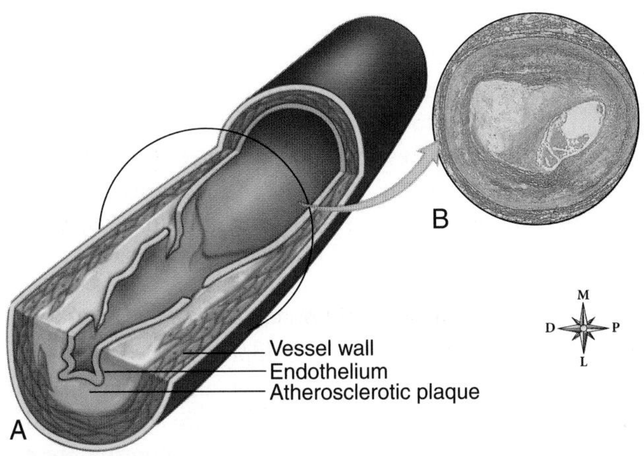

Figure 1-18 Partial blockage of an artery in atherosclerosis. **A,** Atherosclerotic plaque develops from the deposition of fats and other substances in the wall of the artery—a classic symptom of peripheral vascular disease. **B,** Photograph of a cross section of an artery showing partial blockage of lumen by atherosclerotic plaque.

Vessel wall
Endothelium
Atherosclerotic plaque

Box **1-1**	Possible Causes of Myocardial Ischemia
Inadequate Oxygen Supply	**Increased Myocardial Oxygen Demand**
• Anemia • Coronary artery narrowing caused by a clot, vessel spasm, or rapid progression of atherosclerosis • Hypoxemia	• Aortic stenosis • Cocaine, amphetamines • Eating a heavy meal • Emotional stress • Exercise • Exposure to cold weather • Fever • Heart failure • Hypertension • Obstructive cardiomyopathy • Pheochromocytoma • Rapid heart rate • Smoking • Thyrotoxicosis

as dyspnea, shoulder or back pain, weakness, fatigue, a change in mental status, syncope, unexplained nausea, and abdominal or epigastric discomfort. They are also more likely to present with more severe preexisting conditions, such as hypertension, heart failure, or a previous acute MI than a younger patient. Diabetic individuals may present atypically because of autonomic dysfunction. Common signs and symptoms include generalized weakness, syncope, lightheadedness, or a change in mental status. Women who experience an ACS report acute symptoms including chest discomfort, unusual fatigue, sleep disturbances, dyspnea, nausea or vomiting, indigestion, dizziness or fainting, sweating, arm or shoulder pain, and weakness. The location of the discomfort is often in the back, arm, shoulder, or neck. Some women have vague chest discomfort that tends to come and go with no known aggravating factors.

CLINICAL CORRELATION

The extent of arterial narrowing and the amount of reduction in blood flow are critical determinants of coronary artery disease (CAD).

Ischemia can occur because of increased myocardial oxygen demand (i.e., demand ischemia), reduced myocardial oxygen supply (i.e., supply ischemia), or both. If the cause of the ischemia is not reversed and blood flow restored to the affected area of the heart muscle, ischemia may lead to cellular injury and, ultimately, infarction. Ischemia can quickly resolve by reducing the heart's oxygen demand, by resting or slowing the heart rate with medications such as beta-blockers, or by increasing blood flow by dilating the coronary arteries with drugs such as nitroglycerin (NTG). Early assessment that includes a focused medical history as well as emergency care are essential to prevent worsening ischemia.

Ischemia prolonged more than just a few minutes results in myocardial *injury*. *Myocardial injury* refers to myocardial tissue that has been cut off from or experienced a severe reduction in its blood and oxygen supply. Injured myocardial cells are still alive but will die (i.e., *infarct*) if the ischemia is not quickly corrected. An MI occurs when blood flow to the heart muscle stops or is suddenly decreased long enough to cause cell death. The symptoms that accompany an MI are often more intense than those associated with angina and last more than 15 to 20 minutes.[2] If the blocked coronary vessel can be quickly opened to restore blood flow and oxygen to the injured area, no tissue death occurs. Methods to restore blood flow may include giving clot-busting drugs (i.e., fibrinolytics), performing coronary angioplasty, or performing a coronary artery bypass graft (CABG), among others.

CLINICAL CORRELATION

When myocardial cells die, such as during a myocardial infarction (MI), substances in intracardiac cells pass through broken cell membranes and leak into the bloodstream. These substances, which are called *inflammatory markers, cardiac biomarkers,* or *serum cardiac markers*, include creatine kinase (CK), creatine kinase myocardial band (CK-MB), myoglobin, troponin I (TnI), and troponin T (TnT). The presence of these substances in the blood can subsequently be measured by means of blood tests to verify the presence of an infarction. The diagnosis of an acute coronary syndrome (ACS) is made on the basis of the patient's assessment findings and his or her symptoms, history, presence of cardiovascular risk factors, serial electrocardiogram results, blood test results (i.e., cardiac biomarkers), and other diagnostic tests.

Coronary Veins

The coronary (cardiac) veins travel alongside the arteries. Blood that has passed through the myocardial capillaries is drained by branches of the cardiac veins that join the coronary sinus. The coronary sinus is the largest vein that drains the heart (see Figure 1-17). It lies in the groove (sulcus) that separates the atria from the ventricles. The coronary sinus receives blood from the great, middle, and small cardiac veins; a vein of the left atrium; and the posterior vein of the left ventricle. The coronary sinus drains into the right atrium. The anterior cardiac veins do not join the coronary sinus but empty directly into the right atrium.

The Heart's Nerve Supply

[Objective 11]

The myocardium is able to produce its own electrical impulses without signals from an outside source, such as a nerve. Because there are times when the body needs to increase or decrease its heart rate and/or force of contraction, it is beneficial that both divisions of the autonomic nervous system send fibers to the heart (Figure 1-19). The sympathetic division prepares the body to function under stress (i.e., the "fight-or-flight" response). The parasympathetic division conserves and restores body resources (i.e., the "feed-and-breed" or "rest and digest" response).

Sympathetic Stimulation

Sympathetic (accelerator) nerves supply specific areas of the heart's electrical system, atrial muscle, and the ventricular myocardium. When sympathetic nerves are stimulated, the neurotransmitters norepinephrine and epinephrine are released. Remember: the job of the sympathetic division is to prepare the body for emergency or stressful situations.

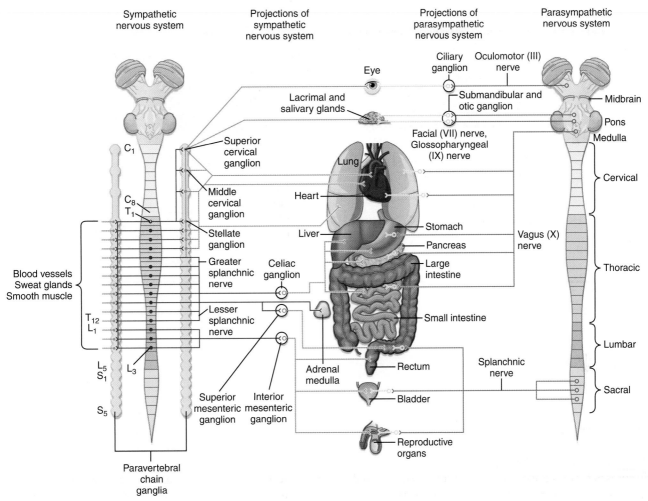

Figure 1-19　Schematic showing the sympathetic and parasympathetic pathways. Sympathetic pathways are shown in red and parasympathetic pathways in blue.

Therefore, the release of norepinephrine and epinephrine results in the following predictable actions:

- Dilation of pupils
- Dilation of smooth muscles of bronchi to improve oxygenation
- Increased heart rate, force of contraction, conduction velocity, blood pressure, and cardiac output
- Increased sweating
- Mobilization of stored energy to ensure an adequate supply of glucose for the brain and fatty acids for muscle activity
- Shunting of blood from skin and blood vessels of internal organs to skeletal muscle

Sympathetic (adrenergic) receptors are located in different organs and have different physiologic actions when stimulated. There are five main types of sympathetic receptors: alpha$_1$, alpha$_2$, beta$_1$, beta$_2$, and dopamine (also called *dopaminergic*).

- Alpha$_1$ receptors are found in the eyes, blood vessels, bladder, and male reproductive organs. Stimulation of alpha$_1$ receptor sites results in constriction.

- Alpha$_2$ receptor sites are found in parts of the digestive system and on presynaptic nerve terminals in the peripheral nervous system. Stimulation results in decreased secretions, peristalsis, and suppression of norepinephrine release.
- Beta receptor sites are divided into beta$_1$ and beta$_2$. Beta$_1$ receptors are found in the heart and kidneys. Stimulation of beta$_1$ receptor sites in the heart results in increased heart rate, contractility, and, ultimately, irritability of cardiac cells (Figure 1-20). Stimulation of beta$_1$ receptor sites in the kidneys results in the release of renin into the blood. Renin promotes the production of angiotensin, a powerful vasoconstrictor. Beta$_2$ receptor sites are found in the arterioles of the heart, lungs, and skeletal muscle. Stimulation results in dilation. Stimulation of beta$_2$ receptor sites in the smooth muscle of the bronchi results in dilation.
- Dopamine receptors are found in the renal, mesenteric, and visceral blood vessels. Stimulation results in dilation.

Sympathetic Effects

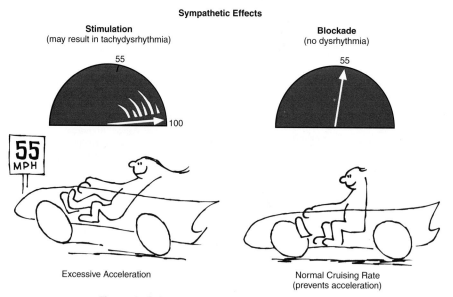

Figure 1-20 Effects of sympathetic stimulation on the heart.

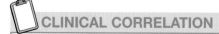

CLINICAL CORRELATION

Remember: Beta₁ receptors affect the heart (you have one heart); beta₂ receptors affect the lungs (you have two lungs).

Parasympathetic Stimulation

Parasympathetic (inhibitory) nerve fibers supply the SA node, atrial muscle, and the AV bundle of the heart by the vagus nerves. Acetylcholine (ACh) is a chemical messenger (neurotransmitter) released when parasympathetic nerves are stimulated. ACh binds to parasympathetic receptors. The two main types of cholinergic receptors are nicotinic and muscarinic receptors. Nicotinic receptors are located in skeletal muscle.

Muscarinic receptors are located in smooth muscle. Parasympathetic stimulation has the following actions:
- Slows the rate of discharge of the SA node (Figure 1-21)
- Slows conduction through the AV node
- Decreases the strength of atrial contraction
- Can cause a small decrease in the force of ventricular contraction

Baroreceptors and Chemoreceptors

Baroreceptors are specialized nerve tissue (sensors). They are found in the internal carotid arteries and the aortic arch. These sensory receptors detect changes in blood pressure. When they are stimulated, they cause a reflex response in either the sympathetic or the parasympathetic

Parasympathetic Effects

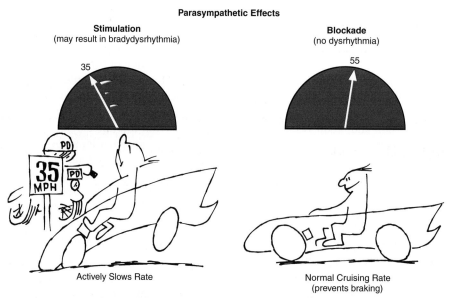

Figure 1-21 Effects of parasympathetic stimulation on the heart.

Table 1-4 Review of the Autonomic Nervous System

	Sympathetic Division	Parasympathetic Division
General effect	Fight or flight	Feed and breed; rest and digest
Primary neurotransmitter	Norepinephrine, epinephrine	Acetylcholine
EFFECTS OF STIMULATION		
Abdominal blood vessels	Constriction (alpha receptors)	No effect
Adrenal medulla	Increased secretion of epinephrine	No effect
Bronchioles	Dilation (beta receptors)	Constriction
Blood vessels of skin	Constriction (alpha receptors)	No effect
Blood vessels of skeletal muscle	Dilation (beta receptors)	No effect
Cardiac muscle	Increased rate and strength of contraction (beta receptors)	Decreased rate; decreased strength of atrial contraction, little effect on strength of ventricular contraction
Coronary blood vessels	Constriction (alpha receptors) Dilation (beta receptors)	Dilation

Box 1-2 Terminology

CHRONOTROPIC EFFECT
- Refers to a change in heart rate.
- A positive chronotropic effect refers to an increase in heart rate.
- A negative chronotropic effect refers to a decrease in heart rate.

INOTROPIC EFFECT
- Refers to a change in myocardial contractility.
- A positive inotropic effect results in an increase in myocardial contractility.
- A negative inotropic effect results in a decrease in myocardial contractility.

DROMOTROPIC EFFECT
- Refers to the speed of conduction through the atrioventricular (AV) junction.
- A positive dromotropic effect results in an increase in AV conduction velocity.
- A negative dromotropic effect results in a decrease in AV conduction velocity.

divisions of the autonomic nervous system. For example, if the blood pressure decreases, the body will attempt to compensate by:
- Constricting peripheral blood vessels
- Increasing heart rate (chronotropy)
- Increasing the force of myocardial contraction (inotropy)

These compensatory responses occur because of a response by the sympathetic division. This is called a *sympathetic or adrenergic response*. If the blood pressure increases, the body will decrease sympathetic stimulation and increase the response by the parasympathetic division. This is called a *parasympathetic or cholinergic response*. The baroreceptors will be "reset" to a new "normal" after a few days of exposure to a specific pressure.

Chemoreceptors in the internal carotid arteries and aortic arch detect changes in the concentration of hydrogen ions (pH), oxygen, and carbon dioxide in the blood. The response to these changes by the autonomic nervous system can be sympathetic or parasympathetic.

A review of the autonomic nervous system can be found in Table 1-4. **Chronotropy**, **inotropy**, and **dromotropy** are terms used to describe effects on heart rate, myocardial contractility, and speed of conduction through the AV node. These terms are explained in Box 1-2.

THE HEART AS A PUMP

The right and left sides of the heart are separated by an internal wall of connective tissue called a **septum**. The *interatrial septum* separates the right and left atria. The *interventricular septum* separates the right and left ventricles. The septa separate the heart into two functional pumps. The right atrium and right ventricle make up one pump. The left atrium and left ventricle make up the other (Figure 1-22).

The right side of the heart is a low-pressure system whose job is to pump unoxygenated blood from the body to and through the lungs to the left side of the heart. This is called the *pulmonary circulation*. The pressure within the right atrium is normally between 2 and 6 mm Hg. The pressure within the right ventricle is normally between 0 and 8 mm Hg when the chamber is at rest (diastole) and between 15 and 25 mm Hg during contraction (systole).

The job of the left heart is to receive oxygenated blood from the lungs and pump it out to the rest of the body. This is called the *systemic circulation*. The left side of the heart is a high-pressure pump. The pressure within the left atrium is normally between 8 and 12 mm Hg. Blood is carried from the heart to the organs of the body through arteries, arterioles, and capillaries. Blood is returned to the right heart through venules and veins.

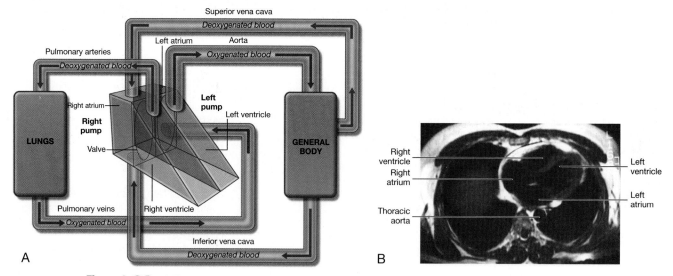

Figure 1-22   A, The heart has two pumps. **B,** Magnetic resonance image of the midthorax showing all four chambers and septa.

The left ventricle is a high-pressure chamber. Its wall is much thicker than the right ventricle (the right ventricle is about 3 to 5 mm thick; the left ventricle is about 13 to 15 mm). This is because the left ventricle must overcome a lot of pressure and resistance from the arteries and contract forcefully in order to pump blood out to the body. The pressure within the left ventricle is normally between 8 and 12 mm Hg when the chamber is at rest (diastole) and between 110 and 130 mm Hg during contraction (systole). Because the wall of the left ventricle is much thicker than the right, the interventricular septum normally bulges to the right.

Cardiac Cycle

[Objectives 12, 13]
The cardiac cycle refers to a repetitive pumping process that includes all of the events associated with blood flow through the heart. The cycle has two phases for each heart chamber: systole and diastole. **Systole** is the period during which the chamber is contracting and blood is being ejected. **Diastole** is the period of relaxation during which the chambers are allowed to fill. The myocardium receives its fresh supply of oxygenated blood from the coronary arteries during ventricular diastole.

The cardiac cycle depends on the ability of the cardiac muscle to contract and on the condition of the heart's conduction system. The efficiency of the heart as a pump may be affected by abnormalities of the cardiac muscle, the valves, or the conduction system.

During the cardiac cycle, the pressure within each chamber of the heart rises in systole and falls in diastole. The heart's valves ensure that blood flows in the proper direction. Blood flows from one heart chamber to another from higher to lower pressure. These pressure relationships depend on the careful timing of contractions. The heart's conduction system (discussed in Chapter 2) provides the necessary timing of events between atrial and ventricular systole.

CLINICAL CORRELATION

In a resting adult, each cardiac cycle lasts approximately 0.8 sec. Atrial systole requires about 0.1 sec. Ventricular systole requires about 0.3 sec. Atrial diastole lasts about 0.7 sec. Ventricular diastole lasts about 0.5 sec during each cardiac cycle. Some processes occur at the same time, such as ventricular systole and atrial diastole. As the heart rate increases, the cardiac cycle length decreases and diastole is shortened relatively more than systole.[4]

Atrial Systole and Diastole
Blood from the tissues of the head, neck, and upper extremities is emptied into the superior vena cava. Blood from the lower body is returned to the inferior vena cava. During atrial diastole, blood from the superior and inferior vena cavae and the coronary sinus enters the right atrium. The amount of blood flowing into the right heart from the systemic circulation is called **venous return**. The right atrium fills and distends. This pushes the tricuspid valve open and the right ventricle fills.

The left atrium receives oxygenated blood from the four pulmonary veins (two from the right lung and two from the left lung). The flaps of the mitral valve open as the left atrium fills. This allows blood to flow into the left ventricle.

The ventricles are 70% filled before the atria contract. Contraction of the atria forces additional blood (about 10% to 30% of the ventricular capacity) into the ventricles (the atrial kick). Thus the ventricles become completely filled with blood during atrial systole. The atria then enter a period of atrial diastole, which continues until the start of the next cardiac cycle.

Ventricular Systole and Diastole
Ventricular systole occurs as atrial diastole begins. As the ventricles contract, blood is propelled through the systemic

and pulmonary circulation and toward the atria. The term *isovolumetric* contraction (meaning, "having the same volume") is used to describe the brief period between the start of ventricular systole and the opening of the SL valves. During this period, the ventricular volume remains constant as the pressure within the chamber rises sharply.

When the right ventricle contracts, the tricuspid valve closes. The right ventricle expels the blood through the pulmonic valve into the pulmonary trunk. The pulmonary trunk divides into a right and left pulmonary artery, each of which carries blood to one lung (i.e., the pulmonary circuit). Blood flows through the pulmonary arteries to the lungs. Blood low in oxygen passes through the pulmonary capillaries. There it comes in direct contact with the alveolar-capillary membrane, where oxygen and carbon dioxide are exchanged. Blood then flows into the pulmonary veins and then to the left atrium.

When the left ventricle contracts, the mitral valve closes to prevent backflow of blood. Blood leaves the left ventricle through the aortic valve to the aorta, which is the main vessel of the systemic arterial circulation. Blood is distributed throughout the body (i.e., the systemic circuit) through the aorta and its branches. Blood continues to move in one direction because pressure pushes it from the high pressure (i.e., arterial) side and valves in the veins prevent backflow on the lower pressure (i.e., venous) side as blood returns to the heart.

Did You Know?

The aorta is composed of four primary parts: the ascending aorta, the aortic arch, the thoracic portion of the descending aorta, and the abdominal portion of the descending aorta.

When the SL valves close, the heart begins a period of ventricular diastole. During ventricular diastole, the ventricles are relaxed and begin to fill passively with blood. The cardiac cycle begins again with atrial systole and the completion of ventricular filling. The cardiac cycle and blood flow through the heart is shown in Figures 1-23 and 1-24.

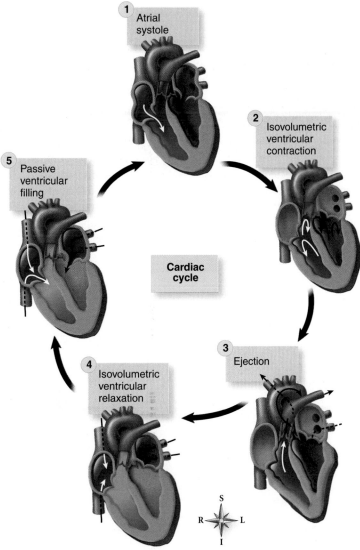

1 Atrial systole

2 Isovolumetric ventricular contraction

5 Passive ventricular filling

Cardiac cycle

4 Isovolumetric ventricular relaxation

3 Ejection

Figure 1-23   The cardiac cycle.

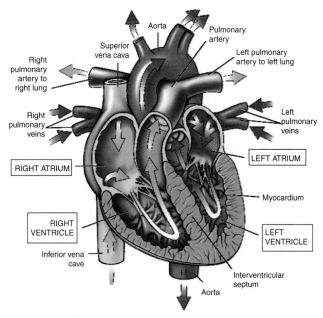

Figure 1-24   Blood flow through the heart.

Did You Know? _____

Both the atria and ventricles have a systolic and diastolic phase. When the term *systole* or *diastole* is used but the area of the heart is not specified, it is assumed that the term refers to *ventricular* systole or diastole.

Blood Pressure

[Objective 14]

The mechanical activity of the heart is reflected by the pulse and blood pressure. **Blood pressure** is the force exerted by the circulating blood volume on the walls of the arteries. The volume of blood in the arteries is directly related to arterial blood pressure.

Blood pressure is equal to cardiac output × peripheral resistance. Cardiac output is discussed below. **Peripheral resistance** is the resistance to the flow of blood determined by blood vessel diameter and the tone of the vascular musculature. **Tone** is a term that may be used when referring to the normal state of balanced tension in body tissues.

Blood pressure is affected by conditions or medications that affect peripheral resistance or cardiac output (Figure 1-25). For example, an increase in either cardiac output or peripheral resistance typically results in an increase in blood pressure. Conversely, a decrease in either will result in a decrease in blood pressure. ▶

Cardiac Output

[Objective 14]

Each ventricle holds about 150 mL of blood when it is full. They normally eject about half this volume (70 to 80 mL) with each contraction. **Cardiac output** is the amount of blood pumped into the aorta each minute by the heart. It is defined as the **stroke volume**, which is the amount of blood ejected from a ventricle with each heartbeat, multiplied by the heart rate. In a healthy average adult, the cardiac output at rest is about 5 L/min (a stroke volume of 70 mL multiplied by a heart rate of 70 beats/min) (Figure 1-26). Because the cardiovascular system is a closed system, the volume of blood leaving one part of the system must equal that entering another part. For example, if the left ventricle normally pumps 5 L/min, the volume flowing through the arteries, capillaries, and veins must equal 5 L/min. Thus, the cardiac output of the right ventricle (pulmonary blood flow) is normally equal to that of the left ventricle on a minute-to-minute basis.

The *percentage* of blood pumped out of a ventricle with each contraction is called the **ejection fraction**. Ejection fraction is used as a measure of ventricular function. A normal ejection fraction is between 50% and 65%. A person is said to have impaired ventricular function when the ejection fraction is less than 40%.

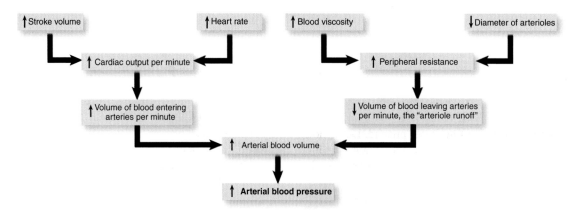

Figure 1-25   Relationship between arterial blood volume and blood pressure. Arterial blood pressure is directly proportional to arterial blood volume. Cardiac output (CO) and peripheral resistance (PR) are directly proportional to arterial blood volume, but for opposite reasons: CO affects blood entering the arteries, and PR affects blood leaving the arteries. If cardiac output increases, the amount of blood entering the arteries increases and tends to increase the volume of blood in the arteries. If peripheral resistance increases, it decreases the amount of blood leaving the arteries, which tends to increase the amount of blood left in them. Thus an increase in either CO or PR results in an increase in arterial blood volume, which increases arterial blood pressure.

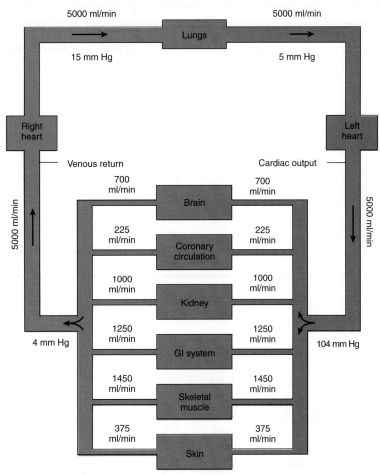

Figure 1-26 Cardiac output. This diagram shows that a typical resting cardiac output (CO) of 5000 mL/min (or 5 L/min) is distributed among the various systems and organs of the body. *GI,* Gastrointestinal.

Stroke Volume

Cardiac output may be increased by an increase in stroke volume *or* heart rate. Stroke volume is determined by the following:

- The degree of ventricular filling when the heart is relaxed (preload)
- The pressure against which the ventricle must pump (afterload)
- The myocardium's contractile state (contracting or relaxing)

Preload, which is also called the *end-diastolic volume,* is the force exerted on the walls of the ventricles at the end of diastole. The volume of blood returning to the heart influences preload. More blood returning to the right atrium (e.g., increased venous return) increases preload. Less blood returning decreases preload. According to the Frank-Starling law of the heart, the greater the stretch of the cardiac muscle (within limits), the greater the resulting contraction. Heart muscle fibers stretch in response to the increased volume (preload) before contracting. Stretching of the muscle fibers allows the heart to eject the additional volume with increased force, thereby increasing stroke volume. So in the normal heart, the greater the preload, the greater the force of ventricular contraction and the greater the stroke volume, resulting in

increased cardiac output. This is important so that the heart can adjust its pumping capacity in response to changes in venous return. For example, during exercise, the heart muscle fibers stretch in response to increased volume (preload) before contracting. If, however, the ventricle is stretched beyond its physiologic limit, cardiac output may fall because of volume overload and overstretching of the muscle fibers. **Heart failure** is a condition in which the heart is unable to pump enough blood to meet the metabolic needs of the body. It may result from any condition that impairs preload, afterload, cardiac contractility, or heart rate.

Afterload is the pressure or resistance against which the ventricles must pump to eject blood. Afterload is influenced by the following:

- Arterial blood pressure
- The ability of the arteries to become stretched (arterial distensibility)
- Arterial resistance

The lower the resistance (lower afterload), the more easily blood can be ejected. Increased afterload (increased resistance) increases the heart's workload. Conditions that contribute to increased afterload include increased thickness of the blood (viscosity) and high blood pressure.

CLINICAL CORRELATION

Abnormal heart rhythms (**dysrhythmias**) such as atrial flutter and atrial fibrillation (discussed in Chapter 4), negatively affect normal atrial contraction. Ineffectual atrial contraction can result in a loss of atrial kick, decreased stroke volume, and a subsequent decrease in cardiac output.

Heart Rate

Remember that cardiac output may be increased by an increase in stroke volume *or* heart rate. Increases in heart rate shorten all phases of the cardiac cycle. The most important is that the time the heart spends relaxing is less. If the length of time for ventricular relaxation is shortened, there is less time for them to fill adequately with blood. If the ventricles do not have time to fill, the following occur:

- The amount of blood sent to the coronary arteries is reduced
- The amount of blood pumped out of the ventricles will decrease (i.e., cardiac output)
- Signs of myocardial ischemia may be seen

The concentrations of extracellular ions also affect heart rate. Excess potassium (i.e., hyperkalemia) causes the heart to become dilated and flaccid (limp), slows the heart rate, and can dramatically alter conduction. An increase in calcium (i.e., hypercalcemia) causes almost the exact opposite effect to those of potassium, causing the heart to go into spastic contraction. Decreased calcium levels (i.e., hypocalcemia) cause the heart to become flaccid, similar to the effects of increased potassium levels.

Other factors that influence heart rate include hormone levels (e.g., epinephrine, norepinephrine), medications, stress, anxiety, fear, and body temperature. Heart rate increases when body temperature increases and decreases when body temperature decreases.

An increase in the force of the heart's contractions (and, subsequently, stroke volume) may occur because of many conditions including norepinephrine and epinephrine release from the adrenal medulla, insulin and glucagon release from the pancreas, and medications, such as calcium, digitalis, dopamine, and dobutamine. A decrease in the force of contraction may result from many conditions including severe hypoxia, decreased pH, elevated carbon dioxide levels (hypercapnea), and medications, such as calcium channel blockers and beta-blockers.

Cardiac output varies depending on hormone balance, an individual's activity level and body size, and the body's metabolic needs. Factors that increase cardiac output include increased body metabolism, exercise, and the age and size of the body. Factors that may decrease cardiac output include **shock**, **hypovolemia**, and heart failure. Signs and symptoms of decreased cardiac output appear in Box 1-3. Heart failure may result from any condition that impairs preload, afterload, cardiac contractility, or heart rate. As the heart begins to fail, the body's compensatory mechanisms attempt to improve cardiac output by manipulating one or more of these factors.

Now that we have discussed cardiac output (CO), stroke volume (SV), and heart rate (HR), let us review an important

---

| Box **1-3** | Signs and Symptoms of Decreased Cardiac Output |

- Acute changes in blood pressure
- Acute changes in mental status
- Cold, clammy skin
- Color changes in the skin and mucous membranes
- Crackles (rales)
- Dyspnea
- Dysrhythmias
- Fatigue
- Orthopnea
- Restlessness

point. Remember that cardiac output may be increased by an increase in heart rate or stroke volume. Consider the following examples:

1. A patient has a stroke volume of 80 mL/beat. His heart rate is 70 beats/minute. Is his cardiac output normal, decreased, or increased? Substitute numbers into the formula you already learned: CO = SV × HR. 5600 mL/min = 80 mL/beat × 70 beats/min. Cardiac output is normally between 4 and 8 L/min. This patient's cardiac output is within normal limits.

2. Now, let us see what an increase in heart rate will do. If the patient's heart rate increases to 180 beats/minute and his stroke volume remains at 80 mL/beat, what happens to his cardiac output? Using our formula again (CO = SV × HR) and substituting numbers, we end up with 14,400 mL/min = 80 mL/beat × 180 beats/min. This patient's cardiac output is increased.

3. What happens to cardiac output if the patient's heart rate is 70 beats/min but his stroke volume drops to 50 mL/beat? Using our formula one more time (CO = SV × HR) and substituting numbers, we end up with 3500 mL/min = 50 mL/beat × 70 beats/min. This patient's cardiac output is decreased. If the patient's heart rate increased to 90 beats/min to try to compensate for his failing pump, what would happen to his cardiac output? (4500 mL/min = 50 mL/beat × 90 beats/min). According to our example, the patient's cardiac output would increase—at least temporarily.

REFERENCES

1. Hall JE: The heart. In *Guyton and Hall textbook of medical physiology,* ed 12, Philadelphia, 2011, Saunders, pp 99–156.
2. O'Connor RE, Brady W, Brooks SC, et al: Part 10: acute coronary syndromes: 2010 American Heart Association guidelines for cardiopulmonary resuscitation and emergency cardiovascular care, *Circulation* 122(Suppl 3):S787–S817, 2010.
3. Karve AM, Bossone E, Mehta RH: Acute ST-segment elevation myocardial infarction: critical care perspective, *Crit Care Clin* 23:685–707, 2007.
4. Boulpaep EL: The heart as a pump. In Boron WF, Boulpaep EL, editors: *Medical physiology: a cellular and molecular approach,* updated ed, Philadelphia, 2005, Saunders, pp 508–533.

STOP & REVIEW—CHAPTER 1

Multiple Choice

Identify the choice that best completes the statement or answers the question.

____1. The area in the middle of the thoracic cavity in which the heart lies is the
   a. Mediastinum.
   b. Pleural cavity.
   c. Parietal cavity.
   d. Visceral cavity.

____2. The inferior surface of the heart is formed by the
   a. Right and left atria.
   b. Right and left ventricles.
   c. Left atrium and left ventricle.
   d. Right atrium and right ventricle.

____3. Which of the following statements is correct?
   a. The circumflex artery is a branch of the right coronary artery.
   b. A branch of the right coronary artery supplies the right atrium and right ventricle.
   c. The major branches of the right coronary artery are the septal and diagonal arteries.
   d. The left main coronary artery is another name for the left anterior descending artery.

____4. The right atrium
   a. Pumps blood to the lungs.
   b. Pumps blood to the systemic circulation.
   c. Receives blood from the right and left pulmonary veins.
   d. Receives blood from the superior and inferior vena cavae and the coronary sinus.

____5. Although about 70% of ventricular filling occurs passively, _____ _____ contributes an additional 10% to 30% of blood flow to ventricular filling.
   a. Atrial kick
   b. Stroke volume
   c. Cardiac output
   d. Ventricular systole

____6. Which of the following is the innermost layer of the heart that lines its inner chambers, valves, and is continuous with the innermost layer of the arteries, veins, and capillaries of the body?
   a. Epicardium
   b. Myocardium
   c. Pericardium
   d. Endocardium

____7. When a ventricle relaxes in the normal heart, blood is prevented from flowing back into it by:
   a. The mitral valve.
   b. A semilunar valve.
   c. The tricuspid valve.
   d. An atrioventricular valve.

____8. The right ventricle:
   a. Pumps oxygenated blood into the systemic circulation.
   b. Pumps unoxygenated blood into the pulmonary circulation.
   c. Receives unoxygenated blood from the systemic circulation.
   d. Receives oxygenated blood from the pulmonary circulation.

____9. The _____ pericardium is the inner layer of the pericardium, which is also the outer layer of the heart wall called the _____.
   a. Parietal, myocardium
   b. Visceral, epicardium
   c. Parietal, endocardium
   d. Visceral, endocardium

____10. Which of the following conditions are potentially reversible?
   a. Myocardial ischemia and myocardial injury
   b. Myocardial injury and myocardial infarction
   c. Myocardial ischemia and myocardial infarction

____11. Which of the following statements is true regarding cardiac output?
   a. The higher the afterload, the more easily blood can be ejected from a ventricle.
   b. Stroke volume is the percentage of blood pumped out of a ventricle with each contraction.
   c. An inverse relationship exists between venous return and preload; increased venous return decreases preload.
   d. Within limits, the more blood that is returned to the heart, the greater the volume of blood that will be pumped during the next contraction.

Questions 12 through 14 pertain to the following scenario.
A 65-year-old man presents with a sudden onset of substernal chest pain that radiates to his left arm and jaw, and nausea. He states that his symptoms began while at rest. The patient has a history of coronary artery disease and had a three-vessel coronary artery bypass graft last year. His medications include diltiazem (Cardizem) and nitroglycerin. He has no known allergies.

____12. On the basis of the information presented, this patient is most likely experiencing a(n):
   a. Stroke.
   b. Cardiac arrest.
   c. Valvular prolapse.
   d. Acute coronary syndrome.

_____**13.** Your assessment reveals that the patient is anxious, his skin is pale and sweaty, and his heart rate is faster than normal for his age. The patient's assessment findings are most likely:
    a. The result of a blocked cerebral blood vessel.
    b. The result of the improper closure of one or more heart valves.
    c. Caused by sympathetic stimulation and the release of norepinephrine.
    d. Caused by parasympathetic stimulation and the release of acetylcholine.

_____**14.** This patient's heart rate is faster than normal for his age. Why might this finding be a cause for concern?
    a. Rapid heart rates predispose the patient to valvular heart disease.
    b. Rapid heart rates shorten diastole and can result in decreased cardiac output.
    c. Rapid heart rates lengthen systole but decrease myocardial contractility, which can lead to shock.
    d. Rapid heart rates are usually accompanied by pulmonary congestion, which leads to heart failure.

Matching

a. Right coronary artery
b. Arteriosclerosis
c. Septum
d. Atria
e. Endocardium
f. Atrioventricular
g. Contracts
h. Half moon

i. Stroke volume
j. Aortic
k. Ventricles
l. Pericardium
m. Ischemia
n. Angina pectoris
o. Ejection fraction

_____**15.** A double-walled sac that encloses the heart
_____**16.** A semilunar valve is shaped like a _____.
_____**17.** Decreased supply of oxygenated blood to a body part or organ
_____**18.** Innermost layer of the heart
_____**19.** Lower heart chambers
_____**20.** This type of heart valve separates an atrium and ventricle
_____**21.** Chest discomfort or other related symptoms of sudden onset that may occur because the increased oxygen demand of the heart temporarily exceeds the blood supply
_____**22.** Coronary artery that supplies the SA node and AV node in most of the population
_____**23.** The amount of blood ejected from a ventricle with each heartbeat
_____**24.** Upper chambers of the heart
_____**25.** One of the semilunar valves
_____**26.** The percentage of blood pumped out of a heart chamber with each contraction
_____**27.** An internal wall of connective tissue
_____**28.** When actin and myosin filaments slide together, the cardiac muscle cell _____.
_____**29.** A chronic disease of the arterial system characterized by abnormal thickening and hardening of the vessel walls

STOP & REVIEW ANSWERS

Multiple Choice

1. ANS: A
The heart lies in the space between the lungs (i.e., the mediastinum) in the middle of the chest. The mediastinum contains the heart, great vessels, trachea, and esophagus, among other structures; it extends from the sternum to the vertebral column.
OBJ: Describe the location of the heart.

2. ANS: B
The heart's bottom (inferior) surface is formed by both the right and left ventricles, but mostly the left. The inferior surface of the heart is also called the *diaphragmatic surface.*
OBJ: Identify the surfaces of the heart.

3. ANS: B
A branch of the right coronary artery supplies the right atrium and right ventricle. The left main coronary artery supplies oxygenated blood to its two primary branches: the left anterior descending (LAD) artery and the circumflex artery. The major branches of the LAD are the septal and diagonal arteries.
OBJ: Name the primary branches and areas of the heart supplied by the right and left coronary arteries.

4. ANS: D
The right atrium receives blood low in oxygen from the superior vena cava (which carries blood from the head and upper extremities), the inferior vena cava (which carries blood from the lower body), and the coronary sinus, which is the largest vein that drains the heart. The left atrium receives freshly oxygenated blood from the lungs via the right and left pulmonary veins. The right ventricle pumps blood to the lungs. The left ventricle pumps blood to the systemic circulation.
OBJ: Identify and describe the chambers of the heart and the vessels that enter or leave each.

5. ANS: A
Although about 70% of ventricular filling occurs passively, atrial contraction (also known as the *atrial kick*) contributes an additional 10% to 30% of blood flow to ventricular filling.
OBJ: Explain atrial kick.

6. ANS: D
The endocardium is the heart's innermost layer. It lines the heart's inner chambers, valves, chordae tendineae (tendinous cords), and papillary muscles and is continuous with the innermost layer of the arteries, veins, and capillaries of the body, thereby creating a continuous, closed circulatory system.
OBJ: Identify the three cardiac muscle layers.

7. ANS: B
The semilunar valves prevent backflow of blood from the aorta and pulmonary arteries into the ventricles. When the right ventricle relaxes, blood is prevented from flowing back into it by the pulmonic valve. When the left ventricle relaxes, blood is prevented from flowing back into it by the aortic valve.
OBJ: Identify and describe the location of the atrioventricular and semilunar valves.

8. ANS: B
The right side of the heart is a low-pressure system whose job is to pump unoxygenated blood from the body to and through the lungs to the left side of the heart. The right ventricle receives blood low in oxygen from the right atrium and pumps the blood through the pulmonic valve into the pulmonary trunk, which divides into the right and left pulmonary arteries.
OBJ: Beginning with the right atrium, describe blood flow through the normal heart and lungs to the systemic circulation.

9. ANS: B
The visceral pericardium is the inner layer of the pericardium, which also attaches to the large vessels that enter and exit the heart and covers the outer surface of the heart muscle (i.e., the epicardium).
OBJ: Describe the structure and function of the coverings of the heart.

10. ANS: A
The sequence of events that occurs during an acute coronary syndrome (ACS) results in conditions that range from myocardial ischemia or injury to death (i.e., necrosis) of heart muscle. Ischemia prolonged more than just a few minutes results in myocardial injury. *Myocardial injury* refers to myocardial tissue that has been cut off from or experienced a severe reduction in its blood and oxygen supply. Injured myocardial cells are still alive but will die (i.e., *infarct*) if the ischemia is not quickly corrected. A myocardial infarction occurs when blood flow to the heart muscle stops or is suddenly decreased long enough to cause cell death.
OBJ: Discuss myocardial ischemia, injury, and infarction, indicating which conditions are reversible and which are not.

11. ANS: D

According to the Frank-Starling law of the heart, the greater the stretch of the cardiac muscle (within limits), the greater the resulting contraction. Preload (end-diastolic volume) is the force exerted on the walls of the ventricles at the end of diastole. In the normal heart, the greater the preload, the greater the force of ventricular contraction and the greater the stroke volume, resulting in increased cardiac output. Afterload is the pressure or resistance against which the ventricles must pump to eject blood. The lower the resistance (lower afterload), the more easily blood can be ejected. The percentage of blood pumped out of a ventricle with each contraction is called the *ejection fraction*.

OBJ: Identify and explain the components of blood pressure and cardiac output.

12. ANS: D

On the basis of the information presented, this patient is most likely experiencing an acute coronary syndrome (ACS). ACS refers to distinct conditions caused by a similar sequence of pathologic events—a temporary or permanent blockage of a coronary artery. These conditions are characterized by an excessive demand or inadequate supply of oxygen and nutrients to the heart muscle associated with plaque disruption, thrombus formation, and vasoconstriction.

OBJ: Define and explain acute coronary syndromes.

Matching

15. ANS: L
16. ANS: H
17. ANS: M
18. ANS: E
19. ANS: K
20. ANS: F
21. ANS: N
22. ANS: A

13. ANS: C

This patient's assessment findings are typical of those experiencing an ACS and are most likely caused by sympathetic stimulation and the release of norepinephrine and epinephrine. The sympathetic division of the autonomic nervous system prepares the body to function under stress ("fight-or-flight" response). The effects of norepinephrine and epinephrine include an increased heart rate, force of contraction, blood pressure, and cardiac output; increased sweating, and shunting of blood from the skin and blood vessels of internal organs to skeletal muscle.

OBJ: Compare and contrast the effects of sympathetic and parasympathetic stimulation of the heart.

14. ANS: B

The coronary arteries fill when the aortic valve is closed and the left ventricle is relaxed (i.e., diastole). If the length of time for ventricular relaxation is shortened (as with rapid heart rates), there is less time for them to fill adequately with blood. If the ventricles do not have time to fill, the amount of blood sent to the coronary arteries is reduced, the amount of blood pumped out of the ventricles will decrease (i.e., cardiac output), and signs of myocardial ischemia may be seen.

OBJ: Identify and discuss each phase of the cardiac cycle.

23. ANS: I
24. ANS: D
25. ANS: J
26. ANS: O
27. ANS: C
28. ANS: G
29. ANS: B

Basic Electrophysiology

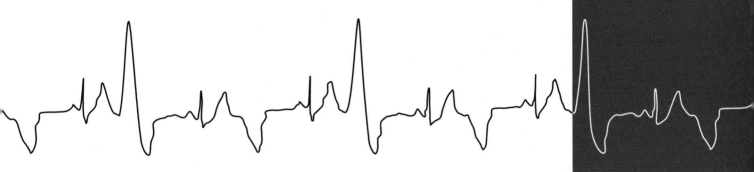

LEARNING OBJECTIVES

After reading this chapter, you should be able to:

1. Describe the two basic types of cardiac cells in the heart, where they are found, and their function.
2. Describe the primary characteristics of cardiac cells.
3. Define the events comprising the cardiac action potential and correlate them with the waveforms produced on the electrocardiogram (ECG).
4. Define the terms *membrane potential, threshold potential, action potential, polarization, depolarization,* and *repolarization.*
5. List the most important ions involved in the cardiac action potential and their primary function in this process.
6. Define the absolute, effective, relative refractory, and supranormal periods and their location in the cardiac cycle.
7. Describe the normal sequence of electrical conduction through the heart.
8. Describe the location, function, and, where appropriate, the intrinsic rate of the following structures: the sinoatrial (SA) node, the atrioventricular (AV) bundle, and the Purkinje fibers.
9. Differentiate the primary mechanisms responsible for producing cardiac dysrhythmias.
10. Describe reentry.
11. Explain the purpose of electrocardiographic monitoring.
12. Identify the limitations of the ECG.
13. Differentiate between the frontal plane and the horizontal plane leads.
14. Describe correct anatomic placement of the standard limb leads, the augmented leads, and the chest leads.
15. Relate the cardiac surfaces or areas represented by the ECG leads.
16. Identify the numeric values assigned to the small and to the large boxes on ECG paper.
17. Identify how heart rates, durations, and amplitudes may be determined from electrocardiographic recordings.
18. Define and describe the significance of each of the following as they relate to cardiac electrical activity: the P wave, the QRS complex, the T wave, the U wave, the PR segment, the TP segment, the ST segment, the PR interval, the QRS duration, and the QT interval.
19. Recognize the changes on the ECG that may reflect evidence of myocardial ischemia, injury, and infarction.
20. Define the term *artifact* and explain methods that may be used to minimize its occurrence.
21. Describe a systematic approach to the analysis and interpretation of cardiac dysrhythmias.

KEY TERMS

Absolute refractory period: Corresponds with the onset of the QRS complex to approximately the peak of the T wave; cardiac cells cannot be stimulated to conduct an electrical impulse, no matter how strong the stimulus

Action potential: A five-phase cycle that reflects the difference in the concentration of charged particles across the cell membrane at any given time

Altered automaticity: A disorder of impulse formation in which cardiac cells fire and initiate impulses before a normal SA node impulse

Amplitude: Height (voltage) of a waveform on the ECG

Arrhythmia: Abnormal heart rhythm

Artifact: Distortion of an ECG tracing by electrical activity that is noncardiac in origin (e.g., electrical interference, poor electrical conduction, patient movement)

Atrioventricular bundle: The bundle of His

Atrioventricular node: A group of cells that conduct an electrical impulse through the heart; located in the floor of the right atrium immediately behind the tricuspid valve and near the opening of the coronary sinus

Augmented limb lead: Leads aVR, aVL, and aVF; these leads record the difference in electrical potential at one location relative to zero potential rather than relative to the electrical potential of another extremity

Automaticity: Ability of cardiac pacemaker cells to spontaneously initiate an electrical impulse without being stimulated from another source (such as a nerve)

AV bundle: The bundle of His

AV node: Specialized cells located in the lower portion of the right atrium; delays the electrical impulse in order to allow the atria to contract and complete filling of the ventricles

Axis: Imaginary line joining the positive and negative electrodes of a lead

Baseline: Straight line recorded on ECG graph paper when no electrical activity is detected

Biphasic: Waveform that is partly positive and partly negative

Bipolar limb lead: ECG lead consisting of a positive and negative electrode

Bundle of His: Fibers located in the upper portion of the interventricular septum that receive an electrical impulse from the AV node and conduct the impulse to the right and left bundle branches

Complex: Several waveforms

Conduction system: A system of pathways in the heart composed of specialized electrical (pacemaker) cells

Conductivity: Ability of a cardiac cell to receive an electrical stimulus and conduct that impulse to an adjacent cardiac cell

Contractility: Ability of cardiac cells to shorten, causing cardiac muscle contraction in response to an electrical stimulus

Depolarization: Movement of ions across a cell membrane, causing the inside of the cell to become more positive; an electrical event expected to result in contraction

Dysrhythmia: Abnormal heart rhythm

Ectopic: Impulse(s) originating from a source other than the SA node

Effective refractory period: Period of the cardiac action potential that includes the absolute refractory period and the first half of the relative refractory period

Electrode: An adhesive pad that contains a conductive gel and is applied at specific locations on the patient's chest wall and extremities and connected by cables to an ECG machine

Electrolytes: Elements or compounds that break into charged particles (ions) when melted or dissolved in water or another solvent

Enhanced automaticity: Abnormal condition in which cardiac cells not normally associated with the property of automaticity begin to depolarize spontaneously or when escape pacemaker sites increase their firing rate beyond that considered normal

Excitability: The ability of cardiac muscle cells to respond to an outside stimulus

Ground electrode: Third ECG electrode (the first and second are the positive and negative electrodes), which minimizes electrical activity from other sources

His-Purkinje system: Portion of the conduction system consisting of the bundle of His, bundle branches, and Purkinje fibers

Indicative changes: ECG changes observed in leads that look directly at the affected area of the heart; indicative changes are significant when they are seen in two anatomically contiguous leads.

Inherent: Natural, intrinsic

Interval: Waveform and a segment; in pacing, the period, measured in milliseconds, between any two designated cardiac events

Intrinsic rate: Rate at which a pacemaker of the heart normally generates impulses

Ion: Electrically charged particle

Isoelectric line: Absence of electrical activity; observed on the ECG as a straight line

J point: Point where the QRS complex and ST segment meet

Lead: Electrical connection attached to the body to record electrical activity

Membrane potential: Difference in electrical charge across the cell membrane

Millivolt (mV): Difference in electrical charge between two points in a circuit

Myocardial cells: Working cells of the myocardium that contain contractile filaments and form the muscular layer of the atrial walls and the thicker muscular layer of the ventricular walls

Pacemaker cells: Specialized cells of the heart's electrical conduction system, capable of spontaneously generating and conducting electrical impulses

Permeability: Ability of a membrane channel to allow passage of electrolytes once it is open

Polarized state: Period after repolarization of a myocardial cell (also called the *resting state*) when the outside of the cell is positive and the interior of the cell is negative

PR interval: P wave plus the PR segment; reflects depolarization of the right and left atria (P wave) and the spread of the impulse through the AV node, AV bundle, right and left bundle branches, and the Purkinje fibers (PR segment)

Purkinje fibers: Fibers found in both ventricles that conduct an electrical impulse through the heart

P wave: First wave in the cardiac cycle; represents atrial depolarization and the spread of the electrical impulse throughout the right and left atria

QRS complex: Several waveforms (i.e., the Q wave, the R wave, and the S wave) that represent the spread of an electrical impulse through the ventricles (i.e., ventricular depolarization)

R wave: On an ECG, the first positive deflection in the QRS complex, representing ventricular depolarization; in pacing, R wave refers to the entire QRS complex, denoting an intrinsic ventricular event

Reciprocal change: ECG changes observed in leads in leads opposite the affected area of the heart; also called *mirror image changes*

Reentry: Spread of an impulse through tissue already stimulated by that same impulse.

Refractoriness: Period of recovery that cells need after being discharged before they are able to respond to a stimulus

Relative refractory period: Corresponds with the downslope of the T wave; cardiac cells can be stimulated to depolarize if the stimulus is strong enough.

Repolarization: Movement of ions across a cell membrane in which the inside of the cell is restored to its negative charge

Segment: Line between waveforms; named by the waveform that precedes and follows it

Sinoatrial node: Normal pacemaker of the heart that normally discharges at a rhythmic rate of 60 to 100 beats/min

ST segment: Portion of the ECG representing the end of ventricular depolarization (end of the R wave) and the beginning of ventricular repolarization (T wave)

Supranormal period: Period during the cardiac cycle when a weaker than normal stimulus can cause cardiac cells to depolarize; extends from the end of phase 3 to the beginning of phase 4 of the cardiac action potential

T wave: Waveform that follows the QRS complex and represents ventricular repolarization

TP segment: Interval between two successive PQRST complexes during which electrical activity of the heart is absent; begins with the end of the T wave through the onset of the following P wave and represents the period from the end of ventricular repolarization to the onset of atrial depolarization

Triggered activity: A disorder of impulse formation that occurs when escape pacemaker and myocardial working cells fire more than once after stimulation by a single impulse resulting in atrial or ventricular beats that occur alone, in pairs, in runs, or as a sustained ectopic rhythm.

Unipolar lead: Lead that consists of a single positive electrode and a reference point

Voltage: Difference in electrical charge between two points

Waveform: Movement away from the baseline in either a positive or negative direction

CARDIAC CELLS

Types of Cardiac Cells

[Objective 1]

In general, cardiac cells have either a mechanical (i.e., contractile) or an electrical (i.e., pacemaker) function. **Myocardial cells** are also called *working cells* or *mechanical cells*, and they contain contractile filaments. When these cells are electrically stimulated, these filaments slide together and cause the myocardial cell to contract. These myocardial cells form the thin muscular layer of the atrial walls and the thicker muscular layer of the ventricular walls (i.e., the myocardium). These cells do not normally generate electrical impulses, and they rely on pacemaker cells for this function.

Pacemaker cells are specialized cells of the electrical conduction system. Pacemaker cells also may be referred to as *conducting cells* or *automatic cells*. They are responsible for the spontaneous generation and conduction of electrical impulses.

Properties of Cardiac Cells

[Objective 2]

When a nerve is stimulated, a chemical (i.e., a neurotransmitter) is released. The chemical crosses the space between the end of the nerve and the muscle membrane (i.e., the neuromuscular junction). The chemical binds to receptor sites on the muscle membrane and stimulates the receptors. An electrical impulse develops and travels along the muscle membrane, resulting in contraction; thus a skeletal muscle normally contracts only after it is stimulated by a nerve.

The heart is unique because it has pacemaker cells that can generate an electrical impulse without being stimulated by a nerve. The ability of cardiac pacemaker cells to create an electrical impulse without being stimulated from another source is called **automaticity**. The heart's normal pacemaker is the SA node because it is capable of self-excitation at a rate quicker than that of other pacemaker sites in the heart. Normal concentrations of sodium ($Na+$), potassium ($K+$), and calcium ($Ca++$) are important in maintaining automaticity. Increased blood concentrations of these electrolytes decrease automaticity. Decreased concentrations of $K+$ and $Ca++$ in the blood increase automaticity.

Cardiac muscle is electrically irritable because of an ionic imbalance across the membranes of cells. **Excitability** (i.e., irritability) is the ability of cardiac muscle cells to respond to an external stimulus, such as that from a chemical, mechanical, or electrical source. **Conductivity** is the ability of a cardiac cell to receive an electrical impulse and conduct it to an adjoining cardiac cell. All cardiac cells possess this characteristic. The intercalated disks present in the membranes of cardiac cells are responsible for the property of conductivity. They allow an impulse in any part of the myocardium to spread throughout the heart. The speed with which the impulse is conducted can be altered by factors such as sympathetic and parasympathetic stimulation and medications. **Contractility** (i.e., inotropy) is the ability of myocardial cells to shorten, thereby causing cardiac muscle contraction in response to an electrical stimulus. The heart normally contracts in response to an impulse that begins in the SA node. The strength of the heart's contraction can be improved with certain medications, such as digitalis, dopamine, and epinephrine.

CARDIAC ACTION POTENTIAL

[Objectives 3, 4, 5]

Before the following discussion of the cardiac action potential, think about how a battery releases energy. A battery has two terminals; one terminal is positive and the other is negative. Charged particles exert forces on each other, and opposite charges attract. Electrons, which are negatively charged particles, are produced by a chemical reaction inside the battery. If a wire is connected between the two terminals, the circuit is completed and the stored energy is released, allowing electrons to flow quickly from the negative terminal along the wire to the positive terminal. If no wire is connected between the terminals, the chemical reaction does not take place and no current flow occurs. **Current** is the flow of electrical charge from one point to another.

Separated electrical charges of opposite polarity (i.e., positive versus negative) have potential energy. The measurement of this potential energy is called **voltage**. Voltage is measured between two points. In the battery example, the current flow is caused by the voltage, or potential difference, between the two terminals. Voltage is measured in units of volts or millivolts.

Human body fluids contain **electrolytes**, which are elements or compounds that break into charged particles (**ions**) when melted or dissolved in water or another solvent. Differences in the composition of ions between the intracellular and extracellular fluid compartments are important for normal body function, including the activity of the heart. Body fluids that contain electrolytes conduct an electric current in much the same way as the wire in the battery example. Electrolytes move about in body fluids and carry a charge, just as electrons moving along a wire conduct a current.

CLINICAL CORRELATION

The main electrolytes that affect the function of the heart are $Na+$, $K+$, $Ca++$, and chloride ($Cl-$). Disorders that affect the concentration of these important electrolytes can have serious consequences. For example, an imbalance of $K+$ can cause life-threatening disturbances in the heart's rhythm.

In the body, ions spend a lot of time moving back and forth across cell membranes (Figure 2-1). When a pathway exists for transfer of a substance across a membrane, the membrane is said to be **permeable** to that substance.[1] As a result, a slight difference in the concentrations of charged particles across the membranes of cells is normal; thus potential energy (i.e., voltage) exists because of the imbalance of charged particles and this imbalance makes the cells excitable. The voltage (i.e., the difference in electrical charges) across the cell membrane is the **membrane potential**.

Electrolytes are quickly moved from one side of the cell membrane to the other by means of pumps (Figure 2-2). These pumps require energy in the form of adenosine triphosphate (ATP) when movement occurs against a concentration gradient. The energy expended by the cells to move electrolytes across the cell membrane creates a flow of current. This flow of current is expressed in volts.

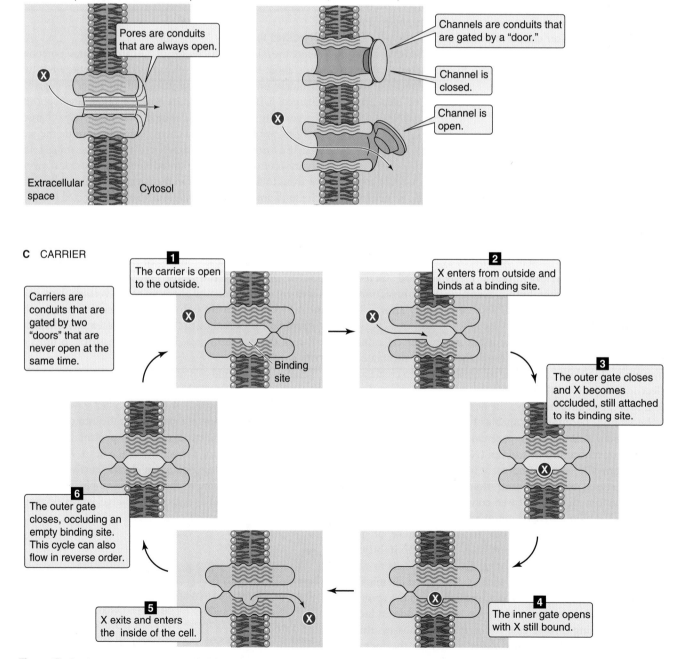

Figure 2-1   Cell membranes contain pathways through which specific ions or other small, water-soluble molecules can cross. Three types of passive transport through a cell membrane are shown.

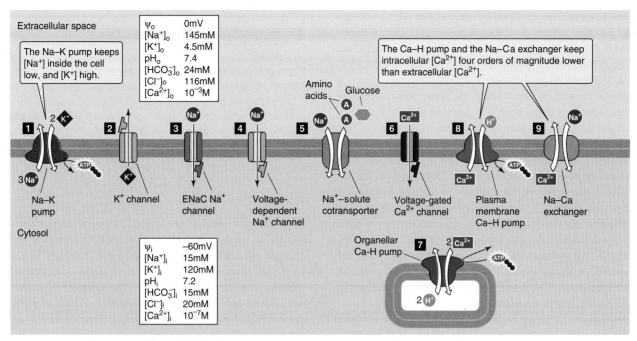

Figure 2-2   Examples of ion concentrations, channels, and transporters in a typical cell.

Voltage appears on an ECG as spikes or waveforms, thus an ECG is actually a sophisticated voltmeter.

Polarization

When a cell is at rest, K+ leaks out of it. Large molecules such as proteins and phosphates remain inside the cell because they are too big to pass easily through the cell membrane. These large molecules carry a negative charge. This results in more negatively charged ions on the inside of the cell. When the inside of a cell is more negative than the outside, it is said to be in a **polarized state** (Figure 2-3).

Depolarization

For a pacemaker cell to "fire" (i.e., produce an impulse), a flow of electrolytes across the cell membrane must exist. When a cell is stimulated, the cell membrane changes and becomes permeable to Na+ and K+, allowing the passage of electrolytes once it is open. Na+ rushes into the cell through

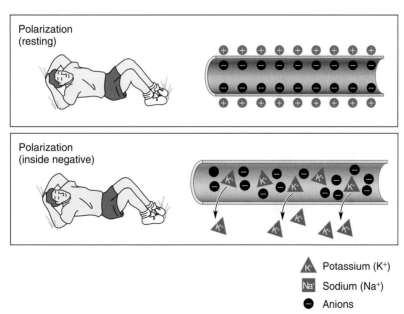

Figure 2-3   Polarization. When the inside of a cell is more negative than the outside it is said to be polarized.

Na+ channels. This causes the inside of the cell to become more positive relative to the outside. A spike (i.e., a waveform) is then recorded on the ECG. The stimulus that alters the electrical charges across the cell membrane may be electrical, mechanical, or chemical.

As described in the battery example, when opposite charges come together, energy is released. When the movement of electrolytes changes the electrical charge of the inside of the cell from negative to positive, an impulse is generated. The impulse causes channels to open in the next cell membrane and then the next. The movement of charged particles across a cell membrane causing the inside of the cell to become positive is called **depolarization** (Figure 2-4). Depolarization occurs because of the movement of Na+ into the cell and proceeds from the innermost layer of the heart (i.e., the endocardium) to the outermost layer (i.e., the epicardium). Depolarization, which is an electrical event, must take place before the heart can contract and pump blood, which is a mechanical event.

An impulse normally begins in the pacemaker cells found in the SA node of the heart. A chain reaction occurs from cell to cell in the heart's electrical conduction system until all the cells have been stimulated and depolarized. This chain reaction is a *wave of depolarization*. The chain reaction is made possible because of gap junctions that exist between the cells. Eventually the impulse is spread from the pacemaker cells to the working myocardial cells, which contract when they are stimulated. When the atria are stimulated, a P wave is recorded on the ECG; thus, the P wave represents atrial depolarization. When the ventricles are stimulated, a QRS complex is recorded on the ECG; thus, the QRS complex represents ventricular depolarization.

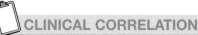
CLINICAL CORRELATION

Depolarization is not the same as contraction. Depolarization is an electrical event that is expected to result in contraction, which is a mechanical event. It is possible to see organized electrical activity on the cardiac monitor, even when the assessment of the patient reveals no palpable pulse. This clinical situation is called *pulseless electrical activity* (PEA).

Repolarization

After the cell depolarizes, it quickly begins to recover and restore its electrical charges to normal. The movement of charged particles across a cell membrane in which the inside of the cell is restored to its negative charge is called **repolarization**. The cell membrane stops the flow of Na+ into the cell and allows K+ to leave it. Negatively charged particles are left inside the cell, thus the cell is returned to its resting state (Figure 2-5). This causes contractile proteins in the working myocardial cells to separate (i.e., relax). The cell can be stimulated again if another electrical impulse arrives at the cell membrane. Repolarization proceeds from the epicardium to the endocardium. On the ECG, the ST segment and T wave represent ventricular repolarization.

Phases of the Cardiac Action Potential

The **action potential** of a cardiac cell reflects the rapid sequence of voltage changes that occur across the cell membrane during the electrical cardiac cycle. The configuration

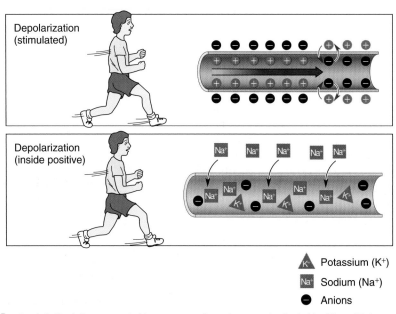

Figure 2-4 Depolarization is the movement of ions across a cell membrane causing the inside of the cell to become more positive.

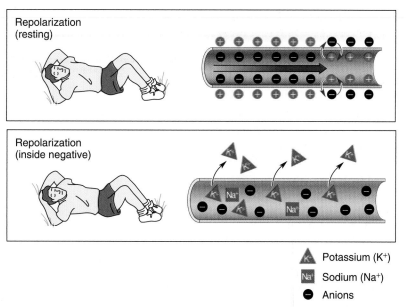

Repolarization
(resting)

Repolarization
(inside negative)

▲ K⁺ Potassium (K⁺)

Na⁺ Sodium (Na⁺)

● Anions

Figure 2-5   Repolarization is the movement of charged particles across a cell membrane in which the inside of the cell is restored to its negative charge.

of the action potential varies depending on the location, size, and function of the cardiac cell.

There are two main types of action potentials in the heart (Figure 2-6). The first type, the fast response action potential, occurs in normal atrial and ventricular myocardial cells and in the **Purkinje fibers**, which are specialized conducting fibers found in both ventricles that conduct an electrical impulse through the heart. The fast response action potential is divided into five phases. Phase 0, called the *upstroke*, *spike*, or *overshoot*, begins when the cell receives an impulse. Na+ moves rapidly into the cell through the Na+ channels, K+ leaves the cell, and Ca++ moves slowly into the cell through Ca++ channels (Figure 2-7). The cell depolarizes and cardiac contraction begins. The upstroke is followed by a period of repolarization, which is divided into three phases. Phases 1, 2, and 3 have been referred to as *electrical systole*. During phase 1 (i.e., initial repolarization), the Na+ channels partially close, slowing the flow of Na+ into the cell. At the same time, Cl− enters the cell and K+ leaves it through K+ channels. The result is a decrease in the number of positive electrical charges within the cell. This produces a small negative deflection in the action potential. The cells of the atria, ventricles, and Purkinje fibers have many calcium channels. During phase 2 (i.e., the plateau phase), Ca++ slowly enters the cell through Ca++ channels. K+ continues to leave the cell slowly through K+ channels. Phase 3 (i.e., repolarization) begins with the downslope of the action potential. The cell rapidly completes repolarization as K+ quickly flows out of the cell. Na+ and Ca++ channels close, stopping the entry of Na+ and Ca++. The rapid movement of K+ out of the cell causes the inside to become progressively more electrically negative. The cell gradually becomes more sensitive to external stimuli until its original sensitivity is restored. Repolarization is complete by the end of phase 3.

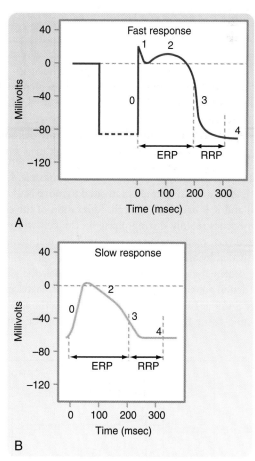

Figure 2-6   Action potentials of fast-response **(A)** and slow-response **(B)** cardiac fibers. The phases of the action potentials are labeled. The effective refractory period (ERP) and the relative refractory period (RRP) are labeled. Note that when compared with fast-response fibers, the resting potential of slow fibers is less negative, the upstroke (phase 0) of the action potential is less steep, the amplitude of the action potential is smaller, phase 1 is absent, and the RRP extends well into phase 4 after the fibers have fully repolarized.

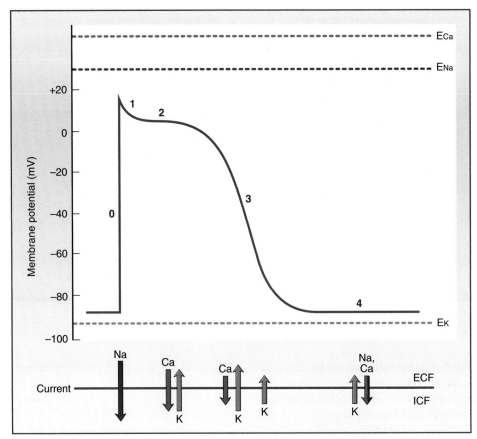

Figure 2-7 Currents responsible for ventricular action potential. The length of the arrows shows the relative size of each ionic current. E, equilibrium potential; ECF, extracellular fluid; ICF, intracellular fluid.

Phase 4 is the resting membrane potential (i.e., return to resting state); this period is called *electrical diastole*. During phase 4, the Na+/K+ pump is activated to move Na+ out of the cell and K+ back into the cell. Relaxation of the cardiac muscle occurs mainly during phase 4. The cell will remain polarized (i.e., ready for discharge) until the cell membrane is reactivated by another stimulus.

The second type of cardiac action potential, the slow response action potential, occurs in the heart's normal pacemaker (i.e., the SA node) and in the AV node, which is the specialized conducting tissue that carries an electrical impulse from the atria to the ventricles (Figure 2-8). The SA and AV nodes of the heart have relatively few sodium channels. Therefore, phase 0, the upstroke, of the slow response action potential is largely the result of the entry of Ca++ into the cell. (Calcium also triggers contraction in all myocardial working cells.) The upstroke is not as rapid or steep as in the atrial, ventricular, and Purkinje fibers. This finding reflects that the action potential is spread more slowly in the SA and AV nodes and conduction of the impulse is more likely to be blocked than in fast-response cardiac tissue.[2] Phase 1 is absent in the slow-response action potential, and the transition from the plateau phase to

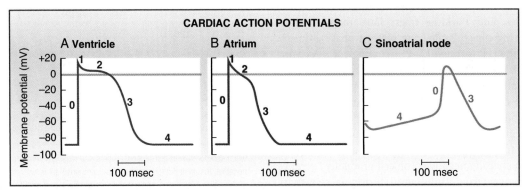

Figure 2-8 Cardiac action potentials in the ventricle, atrium, and sinoatrial node. **A–C,** The numbers correspond to the phases of the action potentials.

repolarization (i.e., phase 3) is less distinct. As in the other cardiac tissues, repolarization is dependent on K+. Changes in the movement of K+ and Ca++ produce activity in pacemaker cells during phase 4. For example, phase 4 is the longest portion of the SA node action potential and accounts for the ability of the cells in the SA node to spontaneously generate an action potential without requiring stimulation by a nerve (automaticity). The rate of phase 4 depolarization affects heart rate.[3] For example, an increase in the rate of phase 4 depolarization results in the SA node firing more action potentials per time, increasing heart rate. In contrast, a decrease in the rate of phase 4 depolarization results in the SA node firing fewer action potentials per time, decreasing heart rate.

CLINICAL CORRELATION

The heart typically beats at a regular rate and rhythm. If this pattern is interrupted, an abnormal heart rhythm can result. Healthcare professionals use the terms **arrhythmia** and **dysrhythmia** interchangeably to refer to an abnormal heart rhythm. Medications used to correct irregular heartbeats and slow down hearts that beat too fast are called *antiarrhythmics*. Although there is no universally accepted classification scheme for antiarrhythmic agents, a commonly used system is to classify the medications by their effects on the cardiac action potential. For example, class I antiarrhythmic medications such as procainamide and lidocaine block sodium channels, interfering with phase 0 depolarization. Class IV antiarrhythmics (Ca++ channel blockers) such as verapamil and diltiazem slow the rate at which calcium passes through the cells, interfering with phase 2 in the cells of the atria, ventricles, and Purkinje fibers.

Refractory Periods

[Objective 6]

Refractoriness is a term that is used to describe the period of recovery that cells need after being discharged before they are able to respond to a stimulus. During the **absolute refractory period** (ARP), the cell will not respond to further stimulation within itself (Figure 2-9). This means that the myocardial working cells cannot contract and that the cells of the electrical conduction system cannot conduct an electrical impulse, no matter how strong the internal electrical stimulus. As a result, tetanic (i.e., sustained) contractions cannot be provoked in the cardiac muscle. The ARP corresponds to the time needed for the reopening of channels that allow the entry of sodium and calcium into the cell.[4] In a fast-response myocardial fiber, the ARP includes phases 0, 1, 2, and part of phase 3 of the cardiac action potential. Slow-response fibers become absolutely refractory at the beginning of the upstroke.[5] The **effective refractory period** includes the ARP and the first half of the relative refractory period. "The distinction between the absolute and effective refractory periods is that *absolute* means *absolutely* no stimulus is large enough to generate another action potential; *effective* means that a *conducted* action potential cannot be generated (i.e., there is not enough inward current to conduct to the next site)."[3]

The **relative refractory period** (RRP) begins at the end of the ARP and ends when the cell membrane is almost fully repolarized. During the RRP, some cardiac cells have repolarized to their threshold potential and thus can be stimulated to respond (i.e., depolarize) to a stronger-than-normal stimulus. After the RRP is a **supranormal period**. A weaker-than-normal

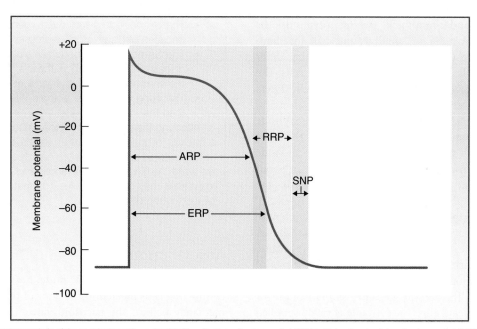

Figure 2-9 Refractory periods of the ventricular action potential. The effective refractory period (ERP) includes the absolute refractory period (ARP) and the first half of the relative refractory period (RRP). The RRP begins when the absolute refractory period ends and includes the last portion of the effective refractory period. The supranormal period (SNP) begins when the relative refractory period ends.

stimulus can cause cardiac cells to depolarize during this period. The supranormal period extends from the end of phase 3 to the beginning of phase 4 of the cardiac action potential. Because the cell is more excitable than normal, dysrhythmias can develop during this period (see Figure 2-9).

ECG Pearl

The duration of the action potential determines the length of the refractory periods. The longer the action potential, the longer the cell is refractory to firing another action potential.[3] The action potential, and, consequently, the refractory period, in cells of the atria (i.e., 150 msec), ventricles (i.e., 250 msec), and Purkinje system (i.e., 300 msec) is long compared with other excitable tissues in the heart because of a sustained period of depolarization (i.e., plateau).

CONDUCTION SYSTEM

[Objectives 7, 8]

The specialized electrical (i.e., pacemaker) cells in the heart are arranged in a system of pathways called the **conduction system**. In the normal heart, the cells of the conduction system are interconnected. The conduction system makes sure that the chambers of the heart contract in a coordinated fashion.

Sinoatrial Node

The SA node is specialized conducting tissue located in the upper posterior part of the right atrium where the superior vena cava and the right atrium meet. It lies less than 1 mm from the epicardial surface. In an adult, the SA node is about 8 mm long and 2 mm thick. Two main types of cells exist within the SA node: (1) small, round cells that have few myofibrils, and (2) slender, elongated cells that differ from the round cells and typical atrial myocardial cells. The round cells are thought to be pacemaker cells and the others are thought to be responsible for conducting the electrical impulse within the SA node and to its borders. The SA node receives its blood supply from the SA node artery that runs lengthwise through the center of the node. The SA node artery originates from the right coronary artery in about 60% of people and from the circumflex artery in the remaining 40%.

The normal heartbeat is the result of an electrical impulse (i.e., an action potential) that begins in the SA node. The SA node is normally the primary pacemaker of the heart because it has the fastest firing rate (specifically, the fastest rate of phase 4 depolarization) of all of the heart's normal pacemaker sites (Figure 2-10). The built-in (i.e., intrinsic) rate of the SA node is 60 to 100 beats/min. The SA node is richly supplied by sympathetic and parasympathetic nerve fibers. Although the SA node normally fires at a rate of 60 to 100 beats/min, this rate can increase to about 180 beats/min, primarily through sympathetic stimulation. Heart rates faster than 150 beats/min can be problematic because: (1) the duration of diastole shortens as heart rate increases, reducing ventricular filling time and, potentially, stroke volume, and (2) the heart's workload and oxygen requirements are increased, but the time for coronary artery filling, which occurs during diastole, is decreased.[6]

As the impulse leaves the SA node, it is spread from cell to cell in wavelike form across the atrial muscle. As the impulse spreads, it stimulates the right atrium, the interatrial septum, and travels along a special pathway called *Bachmann's bundle* to stimulate the left atrium. This results in contraction of the right and left atria at almost the same time. Because a fibrous skeleton separates the atrial myocardium from the ventricular myocardium, the electrical stimulus affects only the atria.

CLINICAL CORRELATION

Areas of the heart other than the sinoatrial (SA) node can initiate beats (i.e., intrinsic automaticity) and assume pacemaker responsibility under special circumstances. The terms **ectopic**, which means out of place, or *latent* are used to describe an impulse that originates from a source other than the SA node. Ectopic pacemaker sites include the cells of the atrioventricular (AV) bundle and Purkinje fibers, although their intrinsic rates are slower than that of the SA node. Although an ectopic pacemaker normally is prevented from discharging because of the dominance of the SA node's rapidly firing pacemaker cells (i.e., overdrive suppression), an ectopic site may assume pacemaker responsibility in the following circumstances:

- The SA node fires too slowly because of vagal stimulation or suppression by medications.
- The SA node fails to fire (i.e., generate an impulse) because of disease or suppression by medications.
- The SA node action potential is blocked because of disease in conducting pathways, failing to activate the surrounding atrial myocardium.
- The firing rate of the ectopic site becomes faster than that of the SA node.

Although the presence of ectopic pacemakers provides a backup or safety mechanism in the event of SA node failure, ectopic pacemaker sites can be problematic if they fire while the SA node is still functioning. For example, ectopic sites may cause early (i.e., premature) beats or sustained rhythm disturbances.

Atrioventricular Node and Bundle

Conduction through the **AV node**, a group of specialized conducting cells located in the floor of the right atrium immediately behind the tricuspid valve, begins before atrial depolarization is completed. The AV node is supplied by the right coronary artery in 85% to 90% of the population. In the remainder, the circumflex artery provides the blood supply.

A   CONDUCTION PATHWAYS THROUGH HEART

B   CARDIAC ACTION POTENTIALS

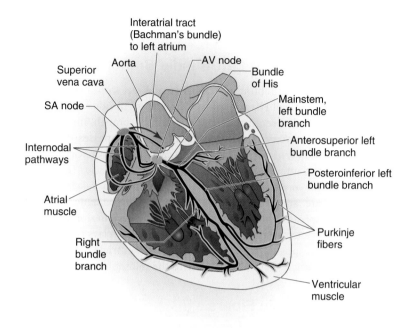

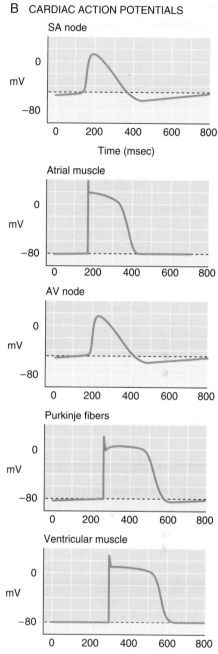

Figure 2-10   Electrical activity in heart tissue. **A,** Conduction pathways through the heart. A section through the long axis of the heart is shown. **B,** Cardiac action potentials. The distinctive shapes of action potentials at five sites along the spread of excitation are shown. AV, atrioventricular; SA, sinoatrial.

The AV node is supplied by both sympathetic and parasympathetic nerve fibers.

The impulse is spread to the AV node by three internodal pathways. These pathways are made up of a mixture of working myocardial cells and specialized conducting fibers. The internodal pathways merge gradually with the cells of the AV node. The AV node has been divided into three functional regions according to their action potentials and responses to electrical and chemical stimulation: (1) the atrionodal (AN) (also called the *transitional zone*) located between the atrium and the rest of the node; (2) the nodal (N) region, the

midportion of the AV node; and (3) the nodal-His (NH) or lower region where the fibers of the AV node gradually merge with the bundle of His (Figure 2-11).

As the impulse enters the AV node through the internodal pathways, conduction is markedly slowed in the AN and N areas of the AV node before the impulse reaches the ventricles. This delay occurs in part because the fibers in the AV node are smaller than those of atrial muscle and have few gap junctions. If this delay did not occur, the atria and the ventricles would contract at about the same time. The delay in conduction allows both atrial chambers to contract and

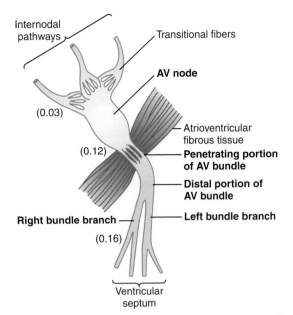

Internodal pathways
Transitional fibers
AV node
(0.03)
Atrioventricular fibrous tissue
(0.12)
Penetrating portion of AV bundle
Distal portion of AV bundle
Right bundle branch
Left bundle branch
(0.16)
Ventricular septum

Figure 2-11   Organization of the atrioventricular (AV) node and AV bundle. The numbers represent the interval of time in fractions of a second from the origin of the impulse in the sinus node.

empty blood into the ventricles before the next ventricular contraction begins. This increases the amount of blood in the ventricles, increasing stroke volume.

ECG Pearl

Because depolarization and repolarization are slow in the AV node, this area is vulnerable to blocks in conduction (AV blocks).

The **bundle of His**, also called the *common bundle* or the **AV bundle**, is located in the upper portion of the interventricular septum and connects the AV node with the bundle branches. Normally, the atria and ventricles are separated by a continuous barrier of fibrous tissue, which acts as an insulator to prevent passage of an electrical impulse through any route other than the AV node and bundle. When the AV node and bundle are bypassed by an abnormal pathway, the abnormal route is called an **accessory pathway**.

The AV bundle has pacemaker cells that have an intrinsic rate of 40 to 60 beats/min. The bundle receives a dual blood supply from branches of the left anterior and posterior descending coronary arteries. Because of this dual blood supply, the bundle is less vulnerable to ischemia. The AV node and the AV bundle are called the *AV junction*. The term **His-Purkinje system** or *His-Purkinje network* refers to the bundle of His, bundle branches, and Purkinje fibers. In the heart's conduction system, the speed of impulse conduction is fastest in the His-Purkinje system and it is slowest in the SA and AV nodes.

Did You Know?

Abnormal cardiac rhythms that develop near or within the AV node are called *junctional dysrhythmias*. Those that develop above the bundle of His or activate the ventricles through an accessory pathway are called *supraventricular dysrhythmias*. Dysrhythmias that develop below the bundle of His are called *ventricular dysrhythmias*.

Right and Left Bundle Branches

The right bundle branch is a direct continuation of the bundle of His and is located on the right side of the interventricular septum. The right bundle branch innervates the right ventricle. The left bundle branch passes through the interventricular septum and carries the electrical impulse to the interventricular septum and left ventricle. The left bundle branch divides into divisions called **fascicles**, which are small bundles of nerve fibers. The anterior fascicle spreads the electrical impulse to the anterior portions of the left ventricle. The posterior fascicle relays the impulse to the posterior portions of the left ventricle, and the septal fascicle relays the impulse to the midseptum.

Purkinje Fibers

The right and left bundle branches divide into smaller and smaller branches and then into a special network of fibers called the **Purkinje fibers**. These fibers spread from the interventricular septum into the papillary muscles. They continue downward to the apex of the heart, making up an elaborate web that penetrates about one third of the way into the ventricular muscle mass. The fibers then become continuous with the muscle cells of the right and left ventricles. The Purkinje fibers have pacemaker cells that have an intrinsic rate of 20 to 40 beats/min. The electrical impulse spreads rapidly through the right and left bundle branches and the Purkinje fibers to reach the ventricular muscle. The electrical impulse spreads from the endocardium to the myocardium, finally reaching the epicardial surface. The ventricular walls are stimulated to contract in a twisting motion that wrings blood out of the ventricular chambers and forces it into arteries. A summary of the conduction system is shown in Table 2-1.

CAUSES OF DYSRHYTHMIAS

[Objective 9]
Dysrhythmias result from disorders of impulse formation, disorders of impulse conduction, or both.

Disorders of Impulse Formation

Enhanced Automaticity
Enhanced automaticity is an abnormal condition in which one of the following occurs: (1) Cardiac cells that are not

Table 2-1	Summary of the Conduction System				
Structure	Location	Function	Intrinsic Pacemaker (beats/min)	Time Lapse from SA Node (seconds)
Sinoatrial (SA) node	Right atrial wall just inferior to opening of superior vena cava	Primary pacemaker; initiates impulse that is normally conducted throughout the left and right atria	60 to 100	0
Atrioventricular (AV) node	Floor of the right atrium immediately behind the tricuspid valve and near the opening of the coronary sinus	Receives impulse from SA node and delays relay of the impulse to the bundle of His, allowing time for the atria to empty their contents into the ventricles before the onset of ventricular contraction.		0.03
Bundle of His (AV bundle)	Superior portion of interventricular septum	Receives impulse from AV node and relays it to right and left bundle branches	40 to 60	0.04
Right and left bundle branches	Interventricular septum	Receives impulse from bundle of His and relays it to Purkinje fibers		0.17
Purkinje fibers	Ventricular myocardium	Receives impulse from bundle branches and relays it to ventricular myocardium	20 to 40	0.20 to 0.22

normally associated with a pacemaker function begin to depolarize spontaneously *or* (2) a pacemaker site other than the SA node increases its firing rate beyond that which is considered normal.

Possible causes for enhanced automaticity include ischemia, hypoxia, electrolyte abnormalities, and exposure to chemicals or toxic substances, among others. Examples of rhythms associated with enhanced automaticity include premature beats, accelerated idioventricular rhythm, accelerated junctional rhythm, and some forms of ventricular tachycardia.

Triggered Activity

Triggered activity results from abnormal electrical impulses that sometimes occur during repolarization, when cells are normally quiet. These abnormal electrical impulses are called *afterdepolarizations*. Triggered activity requires a stimulus to begin depolarization. It occurs when pacemaker cells from a site other than the SA node and myocardial working cells depolarize more than once after being stimulated by a single impulse.

Causes of triggered activity include hypoxia, excessive catecholamines, myocardial ischemia or injury, digitalis toxicity, and medications that prolong repolarization. Triggered activity can result in atrial or ventricular beats that occur alone, in pairs, in "runs" (three or more beats), or as a sustained ectopic rhythm.

Disorders of Impulse Conduction

Conduction Blocks

Blocks of impulse conduction may be partial or complete. They may occur because of trauma, drug toxicity, electrolyte disturbances, myocardial ischemia, or infarction.

A partial conduction block may be slowed or intermittent. In slowed conduction, all impulses are conducted but it takes longer than normal to do so. When an intermittent block occurs, some (but not all) impulses are conducted. When a complete block exists, no impulses are conducted through the affected area. Examples of rhythms associated with disturbances in conduction include AV blocks.

Reentry
[Objective 10]

An impulse normally spreads through the heart only once after it is initiated by pacemaker cells. **Reentry** is the spread of an impulse through tissue already stimulated by that same impulse. An electrical impulse is delayed, blocked, or both, in one or more areas of the conduction system while the impulse is conducted normally through the rest of the conduction system. This results in the delayed electrical impulse entering cardiac cells that have just been depolarized by the normally conducted impulse. Reentry requires the following three conditions (Figure 2-12): (1) A potential conduction circuit or circular conduction pathway, (2) a block within part of the circuit, and (3) delayed conduction with the remainder of the circuit.

If the area the delayed impulse stimulates is relatively refractory, the impulse can cause depolarization of those cells, producing a single premature beat or repetitive electrical impulses. This can result in short periods of an abnormally fast heart rate. Possible causes of reentry include hyperkalemia, myocardial ischemia, and some antiarrhythmic medications. Examples of rhythms associated with reentry are AV reentrant tachycardia and atrial flutter.

CONDITIONS REQUIRED FOR REENTRY

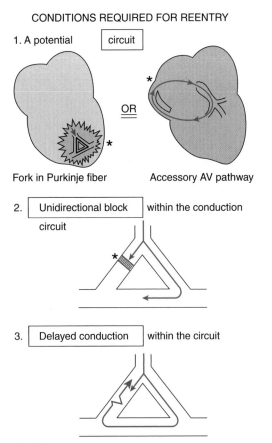

1. A potential circuit

OR

Fork in Purkinje fiber   Accessory AV pathway

2.   Unidirectional block   within the conduction
      circuit

3.   Delayed conduction   within the circuit

Figure 2-12   Reentry requires (1) a potential conduction circuit or circular conduction pathway, (2) a block within part of the circuit, and (3) delayed conduction with the remainder of the circuit.

THE ELECTROCARDIOGRAM

[Objectives 11, 12]

The ECG is a graphic display of the heart's electrical activity. The first ECG was introduced by Willem Einthoven, a Dutch physiologist, in the early 1900s. When electrodes are attached to the patient's limbs or chest and connected by cables to an ECG machine, the ECG machine functions as a voltmeter, detecting and recording the changes in voltage (action potentials) generated by depolarization and repolarization of the heart's cells. The voltage changes are displayed as specific waveforms and complexes (Figure 2-13).

ECG monitoring may be used for the following purposes:
- To monitor a patient's heart rate.
- To evaluate the effects of disease or injury on heart function.
- To evaluate pacemaker function.
- To evaluate the response to medications (e.g., antiarrhythmics).
- To obtain a baseline recording before, during, and after a medical procedure.
- To evaluate for signs of myocardial ischemia, injury, and infarction.

The ECG *can* provide information about the following:
- The orientation of the heart in the chest
- Conduction disturbances
- Electrical effects of medications and electrolytes
- The mass of cardiac muscle
- The presence of ischemic damage

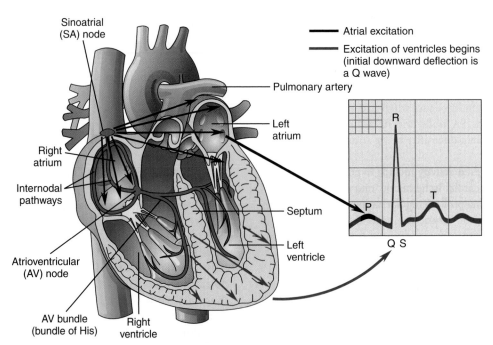

Figure 2-13   Schematic drawing of the conducting system of the heart. An impulse normally is generated in the sinoatrial node and travels through the atria to the atrioventricular (AV) node, down the bundle of His and Purkinje fibers, and to the ventricular myocardium. Recording of the depolarizing and repolarizing currents in the heart with electrodes on the surface of the body produces characteristic waveforms.

The ECG does *not* provide information about the mechanical (contractile) condition of the myocardium. To evaluate the effectiveness of the heart's mechanical activity, the patient's pulse and blood pressure are assessed.

Electrodes

Electrode refers to an adhesive pad containing a conductive substance in the center and that is applied to the patient's skin. The conductive media of the electrode conducts skin surface voltage changes through wires to a cardiac monitor (electrocardiograph). Electrodes are applied at specific locations on the patient's chest wall and extremities to view the heart's electrical activity from different angles and planes.

It is desirable to remove oil and dead cells from the patient's skin before applying electrodes. Skin oil and dead cells may be removed by a variety of techniques, such as a brisk dry rub of the skin. Many electrode manufacturers include an abrasive area on the disposable backing of the electrode for this purpose, but a gauze pad or terrycloth washcloth work well too. In some circumstances, small areas may need to be shaved or chest hair cut if the electrode(s) will not stick. To minimize distortion (artifact), be sure the conductive jelly in the center of the electrode is not dry, and avoid placing the electrodes directly over bony areas (Skill 2-1).

SKILL 2-1   ECG Monitoring

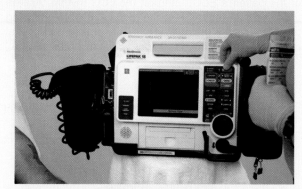

Step 1 Explain the procedure to the patient while checking your equipment. Make sure there are no loose pins in the end of the electrocardiogram (ECG) cable and no frayed or broken cable or lead wires. Make sure the monitor has an adequate paper supply. Connect the ECG cable to the machine. Connect the lead wires to the ECG cable (if not already connected). Turn the power on to the monitor. Adjust the contrast on the screen if necessary.

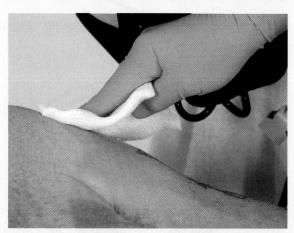

Step 3 Prepare the patient's skin to minimize distortion of the ECG tracing. Do this by briskly rubbing the skin with a dry gauze pad. Do not use alcohol, tincture of benzoin, or antiperspirant when prepping the skin. If electrodes will be applied to the patient's chest instead of limbs, shave small amounts of chest hair if needed before applying electrodes to ensure good contact.

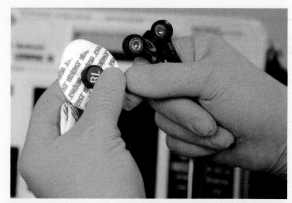

Step 2 Open a package of ECG electrodes. Make sure the electrode gel in the electrodes to be used is moist. Attach an electrode to each lead wire.

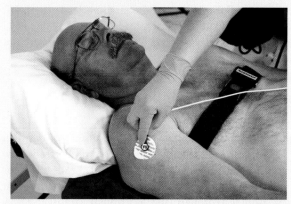

Step 4 One at a time, remove the backing from each electrode and apply them to the patient. Limb lead electrodes usually are placed on the wrists and ankles but may be positioned anywhere on the appropriate limb. To reduce muscle tension, make sure the patient's limbs are resting on a supportive surface. Do not apply electrodes over bony areas, broken skin, joints, skin creases, scar tissue, burns, or rashes.

Continued

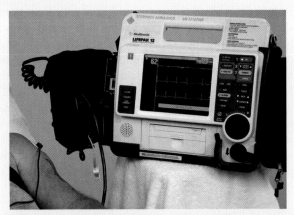

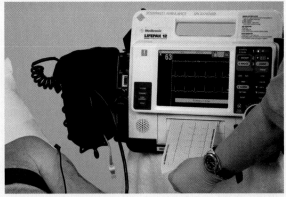

Step 5 Coach the patient to relax. Select the desired lead on the cardiac monitor. Adjust the ECG size if necessary. If the ECG size is set too low, the monitor will not detect QRS complexes and the heart rate display will be incorrect. Feel the patient's pulse and compare it with the heart rate indicator on the monitor. If not already preset, set the heart rate alarms on the monitor according to your agency's policy.

Step 6 Select the print or record button to obtain a copy of the patient's ECG. Interpret the ECG rhythm. Assess the patient to find out how the rate and rhythm are being tolerated. Attach the rhythm strip to the patient's hospital record or prehospital care report. Continue patient care.

One end of a monitoring cable, which is also called a *lead wire*, is attached to the electrode and the other end to an ECG machine. The cable conducts current back to the cardiac monitor. Three-lead wire systems are often used with portable monitor defibrillators (Figure 2-14, A). Five-lead wire systems allow viewing of the six limb leads (I, II, III, aVR, aVL, or aVF) and one chest lead (Figure 2-14, B). ECG cables may be color, symbol, or letter coded. Colors are not standard and often vary.

Leads

[Objectives 13, 14, 15]

A **lead** is a record (i.e., tracing) of electrical activity between two electrodes. Each lead records the *average* current flow at a specific time in a portion of the heart. Leads allow for the viewing of the heart's electrical activity in two different planes: frontal (coronal) and horizontal (transverse). A 12-lead ECG provides views of the heart in both the frontal and horizontal planes and views the surfaces of the left ventricle from 12 different angles. From this, ischemia, injury, and infarction affecting any area of the heart can be identified.

Frontal Plane Leads

Frontal plane leads view the heart from the front of the body as if it were flat (Figure 2-15). Directions in the frontal plane are superior, inferior, right, and left. Six leads view the heart in the frontal plane. Leads I, II, and III are called *standard limb leads*. Leads aVR, aVL, and aVF are called *augmented limb leads*.

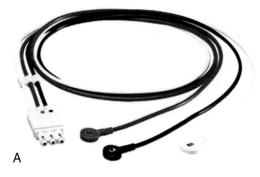

A

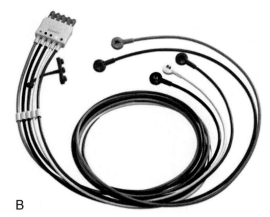

B

Figure 2-14   **A,** Three-lead wire system. **B,** Five-lead wire system.

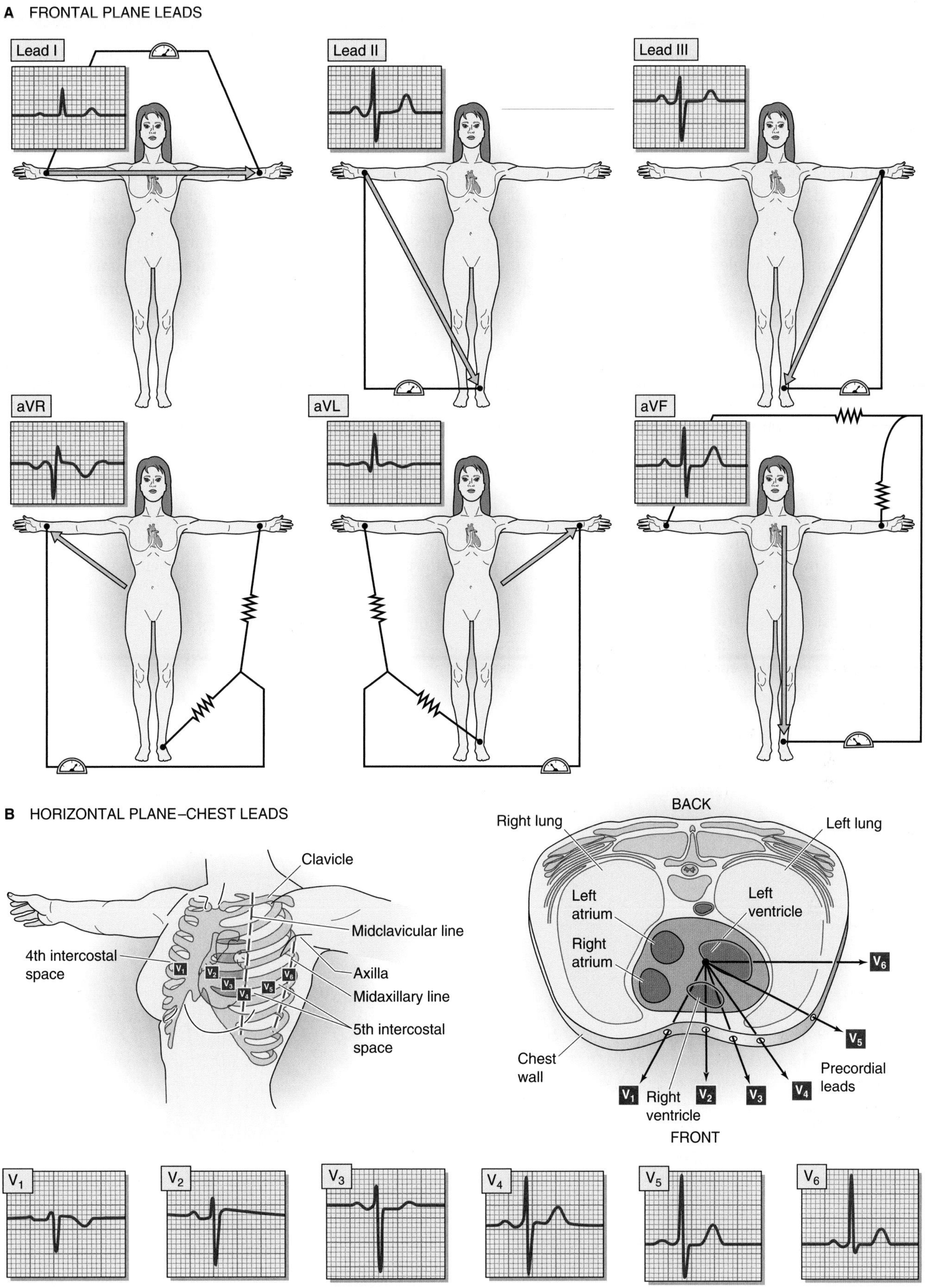

A FRONTAL PLANE LEADS

Lead I

Lead II

Lead III

aVR

aVL

aVF

B HORIZONTAL PLANE–CHEST LEADS

Clavicle

Midclavicular line

Axilla

Midaxillary line

4th intercostal space

5th intercostal space

V_1

V_2 V_3 V_4 V_5 V_6

BACK

Right lung

Left lung

Left atrium

Left ventricle

Right atrium

Chest wall

V_6

V_5

V_1 Right ventricle

V_2

V_3

V_4 Precordial leads

FRONT

V_1

V_2

V_3

V_4

V_5

V_6

Figure 2-15 The electrocardiogram (ECG) leads.

A **bipolar lead** is an ECG lead that has a positive and negative electrode. Each lead records the difference in electrical potential (i.e., voltage) between two selected electrodes. Although all ECG leads are technically bipolar, Leads I, II, and III use two distinct electrodes, one of which is connected to the positive input of the ECG machine and the other to the negative input.[7]

Standard Limb Leads

Leads I, II, and III make up the standard limb leads. If an electrode is placed on the right arm, left arm, and left leg, three leads are formed. The positive electrode is located at the left wrist in lead I, while leads II and III both have their positive electrode located at the left foot. The difference in electrical potential between the positive pole and its corresponding negative pole is measured by each lead.

An imaginary line that joins the positive and negative electrodes of a lead is called the **axis** of the lead. The axes of these three limb leads form an equilateral triangle with the heart at the center, which is called *Einthoven's triangle*. Einthoven's triangle is a way of showing that the two arms and the left leg form apices of a triangle surrounding the heart (Figure 2-16). The two apices at the upper part of the triangle represent the points at which the two arms connect electrically with the fluids around the heart. The lower apex is the point at which the left leg connects with the fluids.[8] Over the

years, electrode placement for leads I, II, and III has been altered and moved to the patient's chest to allow for patient movement and to minimize distortion on the ECG tracing; however, proper electrode positioning for these leads includes placement on the patient's extremities. Where the electrodes are placed on the extremity does not matter as long as bony areas are avoided.

Lead I records the difference in electrical potential between the left arm (+) and right arm (−) electrodes. The positive electrode is placed on the left arm and the negative electrode is placed on the right arm. The third electrode is a ground that minimizes electrical activity from other sources (Figure 2-17). Lead I views the lateral surface of the left ventricle.

Lead II records the difference in electrical potential between the left leg (+) and right arm (−) electrodes. The positive electrode is placed on the left leg and the negative electrode is placed on the right arm. Lead II views the inferior surface of the left ventricle. This lead is commonly used for cardiac monitoring because positioning of the positive and negative electrodes in this lead most closely resembles the normal pathway of current flow in the heart.

Lead III records the difference in electrical potential between the left leg (+) and left arm (−) electrodes. In lead III the positive electrode is placed on the left leg and the negative

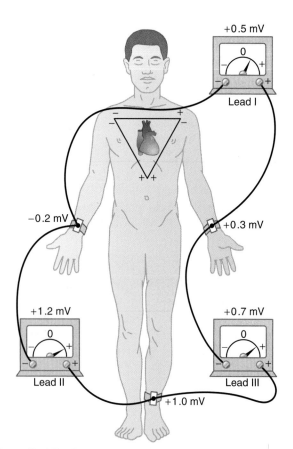

Figure 2-16   Conventional arrangement of electrodes for recording the standard electrocardiographic leads. Einthoven's triangle is superimposed on the chest.

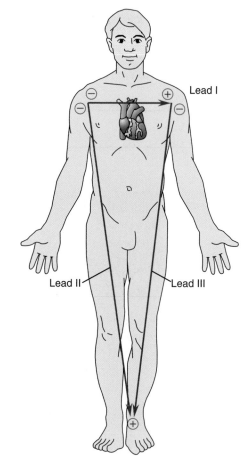

Figure 2-17   Positions of standard limb leads I, II, and III.

electrode is placed on the left arm. Lead III views the inferior surface of the left ventricle. A summary of the standard limb leads can be found in Table 2-2.

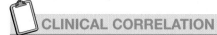

CLINICAL CORRELATION

Leads I, II, III, aVR, aVL, and aVF are obtained from electrodes placed on the patient's arms and legs. The deltoid area is suitable for electrodes attached to the arms and is easily accessible. Either the thigh or lower leg is suitable for the leg electrodes. Use the more convenient site, but keep the electrodes in a similar position. For example, keep the upper extremity electrodes on the deltoids, not one on the upper arm, and one on the inner arm. Be sure that the patient's limbs are resting on a supportive surface. This decreases muscle tension in the patient's arms and legs and helps minimize distortion of the electrocardiogram (ECG) tracing (i.e., artifact). Should circumstances require that the electrodes be placed on the torso, be certain to position them as close to the appropriate limb as possible.

Table 2-2   Standard Limb Leads

Lead	Positive Electrode	Negative Electrode	Heart Surface Viewed
I	Left arm	Right arm	Lateral
II	Left leg	Right arm	Inferior
III	Left leg	Left arm	Inferior

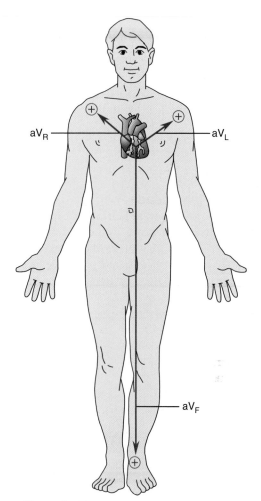

Figure 2-18 Augmented leads aVR, aVL, and aVF.

Augmented Limb Leads

Leads aVR, aVL, and aVF are augmented limb leads that record measurements at a specific electrode with respect to a reference electrode. Frank Norman Wilson and colleagues used the term *central terminal* to describe a reference point that is the average of the limb lead electrical potentials. In the augmented leads, the Wilson central terminal (WCT) is calculated by the ECG machine's computer as an average potential of the electrical currents from the two electrodes other than the one being used as the positive electrode. For example, in lead aVL the positive electrode is located on the patient's left arm. The ECG machine's computer calculates the central terminal by joining the electrical currents obtained from the electrodes on the patient's right arm and left leg. Lead aVL therefore represents the difference in electrical potential between the left arm and the central terminal. The electrical potential of the central terminal is essentially zero.

The electrical potential produced by the augmented leads is normally relatively small. The ECG machine augments (i.e., magnifies) the amplitude of the electrical potentials detected at each extremity by about 50% over those recorded at the standard limb leads. The "a" in aVR, aVL, and aVF refers to augmented. The "V" refers to voltage and the last letter refers to the position of the positive electrode. The "R"

refers to the right arm, the "L" to left arm, and the "F" to left foot (leg). Therefore, the positive electrode in aVR is located on the right arm, aVL has a positive electrode at the left arm, and aVF has a positive electrode positioned on the left leg (Figure 2-18).

Lead aVR views the heart from the right shoulder, which is the positive electrode, and views the base of the heart, which consists primarily of the atria and the great vessels. This lead does not view any wall of the heart. Lead aVL combines views from the right arm and the left leg, with the view being from the left arm and oriented to the lateral wall of the left ventricle. Lead aVF combines views from the right arm and the left arm toward the left leg; it views the inferior surface of the left ventricle from the left leg. A summary of augmented leads can be found in Table 2-3.

Table 2-3   Augmented Limb Leads

Lead	Positive Electrode	Heart Surface Viewed
aVR	Right arm	None
aVL	Left arm	Lateral
aVF	Left leg	Inferior

CLINICAL CORRELATION

Although it may not be immediately obvious, the position of the patient can affect the electrocardiogram (ECG). One reason for differences between tracings obtained in various positions is that although the electrode does not move when the patient changes position, the position of the heart does move relative to that electrode.[9]

Horizontal Plane Leads

Horizontal plane leads view the heart as if the body were sliced in half horizontally. Directions in the horizontal plane are anterior, posterior, right, and left. Six chest (precordial or "V") leads view the heart in the horizontal plane (see Figure 2-15). This allows a view of the front and left side of the heart.

Chest Leads

The chest leads are identified as V_1, V_2, V_3, V_4, V_5, and V_6 (Figure 2-19). Each electrode placed in a "V" position is a positive electrode, measuring electrical potential with respect to the WCT.

CLINICAL CORRELATION

Because their location varies, do not use the nipples as landmarks for chest electrode placement. If your patient is a woman, place the electrodes for leads V_3 through V_6 *under* the breast, rather than *on* the breast.

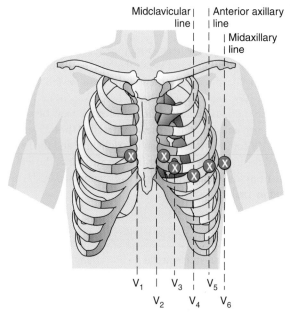

Figure 2-19   Chest (precordial) leads V_1 through V_6.

Lead V_1 is recorded with the positive electrode in the fourth intercostal space, just to the right of the sternum. It important to note that the electrode positions refer to the location of the gel. For example, the gel of the V_1 electrode, not the entire adhesive patch, is positioned in the fourth intercostal space, just to the right of the sternum. Lead V_2 is recorded with the positive electrode in the fourth intercostal space, just to the left of the sternum. Lead V_3 is recorded with the positive electrode on a line midway between V_2 and V_4. Lead V_4 is recorded with the positive electrode in the left midclavicular line in the fifth intercostal space. To evaluate the right ventricle, lead V_4 may be moved to the same anatomic location but on the right side of the chest. The lead is then called V_4R, and it is viewed for ECG changes that are consistent with acute myocardial infarction. Lead V_5 is recorded with the positive electrode in the left anterior axillary line at the same level as V_4. Lead V_6 is recorded with the positive electrode in the left midaxillary line at the same level as V_4. A summary of the chest leads can be found in Table 2-4. Skill 2-2 shows chest lead placement.

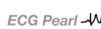

ECG Pearl

Lead V_1 is particularly useful for analyzing dysrhythmias that have a wide QRS complex (e.g., bundle branch blocks, ventricular pacemaker rhythms, wide-QRS tachycardias).

Right Chest Leads

Other chest leads that are not part of a standard 12-lead ECG may be used to view specific surfaces of the heart. Right chest leads are used to evaluate the right ventricle (Figure 2-20). The placement of right chest leads is identical to the placement of the standard chest leads except that it is done on the right side of the chest. A standard 12-lead ECG should be obtained first; the cables for the standard chest leads are then moved to the electrodes repositioned on the right chest for the additional leads. If time does not permit obtaining all of

Table **2-4**	Chest Leads	
Lead	**Positive Electrode Position**	**Heart Surface Viewed**
V_1	Right side of sternum, fourth intercostal space	Septum
V_2	Left side of sternum, fourth intercostal space	Septum
V_3	Midway between V_2 and V_4	Anterior
V_4	Left midclavicular line, fifth intercostal space	Anterior
V_5	Left anterior axillary line; same level as V_4	Lateral
V_6	Left midaxillary line; same level as V_4	Lateral

SKILL 2-2   Chest Lead Placement

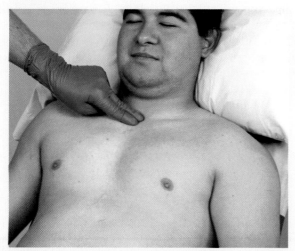

Step 1 An accurate 12-lead electrocardiogram (ECG) requires correctly placing the electrodes. Begin positioning of the chest leads by placing your finger at the notch at the top of the sternum.

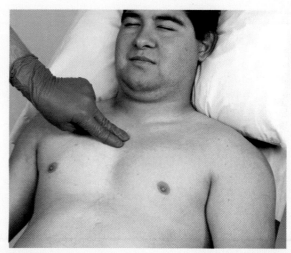

Step 2 Move your finger slowly downward until you feel a slight horizontal ridge or elevation. This is the angle of Louis (sternal angle), where the manubrium joins the body of the sternum.

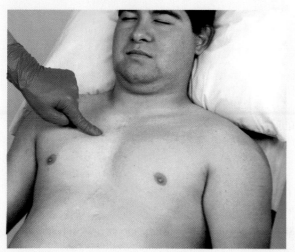

Step 3 Follow the angle of Louis to the patient's right until it articulates with the second rib.

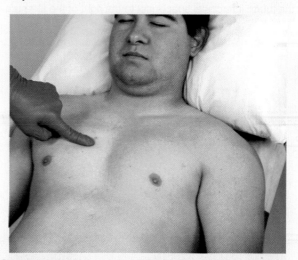

Step 4 Locate the second intercostal space (immediately below the second rib).

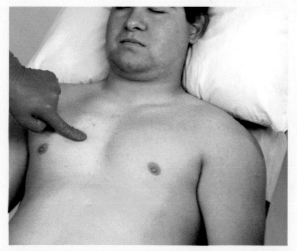

Step 5 From the second intercostal space, the third and fourth intercostal spaces can be found.

Continued

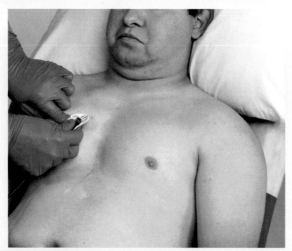

Step 6 V₁ is positioned in the fourth intercostal space just to the right of the sternum. Note: All the electrode positions refer to the location of the gel. For example, the gel of the V₁ electrode, not the entire adhesive patch, is positioned in the fourth intercostal space, just to the right of the sternum.

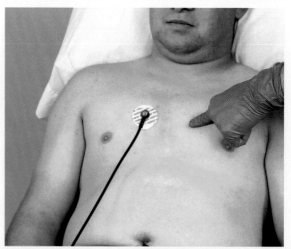

Step 7 From the V₁ position, find the corresponding intercostal space on the left side of the sternum.

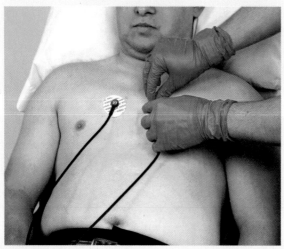

Step 8 Place the V₂ electrode in the fourth intercostal space just to the left of the sternum.

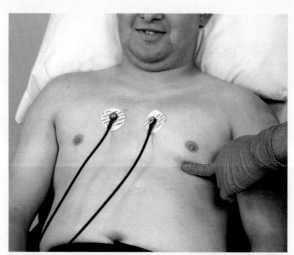

Step 9 From the V₂ position, locate the fifth intercostal space and follow it to the midclavicular line.

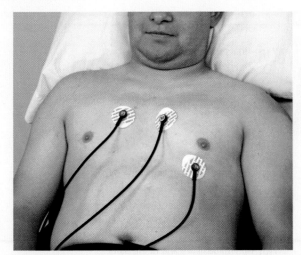

Step 10 Position the V_4 electrode in the fifth intercostals space in the midclavicular line.

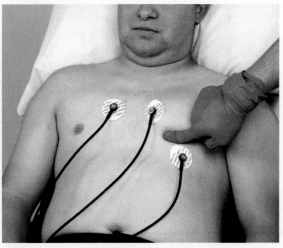

Step 11 V_3 is positioned halfway between V_2 and V_4.

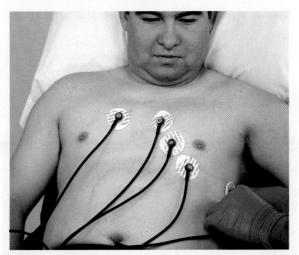

Step 12 V_6 is positioned in the midaxillary line, level with V_4.

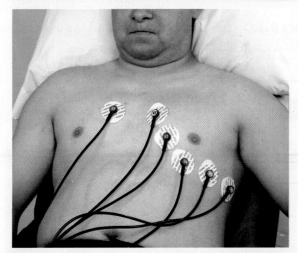

Step 13 V_5 is positioned in the anterior axillary line, level with V_4.

the right chest leads, the lead of choice is V_4R. Skill 2-3 shows placement of the right chest leads.

Posterior Chest Leads

On a standard 12-lead ECG, no leads look directly at the posterior surface of the heart. Additional chest leads may be used for this purpose. These leads are placed further left and toward the back. All of the leads are placed on the same horizontal line as V_4 to V_6. Lead V_7 is placed at the posterior axillary line. Lead V_8 is placed at the angle of the scapula (i.e., the posterior scapular line), and lead V_9 is placed over the left border of the spine. Skill 2-4 shows placement of the posterior chest leads.

CLINICAL CORRELATION

Multiple-lead electrocardiograms (ECGs) are being used with increasing frequency to help spot infarctions of the right ventricle and the posterior wall of the left ventricle. The 15-lead ECG uses all of the leads of a standard 12-lead ECG plus leads V_4R, V_8, and V_9. An 18-lead ECG uses all of the leads of the 15-lead ECG plus leads V_5R, V_6R, and V_7. A 16-lead ECG machine allows recording of two ECGs: (1) a standard 12-lead plus leads V_3R, V_4R, V_5R, and V_6R, and (2) a standard 12-lead plus posterior leads V_7, V_8, and V_9.

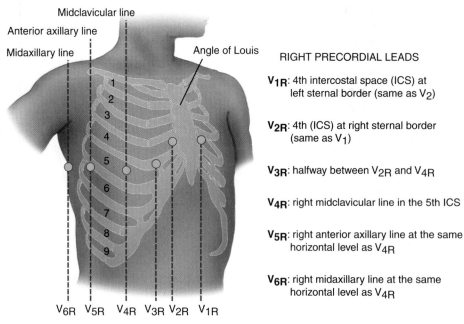

Figure 2-20 Electrode locations for recording a right chest electrocardiogram (ECG). Right chest leads are not a part of a standard 12-lead ECG but are used when a right ventricular infarction is suspected.

RIGHT PRECORDIAL LEADS

V_{1R}: 4th intercostal space (ICS) at left sternal border (same as V_2)

V_{2R}: 4th (ICS) at right sternal border (same as V_1)

V_{3R}: halfway between V_{2R} and V_{4R}

V_{4R}: right midclavicular line in the 5th ICS

V_{5R}: right anterior axillary line at the same horizontal level as V_{4R}

V_{6R}: right midaxillary line at the same horizontal level as V_{4R}

| SKILL 2-3 | Right Chest Lead Placement |

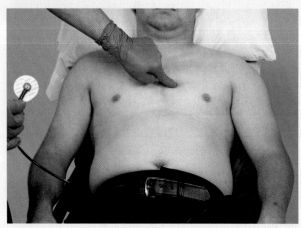

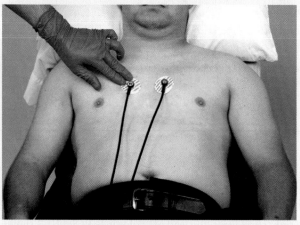

Step 1 A right-sided 12-lead electrocardiogram (ECG) should be obtained when a right ventricular infarction is suspected. Placement of right chest leads is identical to placement of the standard chest leads except it is done on the right side of the chest. When obtaining right-sided and/or posterior leads, obtain a standard 12-lead first. Then move the cables for the standard chest leads to the electrodes for the additional leads. Any chest lead cable can be moved to obtain the right and/or posterior leads. Begin by placing the electrode for V_1R in the fourth intercostal space, just to the left of the sternum.

Step 2 From the V_1R position, find the corresponding intercostal space on the right side of the sternum. This is V_2R. Place the V_2R electrode in the fourth intercostal space, just to the right of the sternum.

SKILL 2-3 | **Right Chest Lead Placement—cont'd**

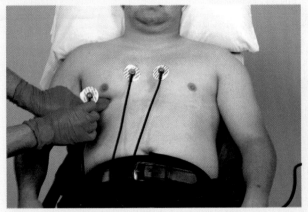

Step 3 From the V₂R position, move your fingers down, find the fifth intercostal space, and follow it to the midclavicular line. Place the V₄R electrode in the fifth intercostal space in the midclavicular line.

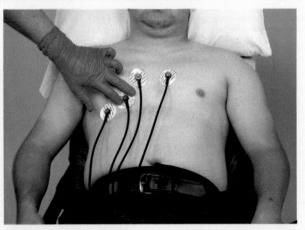

Step 4 Imagine a line between V₂R and V₄R. Position the V₃R electrode halfway between V₂R and V₄R on the imaginary line.

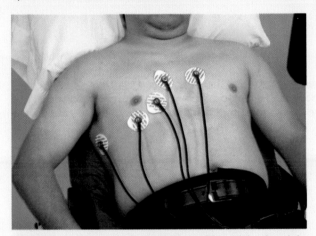

Step 5 The electrode for V₆R is positioned in the right midaxillary line, level with V₄R.

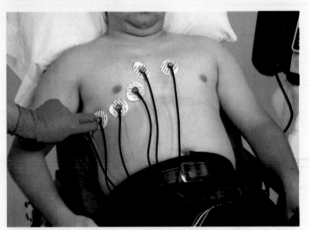

Step 6 Position V₅R in the right anterior axillary line, level with V₄R.

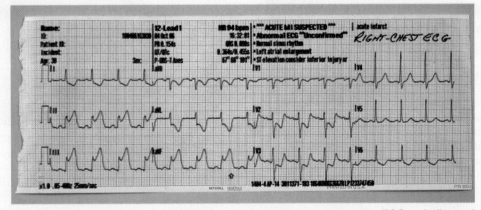

Step 7 Once these leads are printed, the correct lead must be handwritten onto the ECG to indicate the origin of the tracing. Clearly label the upper portion of the ECG tracing "right chest ECG." The computer-generated interpretation also must be disregarded in the event that the cables have been moved.

SKILL 2-4   **Posterior Chest Lead Placement**

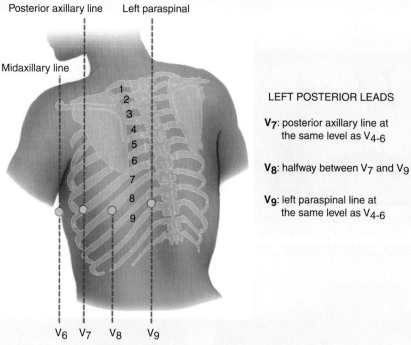

Posterior axillary line   Left paraspinal

Midaxillary line

1
2
3
4
5
6
7
8
9

LEFT POSTERIOR LEADS

V_7: posterior axillary line at the same level as V_{4-6}

V_8: halfway between V_7 and V_9

V_9: left paraspinal line at the same level as V_{4-6}

V_6 V_7 V_8 V_9

Step 1 Posterior chest leads are used when a posterior infarction is suspected. First obtain and print a standard 12-lead electrocardiogram (ECG). Then locate the landmarks for the posterior leads: posterior axillary line, midscapular line, and left border of the spine. Leads V_7, V_8, and V_9 are on the same horizontal line as leads V_4, V_5, and V_6 on the front of the chest.

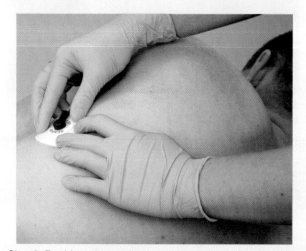

Step 2 Position the patient on his or her side. Find the posterior axillary line. Now locate the fifth intercostal space and place the V_7 electrode. Attach the V_4 lead wire to the V_7 electrode.

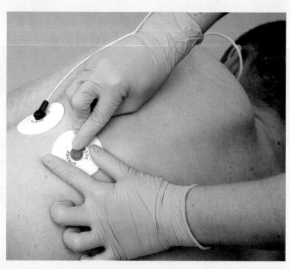

Step 3 Find the left midscapular line and fifth intercostal space. Place the V_8 electrode here. Attach the V_5 lead wire to the V_8 electrode.

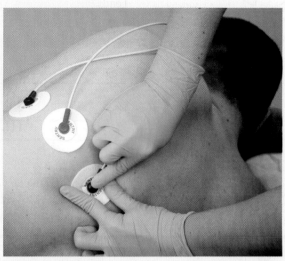

Step 4 Place the electrode for V₉ just left of the spinal column at the fifth intercostal space. Attach the V₆ lead wire to the V₉ electrode.

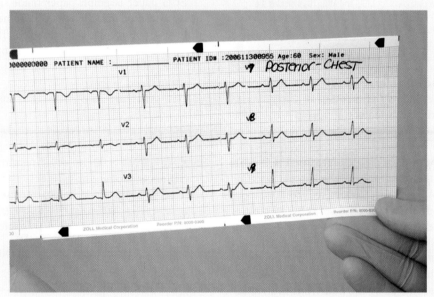

Step 5 Obtain and print the 12-lead ECG. Clearly label the upper portion of the ECG tracing "posterior chest ECG." Remember to relabel lead V₄ on the printout V₇, relabel V₅ to V₈, and V₆ to V₉.

Modified Chest Leads

The modified chest leads (MCL) are bipolar chest leads that are variations of the chest leads. Each modified chest lead consists of a positive and negative electrode applied to a specific location on the chest. Accurate placement of the positive electrode is important.

Lead MCL_1 views the ventricular septum. The negative electrode is placed below the left clavicle toward the left shoulder, and the positive electrode is placed to the right of the sternum in the fourth intercostal space (Figure 2-21). Leads MCL_1 and V_1 are similar but not identical. In V_1, the negative electrode is calculated by the ECG machine at the center of the heart. In MCL_1, the negative electrode is located just below the left clavicle.

Lead MCL_6 is a variation of the chest lead V_6 and views the low lateral wall of the left ventricle. The negative electrode is placed below the left clavicle toward the left shoulder and the positive electrode is placed at the fifth intercostal space, left midaxillary line.

What Each Lead "Sees"[9]

Each positive electrode can be thought of as a camera or an eye looking in at the heart. The particular portion of the heart that each lead "sees" is determined by two factors.

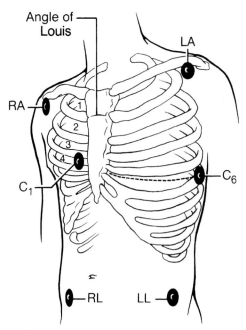

Figure 2-21 Electrode placement for MCL₁ and MCL₆. C₁ indicates the proper position of the chest electrode for monitoring lead V₁, and C₆ indicates the proper position of the chest electrode for monitoring V₆.

The first factor is the dominance of the left ventricle on the ECG, and the second is the position of the positive electrode on the body. Both factors are discussed below, beginning with the dominance of the left ventricle on the ECG.

Because the ECG does not directly measure the heart's electrical activity, it does not "see" all the current flowing through the heart. What the ECG does see from its vantage point on the body's surface is the net result of countless individual currents competing in a tug-of-war. For example, the QRS complex, which represents ventricular depolarization, is not a display of all the electrical activity occurring in the right and left ventricles. It is the net result of a tug-of-war produced by the numerous individual currents in both the right and left ventricles. Because the left ventricle is much more massive than the right, the left overpowers the right. What is seen in the QRS complex is the remaining electrical activity of the left ventricle, that is, the portion not used to cancel out the right ventricle. Therefore, in a normally conducted beat, the QRS complex represents the electrical activity occurring in the left ventricle.

The second factor, position of the positive electrode on the body, determines which portion of the left ventricle is seen by each lead. The view of each lead can be committed to memory, or it can be reasoned easily by remembering where the positive electrode is located. The view of each lead is listed in Table 2-5, while Figure 2-22 demonstrates the portion of the left ventricle that each lead views. Please note that aVR is not included in Table 2-5 or Figure 2-22.

Table **2-5**	What Each Lead "Sees"
Leads	**Heart Surface Viewed**
II, III, aVF	Inferior
V₁, V₂	Septal
V₃, V₄	Anterior
I, aVL, V₅, V₆	Lateral

ELECTROCARDIOGRAPHY PAPER

[Objectives 16, 17]
Remember that the ECG is a graphical representation of the heart's electrical activity. When you place electrodes on the patient's body and connect them to an ECG, the machine records the voltage (i.e., the potential difference) between the electrodes. The needle, or pen, of the ECG moves a specific distance depending on the voltage measured. This recording is made on ECG paper.

ECG paper is graph paper made up of small and large boxes measured in millimeters. The smallest boxes are 1-mm wide and 1-mm high (Figure 2-23). The horizontal axis of the paper corresponds with *time*. Time is used to measure the interval between or duration of specific cardiac events, which is stated in seconds.

ECG paper normally records at a constant speed of 25 mm/sec. Thus, each horizontal unit (i.e., each 1-mm box) represents 0.04 second (25 mm/sec × 0.04 second = 1 mm). Look closely at the boxes in Figure 2-23. You can see that the lines after every five small boxes on the paper are heavier. The heavier lines indicate one large box. Because each large box is the width of five small boxes, a large box represents 0.20 second. Five large boxes, each consisting of five small boxes, represent 1 second; fifteen large boxes equal an interval of 3 seconds; and thirty large boxes represent 6 seconds.

ECG Pearl

The rate at which electrocardiogram (ECG) paper goes through the printer is adjustable. A faster paper speed makes the rhythm appear slower and the QRS wider. Thus, in cases of rapid heart rates, a faster paper speed makes it easier to see the waveforms and analyze the tachycardia. A slower paper speed makes the rhythm appear faster and the QRS narrower.[9]

The vertical axis of the graph paper represents the voltage or amplitude of the ECG waveforms or deflections. Voltage is measured in millivolts (mV). Voltage may appear as a positive or negative value, because voltage is a force with direction as well as amplitude. Amplitude is measured in millimeters (mm). The ECG machine's sensitivity must be calibrated so that a 1-mV electrical signal will produce a deflection that measures exactly 10-mm tall. When properly calibrated, a small box is 1-mm high (i.e., 0.1 mV), and a

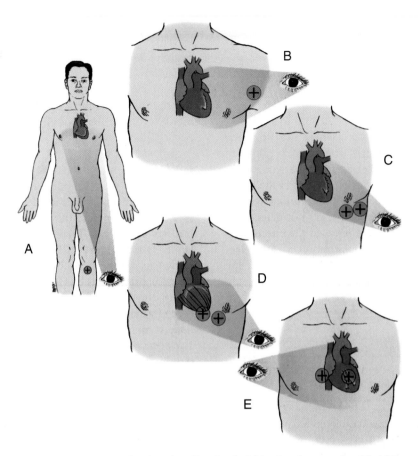

Figure 2-22   **A,** Leads II, III, and aVF each have their positive electrode positioned on the left leg. From the perspective of the left leg, each of them "sees" the inferior wall of the left ventricle. **B,** From their vantage point on the left arm, leads I and aVL "look" in at the lateral wall of the left ventricle. **C,** Leads V₅ and V₆ also "view" the lateral wall because they are positioned on the axillary area of the left chest. **D,** Leads V₃ and V₄ are positioned in the area of the anterior chest. From this perspective, these leads "see" the anterior wall of the left ventricle. **E,** The septal wall is "seen" by leads V₁ and V₂, which are positioned next to the sternum.

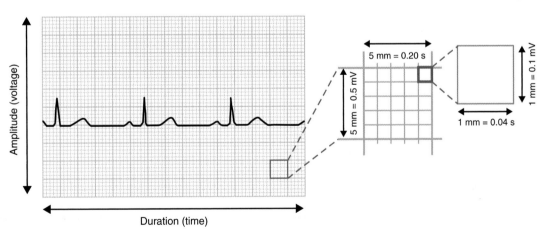

Figure 2-23   Electrocardiographic strip showing the markings for measuring amplitude and duration of waveforms, using a standard recording speed of 25 mm/sec.

large box, which is equal to five small boxes, is 5-mm high (i.e., 0.5 mV). Clinically, the height of a waveform is usually stated in millimeters rather than in millivolts.

Waveforms

[Objective 18]

A **waveform** (i.e., a deflection) is movement away from the baseline in a positive (i.e., upward) or negative (i.e., downward) direction (Box 2-1). Each waveform that you see on an ECG is related to a specific electrical event in the heart. Waveforms are named alphabetically, beginning with P, QRS, T, and U. When electrical activity is not detected, a straight line is recorded. This line is called the **baseline** or **isoelectric line**. If the wave of depolarization (i.e., the electrical impulse) moves toward the positive electrode, the waveform recorded on ECG graph paper will be upright (i.e., a positive deflection) (Figure 2-24). If the wave of depolarization moves away from the positive electrode, the waveform recorded will be inverted (i.e., a downward or negative deflection). A **biphasic** (i.e., partly positive, partly negative) waveform or a straight line is recorded when the wave of depolarization moves perpendicularly to the positive electrode. The term *equiphasic* may be used instead of biphasic to describe a waveform that has no net positive or negative deflection.

P Wave

Activation of the SA node occurs before the onset of the P wave. This event is not recorded on the ECG. However, the spread of that impulse throughout the atria (atrial depolarization) is observed. The first waveform in the cardiac cycle is the *P wave* (Figure 2-25). The beginning of the P wave is recognized as the first abrupt or gradual movement away from the baseline; its end is the point at which the waveform returns to the baseline. The first half of the P wave is recorded when the electrical impulse that originated in the SA node stimulates the right atrium and reaches the AV node. The downslope of the P wave reflects stimulation of the left atrium; thus the P wave represents atrial depolarization and the spread of the electrical impulse throughout the right and left atria. A P wave normally precedes each QRS complex. Normal P wave characteristics are shown in Box 2-2.

The atria contract a fraction of a second after the P wave begins. The atria begin to repolarize at the same time as the ventricles depolarize. A waveform representing atrial repolarization is usually not seen on the ECG because it is small and buried in the QRS complex.

Tall and pointed (i.e., peaked) or wide and notched P waves may be seen in conditions such as chronic obstructive pulmonary disease (COPD), heart failure, or in valvular disease and may be indicative of atrial enlargement (Figure 2-26). Enlargement of the right atrium produces an abnormally tall initial part of the P wave. The latter part of the P wave is prominent in left atrial enlargement.

P waves that begin at a site other than the SA node (i.e., ectopic P waves) may be positive or negative in lead II. If the ectopic pacemaker is in the atria, the P wave will be upright. If the ectopic pacemaker is in the AV bundle, the P wave will be negative (i.e., inverted) in lead II.

QRS Complex

[Objective 19]

A **complex** consists of several waveforms. The QRS complex consists of the Q wave, R wave, and S wave (see Figure 2-25) and represents the spread of the electrical impulse through the ventricles (i.e., ventricular depolarization) and the sum of all ventricular muscle cell depolarizations. Ventricular depolarization normally triggers contraction of ventricular tissue. Thus, shortly after the QRS complex begins, the ventricles contract (Figure 2-27). The QRS complex is significantly larger than the P wave because depolarization of the ventricles involves a considerably greater muscle mass than depolarization of the atria. Atrial repolarization usually

---

Box **2-1**	Terminology

Baseline (isoelectric line): A straight line recorded when electrical activity is not detected
Waveform: Movement away from the baseline in either a positive or negative direction
Segment: A line between waveforms; named by the waveform that precedes or follows it
Complex: Several waveforms
Interval: A waveform and a segment

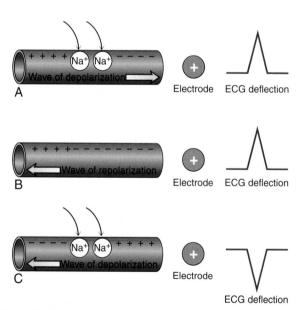

Figure 2-24 Electrocardiographic (ECG) waveforms may be positive (upward) or negative (downward), depending on the location of electrodes on the chest. **A,** A wave of depolarization moving toward a positive electrode results in a positive deflection. **B,** A wave of repolarization moving away from a positive electrode results in a positive deflection. **C,** A wave of depolarization moving away from a positive electrode results in a negative deflection. A biphasic (partly positive, partly negative) waveform or a straight line is recorded when the wave of depolarization moves perpendicularly to the positive electrode.

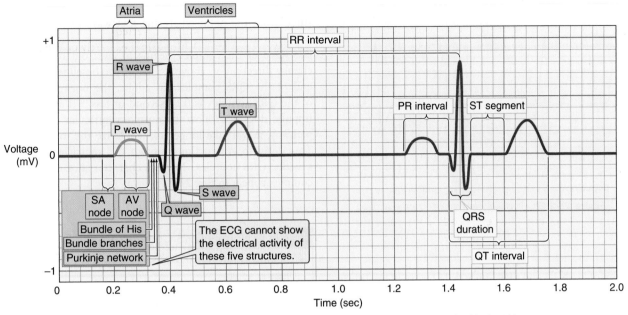

Figure 2-25 Components of the electrocardiogram (ECG) recording. AV, atrioventricular; SA, sinoatrial.

- Smooth and rounded
- No more than 2.5 mm in height
- No more than 0.11 second in duration
- Positive in leads I, II, aVF, and V_2 through V_6

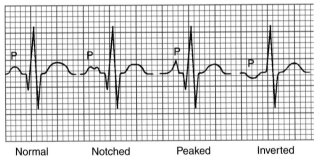

Figure 2-26   Abnormal P waves may be notched, tall and pointed (peaked), or inverted (negative).

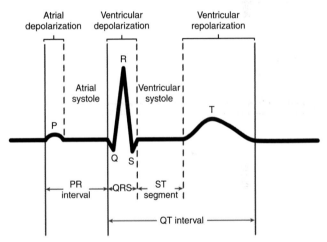

Figure 2-27   Normal electrocardiogram (ECG) waveforms, intervals, and correlation with events of the cardiac cycle. The P wave represents atrial depolarization, followed immediately by atrial systole. The QRS represents ventricular depolarization, followed immediately by ventricular systole. The ST segment corresponds to phase 2 of the action potential, during which time the heart muscle is completely depolarized and contraction normally occurs. The T wave represents ventricular repolarization. The PR interval, measured from the beginning of the P wave to the beginning of the QRS, corresponds to atrial depolarization and impulse delay in the atrioventricular (AV) node. The QT interval, measured from the beginning of the QRS complex to the end of the T wave, represents the time from initial depolarization of the ventricles to the end of ventricular repolarization.

takes place during ventricular depolarization, but the QRS complex overshadows it on the ECG.

A QRS complex normally follows each P wave. One or even two of the three waveforms that make up the QRS complex may not always be present. The QRS complex begins as a downward deflection, the *Q wave.* A Q wave is *always* a negative waveform. The Q wave begins when the ECG leaves the isoelectric line in a downward direction and continues until it returns to the isoelectric line. The Q wave represents depolarization of the interventricular septum, which is activated from left to right. In lead II, the direction of the

current flow is almost perpendicular to it, and more current is moving away from the positive electrode than is moving toward it. In lead MCL_1, depolarization of the interventricular septum will appear as a small, upright R wave. In this lead, this is the first deflection of a normal QRS complex.

It is important to differentiate normal (i.e., a physiologic) Q waves from pathologic Q waves (Figure 2-28). With the

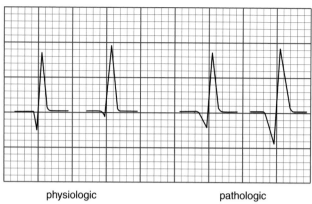

physiologic   pathologic

Figure 2-28 Physiologic and pathologic Q waves.

exception of leads III and aVR, a normal Q wave in the limb leads is less than 0.04 second (i.e., one small box) in duration and less than one third the height of the R wave in that lead. An abnormal (i.e., pathologic) Q wave is more than 0.04 second in duration or more than one third the height of the following R wave in that lead. Myocardial infarction is one possible cause of abnormal Q waves. In the early hours of infarction, an abnormal Q wave may not have developed to its full width or amplitude. Therefore, a single ECG tracing may not identify an abnormal Q wave. In a patient with a suspected MI, be sure to look at Q waves closely. Even if the initial ECG tracings do not show Q waves that are more than 0.04 second in duration or equal to or more than one third of the amplitude of the QRS complex, pathology must be considered if the Q waves become wider or deeper in each subsequent tracing.

The QRS complex continues as a large, upright, triangular waveform known as the *R wave* (see Figure 2-25). The R wave is the first positive (i.e., upright) waveform following the P wave. The S wave is the negative waveform following the R wave. An R wave is *always* positive and an S wave is *always* negative. The R and S waves represent simultaneous depolarization of the right and left ventricles. Because of its greater muscle mass, the QRS complex generally represents the electrical activity occurring in the left ventricle.

The QRS complex may appear predominantly positive, negative, or biphasic, depending on the lead. It is predominantly positive in leads that view the heart from the left (e.g., I, aVL, V_5, V_6) and in leads that look at the heart's inferior surface (e.g., II, III, aVF). In leads that view the heart from the right side, the QRS complex is predominantly negative (e.g., aVR, V_1, V_2). The QRS is normally biphasic in leads V_3, V_4, and sometimes III.

QRS Measurement

The QRS duration is a measurement of the time required for ventricular depolarization. The width of a QRS complex is most accurately determined when it is viewed and measured in more than one lead. The measurement should be taken from the QRS complex with the longest duration and clearest

onset and end. The beginning of the QRS complex is measured from the point where the first wave of the complex begins to deviate from the baseline. The point at which the last wave of the complex begins to level out or distinctly change direction at, above, or below the baseline marks the end of the QRS complex. In adults, the normal duration of the QRS complex is 0.11 second or less.[10] If an electrical impulse does not follow the normal ventricular conduction pathway, it will take longer to depolarize the myocardium. This delay in conduction through the ventricles produces a wider QRS complex. Normal characteristics of the QRS complex appear in Box 2-3.

Box 2-3   Normal QRS Complex Characteristics
• Normal duration of the QRS complex is 0.11 second or less in adults
• With the exception of leads III and aVR, a normal Q wave in the limb leads is less than 0.04 second in duration and less than one third of the amplitude of the R wave in that lead

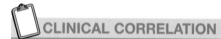

CLINICAL CORRELATION

Einthoven expressed the relationship among leads I, II, and III as the sum of any complex in leads I and III equals that of lead II. Thus, lead I + III = II. Stated another way, the voltage of a waveform in lead I plus the voltage of the same waveform in lead III equals the voltage of the same waveform in lead II. For example, when you look at leads I, II, and III, if the R wave in lead II does not appear to be the sum of the voltage of the R waves in leads I and III, the leads may have been incorrectly applied.

Abnormal QRS Complexes

- In adults, the duration of an abnormal QRS complex is greater than 0.11 second.
- The duration of a QRS caused by an impulse originating in an ectopic pacemaker in the Purkinje network or ventricular myocardium is usually greater than 0.12 second and often 0.16 second or greater.
- If the impulse originates in a bundle branch, the duration of the QRS may be only slightly greater than 0.10 second. For example, a QRS duration between 0.10 and 0.12 second in adults is called an *incomplete* bundle branch block. In adults, a QRS measuring 0.12 second or more is called a *complete* bundle branch block. This is discussed in more detail in Chapter 9.
- Low QRS amplitude is defined as less than 5 mm in all limb leads or less than 10 mm in all chest leads.[11]
- Enlargement of the right ventricle produces an abnormally tall R wave; left ventricular enlargement produces an abnormally deep S wave.

QRS Variations

Although the term *QRS complex* is used, not every QRS complex contains a Q wave, R wave, and S wave. If the QRS complex consists entirely of a positive waveform, it is called an *R wave*. If the complex consists entirely of a negative waveform, it is called a *QS wave*. QS waves may be pathologic. If there are two positive deflections in the same complex, the second is called *R prime* and is written *R'*. If there are two negative deflections following an R wave, the second is called *S prime* and is written *S'*. Capital (i.e., upper case) letters are used to designate waveforms of relatively large amplitude, and small (i.e., lower case) letters are used to label relatively small waveforms (Figure 2-29).

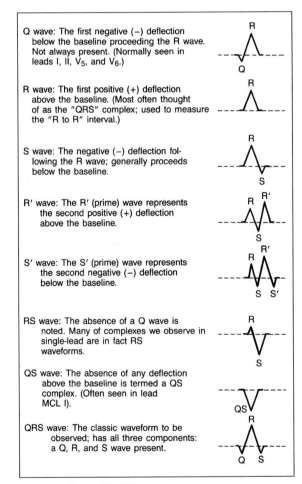

Q wave: The first negative (−) deflection below the baseline proceeding the R wave. Not always present. (Normally seen in leads I, II, V$_5$, and V$_6$.)

R wave: The first positive (+) deflection above the baseline. (Most often thought of as the "QRS" complex; used to measure the "R to R" interval.)

S wave: The negative (−) deflection following the R wave; generally proceeds below the baseline.

R' wave: The R' (prime) wave represents the second positive (+) deflection above the baseline.

S' wave: The S' (prime) wave represents the second negative (−) deflection below the baseline.

RS wave: The absence of a Q wave is noted. Many of complexes we observe in single-lead are in fact RS waveforms.

QS wave: The absence of any deflection above the baseline is termed a QS complex. (Often seen in lead MCL I).

QRS wave: The classic waveform to be observed; has all three components: a Q, R, and S wave present.

Figure 2-29 Various QRS morphologies.

CLINICAL CORRELATION

Lead MCL$_1$ was once used to help differentiate between right and left bundle blocks and distinguish ventricular tachycardia from supraventricular tachycardia with abnormal (i.e., aberrant) ventricular conduction. Because the shape (morphology) of the QRS complex in MCL$_1$ has been shown to differ in 40% of patients with ventricular tachycardia, chest lead V$_1$ should be used instead.[16,17]

T Wave

Ventricular repolarization is represented on the ECG by the T wave (see Figure 2-25). The ARP is still present during the beginning of the T wave. At the peak of the T wave, the RRP has begun. It is during the RRP that a stronger than normal stimulus may produce ventricular dysrhythmias.

In the limb leads, lead II most commonly reveals the tallest T wave. The normal T wave is slightly asymmetric: The peak of the waveform is closer to its end than to the beginning, and the first half has a more gradual slope than the second half (Box 2-4). The beginning of the T wave is identified as the point where the slope of the ST segment appears to become abruptly or gradually steeper. The T wave ends when it returns to the baseline. It may be difficult to clearly determine the onset and end of the T wave. Examples of T waves are shown in Figure 2-30.

The direction of the T wave is normally the same as the QRS complex that precedes it. This is because depolarization begins at the endocardial surface and spreads to the epicardium. Repolarization begins at the epicardium and spreads to the endocardium.

Box 2-4 | Normal T Wave Characteristics

- Slightly asymmetric
- Negative in aVR; may be positive or negative in leads aVL, III, and V$_1$
- Normally upright in leads I, II, and V$_3$ through V$_6$
- Usually 0.5 mm or more in height in leads I and II
- Usually 5 mm or less in height in any limb lead or 10 mm or less in any chest lead

Abnormal T Waves

- A T wave following an abnormal QRS complex is usually opposite in direction of the QRS. In other words, when the QRS complex points down, the T wave points up, and vice versa. This may be seen with ventricular beats or rhythms and in bundle branch block.
- Tall, pointed (i.e., peaked) T waves are commonly seen in hyperkalemia.
- Low-amplitude T waves may be seen in hypokalemia or hypomagnesemia.
- Tall, broad T waves may be seen with internal pacemakers.
- The T wave in leads I, II, aVL, and V$_2$ to V$_6$ should be described as *inverted* when the T-wave amplitude is from −1 mm to −5 mm, as *deep negative* when the amplitude is from −5 mm to −10 mm, and as *giant negative* when the amplitude is more than −10 mm. The T wave may be described as *low* when its amplitude is less than 10% of the R wave amplitude in the same lead and as *flat* when the peak T-wave amplitude is between 1 mm and −1 mm in leads I, II, aVL (with an R wave taller than 3 mm) and V$_4$ to V$_6$.[12]

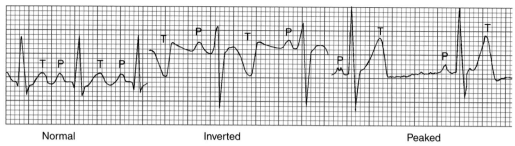

Normal   Inverted   Peaked

Figure 2-30   Examples of T waves.

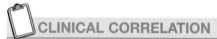

CLINICAL CORRELATION

In a patient experiencing an acute coronary syndrome, T-wave inversion, which may occur simultaneously with ST-segment elevation, suggests the presence of myocardial ischemia. The development of pathologic Q waves provides evidence that tissue death has occurred. A pathologic Q wave indicates the presence of dead myocardial tissue and subsequently, a loss of electrical activity.

U Wave

A U wave is a small waveform that, when seen, follows the T wave. The U wave represents repolarization of the Purkinje fibers in the papillary muscle of the ventricular myocardium.[13,14]

Normal U waves are small, round, and symmetric. U waves are most easily seen when the heart rate is slow and are difficult to identify when the rate exceeds 95 beats/min. When seen, they are generally tallest in leads V_2 and V_3. U waves usually appear in the same direction as the T waves that precede them. The amplitude of the normal U wave is usually proportional to the T wave in the same lead, averaging about 11% of the T wave's amplitude. Negative U waves in V_2 through V_5 are abnormal and may be seen in patients with ischemic heart disease or in the presence of hypertension.

Possible causes of tall U waves include the following:
- Central nervous system disease
- Electrolyte imbalance (e.g., hypokalemia) (Figure 2-31)
- Hyperthyroidism
- Long QT syndrome

- Medications (e.g., amiodarone, digitalis, disopyramide, phenothiazines, procainamide, quinidine)

Segments

[Objectives 18, 19]
A **segment** is a line between waveforms. It is named by the waveform that precedes or follows it.

PR Segment

The PR segment is part of the PR interval—specifically, the horizontal line between the end of the P wave and the beginning of the QRS complex (Figure 2-32). The PR segment is normally isoelectric and represents the spread of the electrical impulse from the AV node, through the AV bundle, right and left bundle branches, and the Purkinje fibers. Atrial repolarization also occurs during this period.

The PR segment normally measures 0.10 second or less but depends on the duration of the P wave and impulse conduction through the AV node, AV bundle, and bundle branches. Most of the conduction delay during the PR segment is a result of slow conduction within the AV node. The PR segment may be depressed in patients with ventricular **hypertrophy** (i.e., an increase in the thickness of a heart chamber because of chronic pressure overload) or chronic pulmonary disease.

TP Segment

The TP segment is the portion of the ECG tracing between the end of the T wave and the beginning of the following P wave during which there is no electrical activity (Figure 2-33).

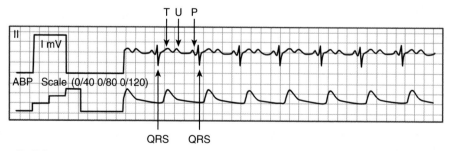

Figure 2-31   Electrocardiogram (ECG) tracing from a patient with a serum potassium of 2.6 mEq/L shows a prominent U wave.

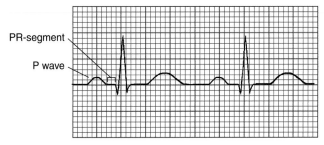

Figure 2-32 The PR segment.

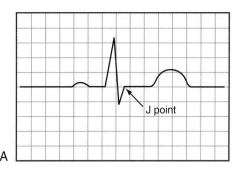

A

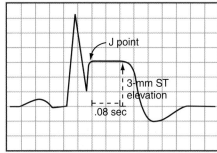

B

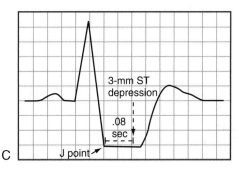

C

Figure 2-34 **A,** Normal position of the J point. **B,** A 3-mm ST segment elevation. **C,** A 3-mm ST segment depression. ST segment changes are measured 0.06 to 0.08 sec after the J point.

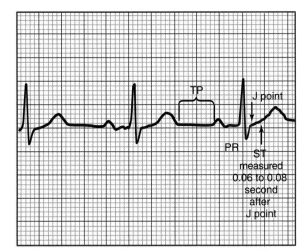

Figure 2-33 The TP segment is used as the reference point for the isoelectric line if the heart rate is slow enough for the TP segment to be clearly seen.

When the heart rate is within normal limits, the TP segment is usually isoelectric and used as the reference point from which to estimate the position of the isoelectric line and determine ST-segment displacement. With rapid heart rates, the TP segment is often unrecognizable because the P wave encroaches on the preceding T wave.

ST Segment

The portion of the ECG tracing between the QRS complex and the T wave is the ST segment (see Figure 2-25). The term *ST segment* is used regardless of whether the final wave of the QRS complex is an R or an S wave. The ST segment represents the early part of repolarization of the right and left ventricles. The normal ST segment begins at the isoelectric line, extends from the end of the S wave, and curves gradually upward to the beginning of the T wave. In the limb leads, the normal ST segment is isoelectric (flat) but may normally be slightly elevated or depressed.

The point where the QRS complex and the ST segment meet is called the *ST junction* or the *J point* (Figure 2-34). The ST segment is considered elevated if the segment is deviated above the baseline and is considered depressed if the segment deviates below it. When looking for ST segment elevation or depression, first locate the J point. Next use the TP segment to estimate the position of the isoelectric line.

Then compare the level of the ST segment to the isoelectric line. Deviation is measured as the number of millimeters of vertical ST-segment displacement from the isoelectric line or from the patient's baseline at a point 0.06 or 0.08 second after the J point.[12,15] It may be difficult to clearly determine the J point in patients with rapid heart rates or hyperkalemia. Some displacement of the ST segment from the isoelectric line is normal and dependent on age, gender, and ECG lead (Table 2-6).

ECG Pearl

Proper machine calibration is critical when analyzing ST segments. The ST segment criteria described here applies *only* when the monitor is adjusted to standard calibration.

Various conditions may cause the displacement of the ST segment from the isoelectric line in either a positive or a negative direction. Myocardial ischemia, injury, and

Table **2-6**	ST-Segment Displacement		
Patient	ECG Lead	Threshold Value for Abnormal J Point Elevation	Threshold Value for Abnormal J Point Depression
Male, 40 years and older	V_2 and V_3	2 mm	0.5 mm
	All other leads	1 mm	1 mm
Male, younger than 40 years	V_2 and V_3	2.5 mm	0.5 mm
	All other leads	1 mm	1 mm
Female	V_2 and V_3	1.5 mm	0.5 mm
	All other leads	More than 1 mm	1 mm
Male, 30 years and older	V_3R and V_4R	0.5 mm	1 mm
Male, younger than 30 years	V_3R and V_4R	1 mm	1 mm
Female	V_3R and V_4R	0.5 mm	1 mm
Male and female	V_7 through V_9	0.5 mm	1 mm

Data from references 7 and 12.

infarction are among the causes of ST-segment deviation. ST-segment elevation in the shape of a "smiley" face (i.e., upward concavity) is usually benign, particularly when it occurs in an otherwise healthy, asymptomatic patient (Figure 2-35). The appearance of coved (i.e., "frowny face") ST-segment elevation is called an *acute injury pattern*. Other causes of ST-segment elevation may represent a normal variant, pericarditis, or ventricular aneurysm, among other causes. Pericarditis causes ST-segment elevation in all or virtually all leads. ST segments are discussed in more detail in Chapter 9.

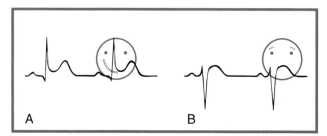

Figure 2-35 **(A)** ST segment elevation in the shape of a "smiley" face (upward concavity) is usually benign, particularly when it occurs in an otherwise healthy, asymptomatic patient. **(B)** ST segment elevation in the shape of a "frowny" face (downward concavity) is more often associated with an acute injury pattern.

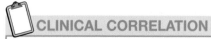

CLINICAL CORRELATION

ST-segment elevation provides the strongest electrocardiogram (ECG) evidence for the early recognition of myocardial infarction. In a patient experiencing an acute coronary syndrome, keep in mind that myocardial injury refers to myocardial tissue that has been cut off from or experienced a severe reduction in its blood and oxygen supply. The tissue is not yet dead and may be salvageable if the blocked vessel can be quickly opened, restoring blood flow and oxygen to the injured area.

Abnormal ST Segments
- ST-segment depression of more than 0.5 mm in leads V_2 and V_3 and more than 1 mm in all other leads is suggestive of myocardial ischemia.
- ST-segment elevation varies and is dependent on patient age, gender, and ECG lead.
- A horizontal ST-segment (i.e., forming a sharp angle with the T wave) is suggestive of ischemia.
- Digitalis causes a depression or scoop of the ST segment that is sometimes referred to as a "dig dip" (Figure 2-36).

CLINICAL CORRELATION

When electrocardiogram (ECG) changes of myocardial ischemia, injury, or infarction occur, they are not found in every lead of the ECG. Findings are considered significant if viewed in two or more leads looking at the same or adjacent area of the heart. If these findings are seen in leads that look directly at the affected area, they are called **indicative changes**. If findings are seen in leads opposite the affected area, they are called **reciprocal changes** (also called *mirror image* changes). Indicative changes are significant when they are seen in two *anatomically contiguous* leads. Two leads are contiguous if they look at the same or adjacent areas of the heart or if they are numerically consecutive chest leads (see Chapter 9).

Intervals

PR Interval
[Objective 18]
An **interval** is made up of a waveform and a segment. The P wave plus the PR segment equals the PR interval (PRI) (Figure 2-37). Remember that the P wave reflects depolarization of the right and left atria. The PR segment represents the spread of the impulse through the AV node, AV bundle, right and left bundle branches, and the Purkinje

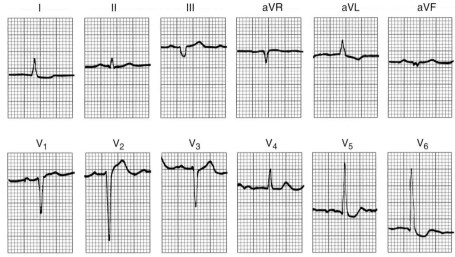

Figure 2-36 Digitalis may produce a characteristic "scooping" of the ST segment, as seen here in leads V₅ and V₆.

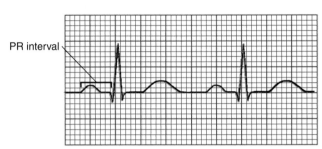

Figure 2-37 The PR interval reflects depolarization of the right and left atria (P wave) and the spread of the impulse through the atrioventricular (AV) node, AV bundle, right and left bundle branches, and the Purkinje fibers (PR segment).

fibers. The PRI does not reflect the duration of conduction from the SA node to the right atrium.

The PRI is measured from the point where the P wave leaves the baseline to the beginning of the QRS complex. The term *PQ interval* is preferred by some, because it is the period that is actually measured unless a Q wave is absent. The PRI changes with heart rate but normally measures 0.12 to 0.20 second in adults (Box 2-5). As the heart rate increases, the duration of the PRI shortens. A PRI is considered *short* if it is less than 0.12 second and *long* if it is more than 0.20 second.

ECG Pearl

Measuring how quickly or slowly an electrical impulse spreads through the heart provides important information about the condition of the heart's conduction system and the muscle itself.

Box **2-5**	Normal PR Interval Characteristics

- Normally measures 0.12 to 0.20 second in adults; may be shorter in children and longer in older adults
- Normally shortens as heart rate increases

Abnormal PR Intervals

Delays in impulse conduction through the atria, AV node, or AV bundle can result in prolongation (greater than 0.20 second) of the PRI. Conditions causing such disturbances may be inflammatory, circulatory, nervous, endocrine, or pharmacological in origin. The P wave associated with a prolonged PRI may be normal or abnormal.

A PRI of less than 0.12 second may be seen when the impulse originates in an ectopic pacemaker in the atria close to the AV node or in the AV bundle. A shortened PRI may also occur if the electrical impulse progresses from the atria to the ventricles through an abnormal conduction pathway that bypasses the AV node and depolarizes the ventricles earlier than usual.

QT Interval
[Objective 18]

The **QT interval** is the period from the beginning of the QRS complex to the end of the T wave. It represents total ventricular activity; this is the time from ventricular depolarization (i.e., activation) to repolarization (i.e., recovery) (see Figure 2-25). When measuring the QT interval, first select a lead with the most clearly defined T-wave end. To ensure meaningful comparisons of later tracings, use the same lead for subsequent measurements. In the absence of a Q wave, the QT interval is measured from the beginning of the R wave to the end of the T wave. The term *QT interval* is used regardless of whether the QRS complex begins with a Q wave or an R wave.

ECG Pearl

The QT interval is usually longest in chest leads V₂, V₃, or V₄.[12,17]

The duration of the QT interval varies in accordance with age, gender, and heart rate. As the heart rate increases, the QT interval shortens (i.e., decreases). As the heart rate decreases, the QT interval lengthens (i.e., increases). To quickly estimate the QT interval, first measure the interval between two consecutive R waves (R-R interval). If the measured QT interval is less than half the R-R interval of that QRS complex and the R wave of the following complex, it is probably normal (provided the patient's heart rate is 95 beats/min or less). A QT interval that is approximately half the R-R interval is probably borderline. A QT interval that is more than half the R-R interval is probably prolonged.

Because of the variability of the QT interval with the heart rate, it can be measured more accurately if it is corrected (i.e., adjusted) for the patient's heart rate. The corrected QT interval is calculated as the QT interval divided by the square root of the R-R interval and noted as QT_c. The QT interval is considered short if it is 0.39 second or less and prolonged if it is 0.46 second or longer in women or 0.45 second or longer in men.[12]

A prolonged QT interval indicates a lengthened RRP. A QT_c of more than 0.50 second in either gender has been correlated with a higher risk for ventricular dysrhythmias (e.g., torsades de Pointes [TdP]). A prolonged QT interval may be congenital or acquired. Myocardial ischemia or infarction, electrolyte disorders, sudden decreases in heart rate, acute neurologic events, and medications (e.g., amiodarone, sotalol) can prolong the QT interval. Digitalis and hypercalcemia shorten the QT interval.

R-R and P-P Intervals

The R-R (R wave-to-R wave) and P-P (P wave-to-P wave) intervals are used to determine the rate and rhythmicity (regularity) of a cardiac rhythm. To evaluate the rhythmicity of the ventricular rhythm on a rhythm strip, the interval between two consecutive R waves is measured (see Figure 2-25). The distance between succeeding R-R intervals is measured and compared. If the ventricular rhythm is regular, the R-R intervals will measure the same. To evaluate the rhythmicity of the atrial rhythm, the same procedure is used but the interval between two consecutive P waves is measured and compared to succeeding P-P intervals.

Artifact

[Objective 20]

Accurate ECG rhythm recognition requires a tracing in which the waveforms and intervals are free of distortion. Distortion of an ECG tracing by electrical activity that is noncardiac in origin is called **artifact**. Because artifact can mimic various cardiac dysrhythmias, including ventricular fibrillation, it is essential to evaluate the patient before initiating any medical intervention.

Artifact may be caused by loose electrodes, broken ECG cables or broken wires, muscle tremor, patient movement, external chest compressions, and 60-cycle interference.

Proper preparation of the patient's skin and evaluation of the monitoring equipment (e.g., electrodes, wires) before use can minimize the problems associated with artifact.

Loose Electrodes

An irregular baseline may be identified by bizarre, irregular deflections of the baseline on the ECG paper. This may be the result of a broken lead wire, poor electrical contact, or a loose electrode (Figure 2-38). When hair is present in large quantities, it may interfere with electrode adhesion. When the gel is in contact with hair instead of skin, penetration will be hindered. A simple disposable razor may be used to remove hair before placing the electrodes, but many prefer to use electric clippers instead. Whatever device is used, it is important to remove the hair in the area where the electrodes will be applied.

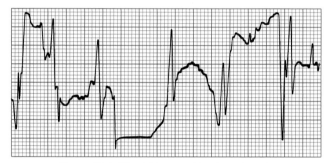

Figure 2-38   Artifact caused by a loose electrode.

Patient Movement/Muscle Activity

A wandering baseline may occur because of normal respiratory movement (particularly when electrodes have been applied directly over the ribs) or because of poor electrode contact with the patient's skin. Seizures, shivering, tense muscles, or Parkinson disease may cause muscle tremor artifact (Figure 2-39). Consider clipping the ECG cable to the patient's clothing to minimize excessive movement.

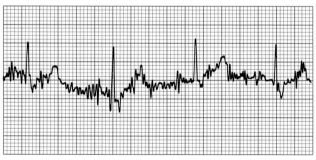

Figure 2-39   Artifact caused by muscle tremors.

60-Cycle (AC) Interference

A phenomenon known as 60-cycle interference may be caused by improperly grounded electrical equipment or other electrical interference (Figure 2-40). If 60-cycle interference is observed, check for crossing of cable wires with

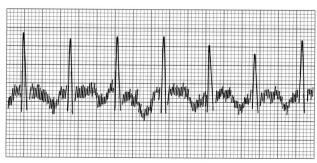

Figure 2-40 Artifact caused by 60-cycle interference.

other electrical wires (such as a bed control) or frayed and broken wires. Verify that all electrical equipment is properly grounded and that the cable electrode connections are clean.

SYSTEMATIC RHYTHM INTERPRETATION

[Objective 21]

A systematic approach to rhythm analysis that is consistently applied when analyzing a rhythm strip is essential (Box 2-6). If you do not develop such an approach, you are more likely to miss something important. Begin analyzing the rhythm strip from left to right.

Assess Rhythmicity

The term *rhythm* is used to indicate the site of origin of an electrical impulse (such as a sinus rhythm or ventricular rhythm) and to describe the regularity or irregularity of waveforms. The waveforms on an ECG strip are evaluated for regularity by measuring the distance between the P waves and QRS complexes. If the ventricular rhythm is regular, the R-R intervals will be equal (measure the same). Similarly, if the atrial rhythm is regular, the P-P intervals will be equal. If the variation between the shortest and longest R-R intervals (or P-P intervals) is not exactly the same—but is less than 0.04 second—the rhythm is termed *essentially regular.*

If the shortest and longest R-R or P-P intervals vary by more than 0.04 second (one small box), the rhythm is considered *irregular.* Various terms may be used to describe an irregular rhythm, which may be normal, fast, or slow. A

> **Box 2-6 Systematic Rhythm Interpretation**
> 1. Assess rhythmicity (atrial and ventricular).
> 2. Assess rate (atrial and ventricular).
> 3. Identify and examine waveforms.
> 4. Assess intervals (e.g., PR, QRS, QT) and examine ST segments.
> 5. Interpret the rhythm and assess its clinical significance.

regularly irregular rhythm is one in which the R-R intervals are not the same, the shortest and longest R-R intervals vary by more than 0.04 second, and there is a repeating pattern of irregularity. A regularly irregular rhythm may be caused by grouped beating (a repeating pattern of irregularity). An *irregularly irregular rhythm* is one in which the R-R intervals are not the same, there is no repeating pattern of irregularity, and the shortest and longest R-R intervals vary by more than 0.04 second. Atrial fibrillation is an example of an irregularly irregular rhythm. An irregularly irregular rhythm may also be called a *grossly irregular rhythm* or *totally irregular rhythm.*

Ventricular Rhythm

To determine if the ventricular rhythm is regular or irregular, measure the distance between two consecutive R-R intervals. Place one point of a pair of calipers, or make a mark on a piece of paper, on an R wave (Figure 2-41). Place the other point of the calipers, or make a second mark on the paper, at an identical point on the R wave of the next QRS complex. Without adjusting the calipers, evaluate each succeeding R-R interval. If paper is used, lift the paper and move it across the rhythm strip. Compare the distance measured with the other R-R intervals. If the ventricular rhythm is regular, the R-R intervals will measure the same. Rhythm and regularity also may be determined by counting the small squares between intervals and comparing the intervals.

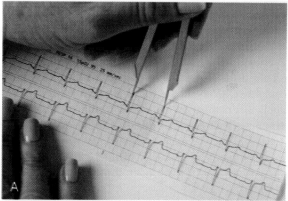
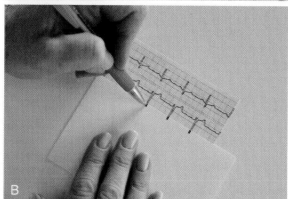

Figure 2-41 **A,** Establishing ventricular rhythmicity with calipers. **B,** Establishing ventricular rhythmicity with paper and pencil.

Atrial Rhythm

To determine if the atrial rhythm is regular or irregular, follow the same procedure previously described for evaluation of ventricular rhythm but measure the distance between two consecutive P-P intervals (instead of R-R intervals) and compare that distance with the other P-P intervals. The P-P intervals will measure the same if the atrial rhythm is regular. For accuracy, the R-R or P-P intervals should be evaluated across an entire 6-second rhythm strip.

Assess Rate

Calculation of the heart rate is important because deviations from normal can affect the patient's ability to maintain an adequate blood pressure and cardiac output. Although the atrial rate and ventricular rate are normally the same, the atrial and ventricular rates differ in some dysrhythmias and therefore both must be calculated.

In adults, a **tachycardia** (tachy = fast) exists if the rate is more than 100 beats per minute. Some dysrhythmias with very rapid ventricular rates (above 150 beats/min) require the delivery of medications or a shock to stop the rhythm. A **bradycardia** exists if the rate is less than 60 beats per minute (brady = slow). Many patients tolerate a heart rate of 50 to 60 beats/min but become symptomatic when the rate drops below 50.

There are several methods used for calculating heart rate. A discussion of each method follows.

Method 1: Six-Second Method

Most ECG paper is printed with 1-second or 3-second markers on the top or bottom of the paper. On ECG paper, 5 large boxes = 1 second, 15 large boxes = 3 seconds, and 30 large boxes = 6 seconds. To determine the ventricular rate, count the number of complete QRS complexes within a period of 6 seconds and multiply that number by 10 to find the number of complexes in 1 minute (Figure 2-42). The 6-second method, also called *the rule of 10*, may be used for regular and irregular rhythms. This is the simplest, quickest, and most commonly used method of rate measurement, but it also is the most inaccurate.

Method 2: Large Boxes

The large box method of rate determination is also called the *rule of 300*. To determine the ventricular rate, count the number of large boxes between an R-R interval and divide into 300 (see Figure 2-42). To determine the atrial rate, count the number of large boxes between a P-P interval and divide into 300 (Table 2-7). This method is best used if the rhythm is regular; however, it may be used if the rhythm is irregular and a rate range (slowest [longest R-R interval] and fastest [shortest R-R interval] rate) is given.

A variation of the large box method is called the *sequence method*. To determine the ventricular rate, select an R wave that falls on a dark vertical line. Number the next six consecutive dark vertical lines as follows: 300, 150, 100, 75, 60, and 50 (Figure 2-43). Note where the next R wave falls in relation to the six dark vertical lines already marked. This is the heart rate.

Method 3: Small Boxes

The small box method of rate determination is also called *the rule of 1500*. Each 1-mm box on the graph paper represents 0.04 second. A total of 1500 boxes represents 1 minute (60 sec/min divided by 0.04 sec/box = 1500 boxes/min). To calculate the ventricular rate, count the number of small boxes between the R-R interval and divide into 1500 (see Figure 2-42). To determine the atrial rate, count the number of small boxes between the P-P interval and divide into 1500. This method is time consuming but accurate. If the rhythm is irregular, a rate range should be given.

Identify and Examine Waveforms

Look to see if the normal waveforms (P, Q, R, S, and T) are present. To locate P waves, look to the left of each QRS complex. Normally one P wave precedes each QRS complex; they occur regularly (P-P intervals are equal); and they look similar in size, shape, and position.

Next, evaluate the QRS complex. Are QRS complexes present? If so, does a QRS follow each P wave? Do the QRS complexes look alike? Assess the T waves. Does a T wave

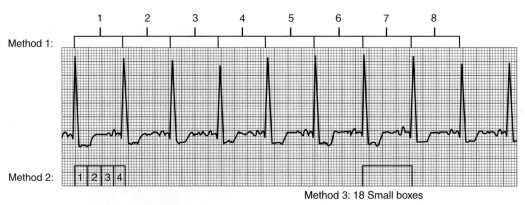

Figure 2-42 Calculating heart rate. Method 1: Number of R-R intervals in 6 seconds × 10 (e.g., 8 ×10 = 80/min). Method 2: Number of large boxes between QRS complexes divided into 300 (e.g., 300 divided by 4 = 75/min). Method 3: Number of small boxes between QRS complexes divided into 1500 (e.g., 1500 divided by 18 = 84/min).

Table 2-7	Heart Rate Determination Based on the Number of Large Boxes	
Number of Large Boxes	Heart Rate (beats/min)
1	300
2	150
3	100
4	75
5	60
6	50
7	43
8	38
9	33
10	30

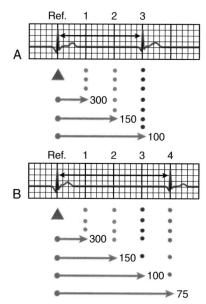

Figure 2-43 Determining heart rate–sequence method. To measure the ventricular rate, find a QRS complex that falls on a heavy dark line. Count 300, 150, 100, 75, 60, and 50 until a second QRS complex occurs. This will be the heart rate. (A) Heart rate = 100 beats/min. (B) Heart rate = 75 beats/min.

follow each QRS complex? Does a P wave follow the T wave? Are the T waves upright and of normal height? Look to see if a U wave is present. If so, note its height and direction (positive or negative).

Assess Intervals and Examine Segments

PR Interval

Intervals are measured to evaluate conduction. Is a PRI present? If so, measure the PRI and determine if they are equal. The PRI is measured from the point where the P wave leaves the baseline to the beginning of the QRS complex. Are the PRIs within normal limits? Remember that a normal PRI measures 0.12 to 0.20 second. If the PRIs are the same, they are said to be constant. If the PRIs are different, is a pattern present? In some dysrhythmias, the duration of the PRI will

increase until a P wave appears with no QRS after it. This is referred to as *lengthening* of the PRI. PRIs that vary in duration and have no pattern are said to be *variable*.

QRS Duration

Identify the QRS complexes and measure their duration. The beginning of the QRS is measured from the point where the first wave of the complex begins to deviate from the baseline. The point at which the last wave of the complex begins to level out at, above, or below the baseline marks the end of the QRS complex. The QRS is considered narrow (i.e., normal) if it measures 0.11 second or less and wide if it measures more than 0.11 second. A narrow QRS complex is presumed to be supraventricular in origin.

QT Interval

To determine the QT interval, measure the interval between two consecutive R waves (R-R interval). If the measured QT interval is less than half the R-R interval of that QRS complex and the R wave of the following complex, it is probably normal (provided the patient's heart rate is 95 beats/min or less). Alternately, count the number of small boxes between the beginning of the QRS complex and the end of the T wave. Then multiply that number by 0.04 second. If no Q wave is present, measure the QT interval from the beginning of the R wave to the end of the T wave. In general, a QT interval of 0.44 second or less is considered normal.

Examine ST Segments

Determine the presence of ST segment elevation or depression. Remember that the TP segment is used as the baseline from which to evaluate the degree of displacement of the ST segment from the isoelectric line. If ST segment displacement is present, note the number of millimeters of deviation from the isoelectric line or from the patient's baseline at a point 0.06 or 0.08 second after the J point.

Interpret the Rhythm

Interpret the rhythm, specifying the site of origin (pacemaker site) of the rhythm (sinus), the mechanism (bradycardia), and the ventricular rate. For example, "Sinus bradycardia at 38 beats/min." Assess the patient to find out how he or she is tolerating the rate and rhythm.

REFERENCES

1. Aronson PS, Boron WF, Boulpaep EL: Physiology of membranes. In Boron WF, Boulpaep EL editors: *Medical physiology: a cellular and molecular approach*, updated ed, Philadelphia, 2005, Saunders, pp 50–86.
2. Koeppen BM, Stanton BA: Elements of cardiac function. In *Berne & Levy physiology*, ed 6, updated ed, Philadelphia, 2010, Saunders, p 292.
3. Costanzo LS. Cardiovascular electrophysiology. In *Physiology*, ed 4, Philadelphia, 2010, Saunders, pp 125–137.

4. McCance KL, Brashers VL: Structure and function of the cardiovascular and lymphatic systems. In Huether SE, McCance KL, Brashers VL, et al: *Understanding pathophysiology*, ed 4, St. Louis, 2008, Mosby, p 576.

5. Levy MN, Pappano A: Electrical activity of the heart. In Levy MN, Koeppen BM, Stanton BA, editors: *Berne & Levy principles of physiology*, ed 4, Philadelphia, 2006, Mosby, pp 208–224.

6. DeBeasi LC: Physiology of the cardiovascular system. In Price SA, Wilson LM, editors: *Pathophysiology: clinical concepts of disease processes*, ed 6, St. Louis, 2003, Mosby, pp 416–428.

7. Wagner GS, Macfarlane P, Wellens H, et al: AHA/ACCF/HRS recommendations for the standardization and interpretation of the electrocardiogram: part VI: acute ischemia/infarction: a scientific statement from the American Heart Association Electrocardiography and Arrhythmias Committee, Council on Clinical Cardiology; the American College of Cardiology Foundation; and the Heart Rhythm Society, *J Am Coll Cardiol* 53:1003–1011, 2009.

8. Hall, JE: The heart. In *Guyton and Hall textbook of medical physiology*, ed 12, Philadelphia, 2011, Saunders, pp 99–156.

9. Phalen T, Aehlert B: Introduction to the 12-lead ECG. In *The 12-lead in acute coronary syndromes*, ed 3, St Louis, 2012, Mosby, pp 21–50.

10. Surawicz B, Childers R, Deal BJ, et al: AHA/ACCF/HRS recommendations for the standardization and interpretation of the electrocardiogram: part III: intraventricular conduction disturbances: a scientific statement from the American Heart Association Electrocardiography and Arrhythmias Committee, Council on Clinical Cardiology; the American College of Cardiology Foundation; and the Heart Rhythm Society, *J Am Coll Cardiol* 53:976–981, 2009.

11. Ganze L, Curtiss E: Electrocardiography. In Goldman L, Ausiello D, editors: *Cecil medicine*, ed 23, Philadelphia, 2008, Saunders, pp 320–326.

12. Rautaharju PM, Surawicz B, Gettes LS: AHA/ACCF/HRS recommendations for the standardization and interpretation of the electrocardiogram: part IV: the ST segment, T and U waves, and the QT interval: a scientific statement from the American Heart Association Electrocardiography and Arrhythmias Committee, Council on Clinical Cardiology; the American College of Cardiology Foundation; and the Heart Rhythm Society, *J Am Coll Cardiol* 53:982–991, 2009.

13. Patton KA, Thibodeau GA: Physiology of the cardiovascular system. In *Anatomy & physiology*, ed 7, St Louis, 2010, Mosby, pp 661–701.

14. Lederer WJ: Cardiac electrophysiology and the electrocardiogram. In Boron WF, Boulpaep EL, editors: *Medical physiology: a cellular and molecular approach*, updated ed, Philadelphia, 2005, Saunders, pp 483–507.

15. Litwin SE: Diagnostic tests and procedures in the patient with cardiovascular disease. In Andreoli TE, Benjamin IJ, Griggs RC, et al: *Andreoli and Carpenter's Cecil essentials of medicine*, ed 8, Philadelphia, 2010, Saunders, pp 46–65.

16. Drew BJ, Scheinman MM: ECG criteria to distinguish between aberrantly conducted supraventricular tachycardia and ventricular tachycardia: practical aspects for the immediate care setting, *Pacing Clin Electrophysiol* 18:2194–2208, 1995.

17. Drew BJ, Califf RM, Funk M, et al: Practice standards for electrocardiographic monitoring in hospital settings: an American Heart Association scientific statement from the Councils on Cardiovascular Nursing, Clinical Cardiology, and Cardiovascular Disease in the Young, *Circulation* 110:2721–2746, 2004.

STOP & REVIEW—CHAPTER 2

True/False

Indicate whether the statement is true or false.

_____ **1.** The cardiac action potential is a reflection of the difference in the concentration of charged particles across a cell membrane at any given time.

_____ **2.** If the wave of depolarization (electrical impulse) moves toward the positive electrode, the waveform recorded on ECG graph paper will be inverted (negative deflection).

_____ **3.** Ventricular depolarization is reflected on the ECG as the T wave.

_____ **4.** Leads V_1 and V_2 view the ventricular septum.

_____ **5.** Enhanced automaticity is a disorder of impulse conduction.

_____ **6.** The effective refractory period is the period of the cardiac action potential that includes the absolute refractory period and the first half of the relative refractory period.

Multiple Choice

Identify the choice that best completes the statement or answers the question.

_____ **7.** The ST segment is measured from:
   a. The end of the QRS complex to the end of the T wave.
   b. The beginning of the QRS complex to the end of the T wave.
   c. The end of the QRS complex to the beginning of the T wave.
   d. The beginning of the QRS complex to the beginning of the T wave.

_____ **8.** Five large boxes, each consisting of five small boxes, represent _____ on ECG paper.
   a. 1 second
   b. 3 seconds
   c. 6 seconds
   d. 10 seconds

_____ **9.** Which part of the conduction system receives an impulse from the SA node but delays relaying that impulse to the bundle of His, allowing time for the atria to empty their contents into the ventricles before the onset of ventricular contraction?
   a. AV node
   b. Right atrium
   c. Left bundle branch
   d. Right bundle branch

_____ **10.** On the ECG, the time necessary for the spread of an electrical impulse through the atria, AV node, bundle of His, right and left bundle branches, and the Purkinje fibers reflected by the
   a. TP segment.
   b. PR interval.
   c. QT interval.
   d. QRS duration.

_____ **11.** The normal duration of the QRS complex is
   a. 0.06 second or less.
   b. 0.11 second or less.
   c. 0.04 to 0.14 second.
   d. 0.20 to 0.38 second.

_____ **12.** The main electrolytes that affect cardiac function are
   a. sodium, potassium, calcium, and chloride.
   b. phosphate, sodium, sulfate, and potassium.
   c. chloride, sulfate, phosphate, and bicarbonate.
   d. bicarbonate, calcium, magnesium, and chloride.

_____ **13.** The portion of the ECG tracing used to determine the degree of ST segment displacement is the
   a. PR interval.
   b. QT interval.
   c. TP segment.
   d. QRS complex.

_____ **14.** In the normal heart, the primary pacemaker is the
   a. AV node.
   b. SA node.
   c. AV bundle.
   d. Purkinje fibers.

_____ **15.** Which of the following surfaces of the heart are not directly viewed when using a standard 12-lead ECG?
   a. Anterior and lateral surfaces of the left ventricle
   b. Lateral and inferior surfaces of the left ventricle
   c. Inferior and posterior surfaces of the left ventricle
   d. Right ventricle and posterior surface of the left ventricle

____**16.** U waves represent:
   a. Atrial depolarization.
   b. Ventricular depolarization.
   c. Repolarization of the bundle of His.
   d. Repolarization of the Purkinje fibers.

____**17.** _____ cells are specialized cells of the electrical conduction system responsible for the spontaneous generation and conduction of electrical impulses.
   a. Working
   b. Pacemaker
   c. Mechanical
   d. Contractile

____**18.** Where is the positive electrode placed in lead III?
   a. Left arm
   b. Right arm
   c. Left leg/foot
   d. Right leg/foot

____**19.** When an ECG machine is properly calibrated, a 1-millivolt (mV) electrical signal will produce a deflection measuring exactly _____ tall.
   a. 1-millimeter
   b. 5-millimeters
   c. 10-millimeters
   d. 20-millimeters

____**20.** Which of the following are horizontal plane leads?
   a. Leads I and aVL
   b. Leads I, II, and III
   c. Leads V_1, V_2, V_3, V_4, V_5, and V_6
   d. Leads I, II, III, aVR, aVL, and aVF

Questions 21 through 26 pertain to the following scenario.

You are caring for a 64-year-old man complaining of chest pain that he rates a 9 on a 0 to 10 scale. He states his symptoms began 20 minutes ago while moving boxes in his garage.

____**21.** You are applying ECG leads to this patient and will be using lead II for continuous monitoring. Lead II is an example of a(n):
   a. Chest lead.
   b. Horizontal lead.
   c. Standard limb lead.
   d. Augmented limb lead.

Completion

Complete each statement.

27. _____ is the spread of an impulse through tissue already stimulated by that same impulse.

28. Distortion of an ECG tracing by electrical activity that is noncardiac in origin is called _____.

____**22.** In lead II, the positive electrode is placed on the:
   a. Left leg.
   b. Right leg.
   c. Right arm.
   d. Left wrist.

____**23.** When analyzing this patient's ECG rhythm, the first areas of the rhythm strip that should be assessed are:
   a. Rhythmicity and rate.
   b. Intervals and segments.
   c. P waves and QRS complexes.
   d. Rate and waveform identification.

____**24.** The patient's ECG shows four large squares between two consecutive R waves. Based on this information, you calculate the patient's heart rate to be _____ beats/min.
   a. 50
   b. 75
   c. 100
   d. 150

____**25.** When analyzing the leads facing the affected area of the heart, ECG evidence of myocardial injury is displayed as:
   a. Inverted P waves.
   b. Pathologic Q waves.
   c. ST segment elevation.
   d. ST segment depression.

____**26.** Which of the following statements is true regarding analysis of the ST segment on this patient's ECG?
   a. ST segment displacement should be measured at a point 0.12 sec after the J point.
   b. ST segment elevation viewed in lead II would be considered clinically significant if also seen in lead III or aVF.
   c. Based on this patient's age, ST segment elevation seen in lead II would be considered clinically significant if elevated more than 0.5 mm.
   d. Use the PR interval as the baseline from which to evaluate the degree of ST segment displacement from the isoelectric line.

29. _____ refers to the ability of cardiac muscle cells to respond to an external stimulus, such as that from a chemical, mechanical, or electrical source.

Matching

Waveforms, Segments, and Intervals

Match the key terms with their definitions by placing the letter of each correct answer in the space provided.

a. 0.04 sec
b. QT
c. 0.11 sec or less
d. Interval
e. Segment
f. 0.5 sec
g. 3 sec

h. Complex
i. 0.06 to 0.08 sec
j. Waveform
k. 0.12 to 0.20 sec
l. J point
m. Millimeters
n. ST segment elevation

_____**30.** A line between waveforms

_____**31.** Several waveforms

_____**32.** Normal duration of the PR interval

_____**33.** The area where the QRS complex and the ST segment meet

_____**34.** This ECG change provides the strongest ECG evidence for the early recognition of myocardial infarction.

_____**35.** The _____ interval represents total ventricular activity.

_____**36.** The amplitude of a waveform is measured in _____.

_____**37.** A corrected QT interval of more than _____ in either gender has been correlated with a higher risk for ventricular dysrhythmias.

_____**38.** On ECG paper, each horizontal 1-mm box represents _____.

_____**39.** Normal duration of the QRS complex

_____**40.** ST segment displacement is measured _____ after the J point.

_____**41.** Movement away from the baseline in either a positive or negative direction

_____**42.** A waveform and a segment

_____**43.** On ECG paper, 15 large boxes represents _____.

The Cardiac Action Potential

Match the key terms in the left column with the definitions in the right column by placing the letter of each correct answer in the space provided.

a. Procainamide and lidocaine
b. Fast-response
c. Depolarization
d. Verapamil and diltiazem

e. Action potential
f. Wave of depolarization
g. Slow-response
h. Repolarization

_____**44.** This type of action potential occurs in the SA and AV nodes.

_____**45.** A chain reaction that occurs from cell to cell in the heart's electrical conduction system until all the cells have been stimulated

_____**46.** The movement of charged particles across a cell membrane in which the inside of the cell is restored to its negative charge

_____**47.** Examples of antiarrhythmics that block sodium channels

_____**48.** The rapid sequence of voltage changes that occur across the cell membrane during the electrical cardiac cycle

_____**49.** This type of action potential occurs in normal atrial and ventricular myocardial cells and in the Purkinje fibers.

_____**50.** The movement of ions across a cell membrane causing the inside of the cell to become more positive

_____**51.** Examples of antiarrhythmics that slow the rate at which calcium passes through the cells

Short Answer

52. Indicate the inherent rates for each of the following pacemaker sites:

Sinoatrial (SA) node: _____

Atrioventricular (AV) bundle: _____

Ventricles: _____

53. List four (4) properties of cardiac cells.
1.
2.
3.
4.

54. List three (3) uses for ECG monitoring.
1.
2.
3.

55. Complete the following chart:

Lead	Positive Electrode	Negative Electrode	Heart Surface Viewed
Lead I	_____	_____	_____
Lead II	_____	_____	_____
Lead III	_____	_____	_____

56. List five (5) steps used in ECG rhythm analysis.
1.
2.
3.
4.
5.

57. What are the R-R and P-P intervals used for in ECG monitoring?

_____

_____

_____

58. List three (3) possible causes of a poor ECG tracing.
1.
2.
3.

BASIC ELECTROPHYSIOLOGY—*PRACTICE RHYTHM STRIPS*

For each of the following rhythm strips determine the atrial and ventricular rates; label the P wave, QRS complex, and T wave; and measure the PR interval, QRS duration, and QT interval. Determine if the atrial and ventricular rhythm for each strip is regular or irregular. *Not all waveforms will be present in each of the following rhythm strips.*

59.

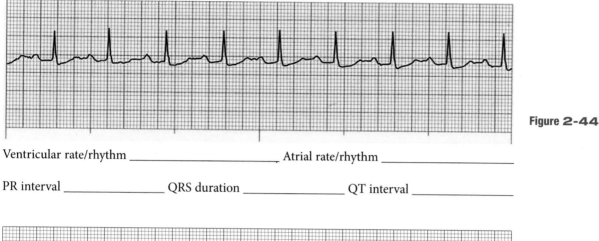

Figure **2-44**

Ventricular rate/rhythm _____ Atrial rate/rhythm _____

PR interval _____ QRS duration _____ QT interval _____

60.

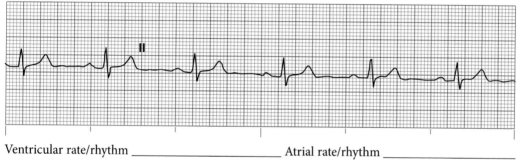

Figure **2-45**

Ventricular rate/rhythm _____ Atrial rate/rhythm _____

PR interval _____ QRS duration _____ QT interval _____

61.

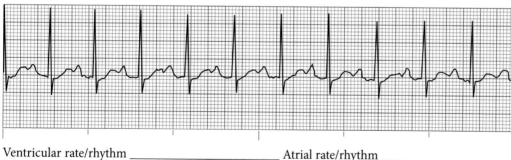

Figure **2-46**

Ventricular rate/rhythm _____ Atrial rate/rhythm _____

PR interval _____ QRS duration _____ QT interval _____

62.

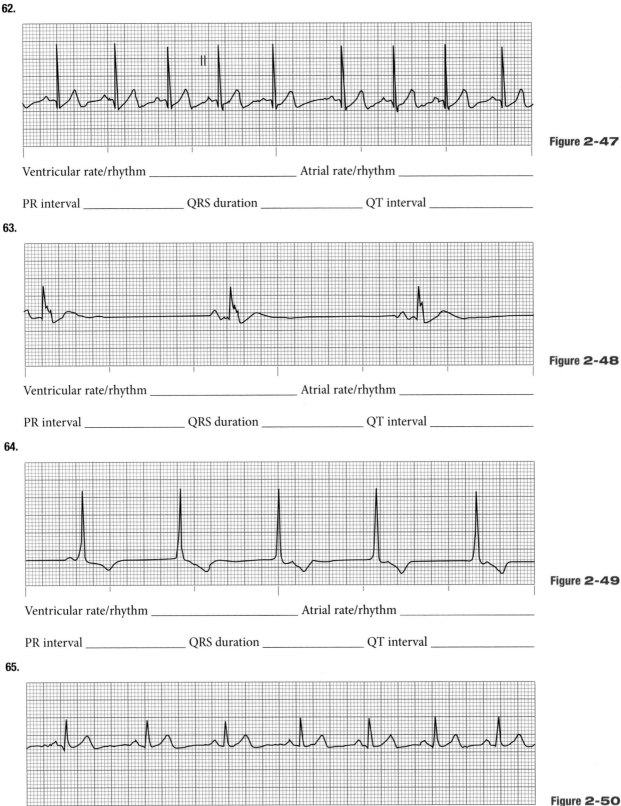

Figure 2-47

Ventricular rate/rhythm _____ Atrial rate/rhythm _____

PR interval _____ QRS duration _____ QT interval _____

63.

Figure 2-48

Ventricular rate/rhythm _____ Atrial rate/rhythm _____

PR interval _____ QRS duration _____ QT interval _____

64.

Figure 2-49

Ventricular rate/rhythm _____ Atrial rate/rhythm _____

PR interval _____ QRS duration _____ QT interval _____

65.

Figure 2-50

Ventricular rate/rhythm _____ Atrial rate/rhythm _____

PR interval _____ QRS duration _____ QT interval _____

66.

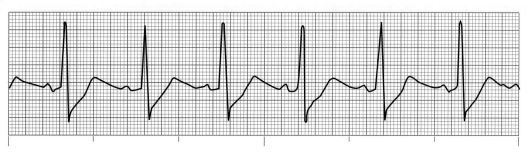

Figure 2-51

Ventricular rate/rhythm _____ Atrial rate/rhythm _____

PR interval _____ QRS duration _____ QT interval _____

67.

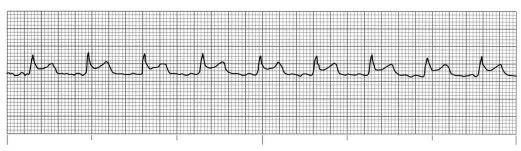

Figure 2-52

Ventricular rate/rhythm _____ Atrial rate/rhythm _____

PR interval _____ QRS duration _____ QT interval _____

68.

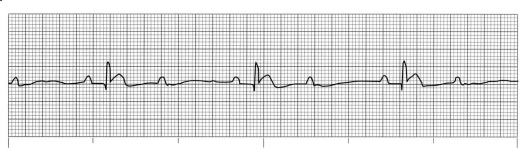

Figure 2-53

Ventricular rate/rhythm _____ Atrial rate/rhythm _____

PR interval _____ QRS duration _____ QT interval _____

STOP & REVIEW ANSWERS

True/False

1. ANS: T

The action potential of a cardiac cell reflects the rapid sequence of voltage changes that occur across the cell membrane during the electrical cardiac cycle. The configuration of the action potential varies depending on the location, size, and function of the cardiac cell.
OBJ: Define the terms *membrane potential*, *threshold potential*, *action potential*, *polarization*, *depolarization*, and *repolarization*.

2. ANS: F

If the wave of depolarization (electrical impulse) moves toward the positive electrode, the waveform recorded on ECG graph paper will be upright (positive deflection).
OBJ: Define the terms *membrane potential*, *threshold potential*, *action potential*, *polarization*, *depolarization*, and *repolarization*.

3. ANS: F

The QRS complex represents ventricular depolarization. Ventricular repolarization is recorded on the ECG as the ST segment and T wave.
OBJ: Define and describe the significance of each of the following as they relate to cardiac electrical activity: P wave, QRS complex, T wave, U wave, PR segment, TP segment, ST segment, PR interval, QRS duration, and QT interval.

Multiple Choice

7. ANS: C

The portion of the ECG tracing between the QRS complex and the T wave is the ST segment. The term *ST segment* is used regardless of whether the final wave of the QRS complex is an R or an S wave. The ST segment represents the early part of repolarization of the right and left ventricles. The normal ST segment begins at the isoelectric line, extends from the end of the S wave, and curves gradually upward to the beginning of the T wave.
OBJ: Define and describe the significance of each of the following as they relate to cardiac electrical activity: P wave, QRS complex, T wave, U wave, PR segment, TP segment, ST segment, PR interval, QRS duration, and QT interval.

8. ANS: A

Five large boxes, each consisting of five small boxes, represent 1 second. Fifteen large boxes equal an interval of 3 sec. Thirty large boxes represent 6 sec.
OBJ: Identify the numeric values assigned to the small and large boxes on ECG paper.

4. ANS: T

OBJ: Relate the cardiac surfaces or areas represented by the electrocardiogram leads.

5. ANS: F

Enhanced automaticity is a disorder of impulse formation in which one of the following occurs:
- Cardiac cells that are not normally associated with a pacemaker function begin to depolarize spontaneously *or*
- A pacemaker site other than the SA node increases its firing rate beyond that which is considered normal.

OBJ: Differentiate the primary mechanisms responsible for producing cardiac dysrhythmias.

6. ANS: T

The effective refractory period is the period of the cardiac action potential that includes the absolute refractory period and the first half of the relative refractory period.
OBJ: Define the absolute, effective, relative refractory, and supranormal periods and their location in the cardiac cycle.

9. ANS: A

As the electrical impulse enters the AV node through the internodal pathways, conduction is markedly slowed before the impulse reaches the ventricles. The delay in conduction allows both atrial chambers to contract and empty blood into the ventricles before the next ventricular contraction begins. This increases the amount of blood in the ventricles, increasing stroke volume.
OBJ: Describe the normal sequence of electrical conduction through the heart.

10. ANS: B

The PR interval is the P wave plus the PR segment. It reflects depolarization of the right and left atria (P wave) and the spread of the impulse through the AV node, AV bundle, right and left bundle branches, and the Purkinje fibers (PR segment).
OBJ: Define and describe the significance of each of the following as they relate to cardiac electrical activity: P wave, QRS complex, T wave, U wave, PR segment, TP segment, ST segment, PR interval, QRS duration, and QT interval.

11. ANS: B

In adults, the normal duration of the QRS complex is 0.11 sec or less. If an electrical impulse does not follow the normal ventricular conduction pathway, it will take longer to depolarize the myocardium. This delay in conduction through the ventricles produces a wider QRS complex.

OBJ: Define and describe the significance of each of the following as they relate to cardiac electrical activity: P wave, QRS complex, T wave, U wave, PR segment, TP segment, ST segment, PR interval, QRS duration, and QT interval.

12. ANS: A

The main electrolytes that affect the function of the heart are sodium, potassium, calcium, and chloride. Disorders that affect the concentration of these important electrolytes can have serious consequences. For example, an imbalance of potassium can cause life-threatening disturbances in the heart's rhythm.

OBJ: List the most important ions involved in the cardiac action potential and their primary function in this process.

13. ANS: C

When the heart rate is within normal limits, the TP segment is usually isoelectric and used as the reference point from which to estimate the position of the isoelectric line and determine ST segment displacement.

OBJ: Define and describe the significance of each of the following as they relate to cardiac electrical activity: P wave, QRS complex, T wave, U wave, PR segment, TP segment, ST segment, PR interval, QRS duration, and QT interval.

14. ANS: B

The SA node is normally the primary pacemaker of the heart because it has the fastest firing rate (specifically, the fastest rate of phase 4 depolarization) of all of the heart's normal pacemaker sites.

OBJ: Describe the normal sequence of electrical conduction through the heart.

15. ANS: D

The right ventricle and posterior surface of the left ventricle are not directly viewed when using a standard 12-lead ECG. Right chest leads and posterior chest leads, respectively, are used for this purpose.

OBJ: Relate the cardiac surfaces or areas represented by the electrocardiogram leads.

16. ANS: D

A U wave is a small waveform that, when seen, follows the T wave. U waves represent repolarization of the Purkinje fibers.

OBJ: Define and describe the significance of each of the following as they relate to cardiac electrical activity: P wave, QRS complex, T wave, U wave, PR segment, TP segment, ST segment, PR interval, QRS duration, and QT interval.

17. ANS: B

Pacemaker cells are specialized cells of the heart's electrical system. Pacemaker cells also may be referred to as conducting cells or automatic cells. They are responsible for spontaneously generating and conducting electrical impulses.

OBJ: Describe the two basic types of cardiac cells in the heart, where they are found, and their function.

18. ANS: C

Lead III records the difference in electrical potential between the left leg (+) and left arm (−) electrodes. In lead III the positive electrode is placed on the left leg and the negative electrode is placed on the left arm.

OBJ: Describe correct anatomic placement of the standard limb leads, augmented leads, and chest leads.

19. ANS: C

An ECG machine's sensitivity must be calibrated so that a 1-mV electrical signal will produce a deflection measuring exactly 10-mm tall. When properly calibrated, a small box is 1-mm high (0.1 mV), and a large box (equal to five small boxes) is 5-mm high (0.5 mV).

OBJ: Identify how heart rates, durations, and amplitudes may be determined from electrocardiographic recordings.

20. ANS: C

Six chest (precordial or "V") leads view the heart in the horizontal plane. The chest leads are identified as V_1, V_2, V_3, V_4, V_5, and V_6.

OBJ: Differentiate between the frontal plane and the horizontal plane leads.

21. ANS: C

Frontal plane leads view the heart from the front of the body as if it were flat. Directions in the frontal plane are superior, inferior, right, and left. Six leads view the heart in the frontal plane. Leads I, II, and III are called *standard limb leads*. Leads aVR, aVL, and aVF are called *augmented limb leads*.

OBJ: Differentiate between the frontal plane and the horizontal plane leads.

22. ANS: A

Lead II records the difference in electrical potential between the left leg (+) and right arm (−) electrodes. The positive electrode is placed on the left leg and the negative electrode is placed on the right arm.

OBJ: Describe correct anatomic placement of the standard limb leads, augmented leads, and chest leads.

23. ANS: A

When analyzing a rhythm strip, begin by assessing rhythmicity (atrial and ventricular) and rate (atrial and ventricular).

OBJ: Describe a systematic approach to the analysis and interpretation of cardiac dysrhythmias.

24. ANS: B
Using the large box (rule of 300) method to calculate heart rate, four large boxes between two consecutive R waves equals a heart rate of 75 beats/min (300 divided by 4).
OBJ: Identify how heart rates, durations, and amplitudes may be determined from electrocardiographic recordings.

25. ANS: C
In a patient experiencing an acute coronary syndrome, ECG evidence of myocardial injury is displayed as ST segment elevation in the leads facing the affected area of the heart.
OBJ: Recognize the changes on the ECG that may reflect evidence of myocardial ischemia, injury, and infarction.

26. ANS: B
The TP segment is used as the baseline from which to evaluate the degree of displacement of the ST segment from the isoelectric line. If ST segment displacement is present, note the number of millimeters of deviation from the isoelectric line or from the patient's baseline at a point 0.06 to 0.08 sec after the J point.

Completion

27. ANS: <u>Reentry</u> is the spread of an impulse through tissue already stimulated by that same impulse.
OBJ: Describe reentry.

28. ANS: Distortion of an ECG tracing by electrical activity that is noncardiac in origin is called <u>artifact</u>.
OBJ: Define the term *artifact* and explain methods that may be used to minimize its occurrence.

Matching

30. ANS: E
31. ANS: H
32. ANS: K
33. ANS: L
34. ANS: N
35. ANS: B
36. ANS: M
37. ANS: F
38. ANS: A
39. ANS: C
40. ANS: I

Short Answer

52. ANS:
SA node: 60 to 100 beats/min
AV bundle: 40 to 60 beats/min
Ventricles: 20 to 40 beats/min
OBJ: Describe the location, function, and (where appropriate), the intrinsic rate of the following structures: Sinoatrial (SA) node, atrioventricular (AV) bundle, and Purkinje fibers.

When ECG changes of myocardial ischemia, injury, or infarction occur, they are not found in every lead of the ECG. Findings are considered significant if viewed in two or more leads looking at the same or adjacent areas of the heart. If these findings are seen in leads that look directly at the affected area, they are called *indicative changes*. Indicative changes are significant when they are seen in two *anatomically contiguous* leads. Two leads are contiguous if they look at the same or adjacent areas of the heart or if they are numerically consecutive chest leads. Remember that leads II, III, and aVF view the inferior wall of the left ventricle. Therefore, in this patient situation, ST segment changes viewed in lead II would be considered clinically significant if elevated more than 1 mm and also seen in lead III or aVF.
OBJ: Recognize the changes on the ECG that may reflect evidence of myocardial ischemia, injury, and infarction.

29. ANS: <u>Excitability</u> (or irritability) refers to the ability of cardiac muscle cells to respond to an external stimulus, such as that from a chemical, mechanical, or electrical source.
OBJ: Describe the primary characteristics of cardiac cells.

41. ANS: J
42. ANS: D
43. ANS: G

44. ANS: G
45. ANS: F
46. ANS: H
47. ANS: A
48. ANS: E
49. ANS: B
50. ANS: C
51. ANS: D

53. ANS:
The four properties of cardiac cells are: (1) automaticity, (2) excitability (or irritability), (3) conductivity, and (4) contractility.
OBJ: Describe the primary characteristics of cardiac cells.

54. ANS:

ECG monitoring may be used for the following purposes:

- Monitor a patient's heart rate
- Evaluate the effects of disease or injury on heart function
- Evaluate pacemaker function
- Evaluate the response to medications (such as antiarrhythmics)
- Obtain a baseline recording before, during, and after a medical procedure
- Evaluate for signs of myocardial ischemia, injury, and infarction

OBJ: Explain the purpose of electrocardiographic monitoring.

55. ANS:

Lead	Positive Electrode	Negative Electrode	Heart Surface Viewed
Lead I	Left arm	Right arm	Lateral
Lead II	Left leg	Right arm	Inferior
Lead III	Left leg	Left arm	Inferior

OBJ: Relate the cardiac surfaces or areas represented by the electrocardiogram leads.

56. ANS:

1. Assess rhythmicity (atrial and ventricular)
2. Assess rate (atrial and ventricular)
3. Identify and examine waveforms
4. Assess intervals (PR, QRS, and QT) and examine ST segments
5. Interpret the rhythm (and assess its clinical significance)

OBJ: Describe a systematic approach to the analysis and interpretation of cardiac dysrhythmias.

57. ANS:

The R-R (R wave-to-R wave) and P-P (P wave-to-P wave) intervals are used to determine the rate and regularity of a cardiac rhythm.

OBJ: Describe a systematic approach to the analysis and interpretation of cardiac dysrhythmias.

58. ANS:

Possible causes of a poor ECG tracing include excessive body hair, loose electrode, muscle tremor, dried electrode gel, improper lead placement, 60-cycle interference, broken ECG cables or wires, poor electrical contact (e.g., diaphoresis), and external chest compressions.

OBJ: Define the term *artifact* and explain methods that may be used to minimize its occurrence.

59.

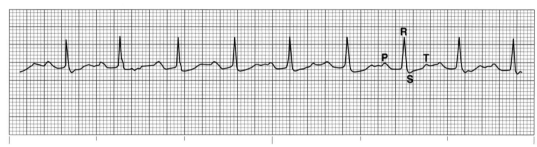

Figure **2-54**

Ventricular rate/rhythm	88 beats/min; regular
Atrial rate/rhythm	88 beats/min; regular
PR interval	0.24 second
QRS duration	0.06 second
QT interval	0.32 second

60.

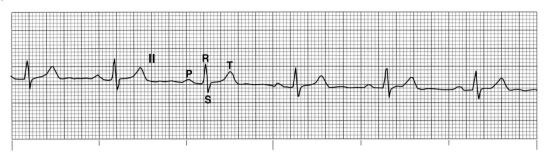

Figure **2-55**

Ventricular rate/rhythm	58 beats/min; regular
Atrial rate/rhythm	58 beats/min; regular
PR interval	0.20 second
QRS duration	0.08 second
QT interval	0.40 second

61.

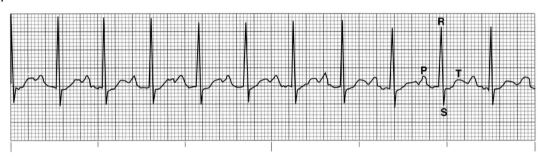

Figure **2-56**

Ventricular rate/rhythm	107 beats/min; regular
Atrial rate/rhythm	107 beats/min; regular
PR interval	0.24 second
QRS duration	0.08 second
QT interval	0.32 second

62.

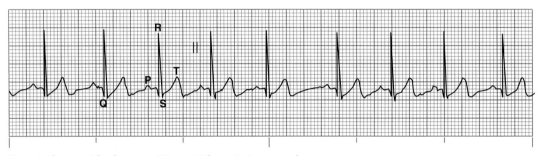

Figure **2-57**

Ventricular rate/rhythm	75 to 100 beats/min; irregular
Atrial rate/rhythm	75 to 100 beats/min; irregular
PR interval	0.14 to 0.16 second
QRS duration	0.08 second
QT interval	0.56 second

63.

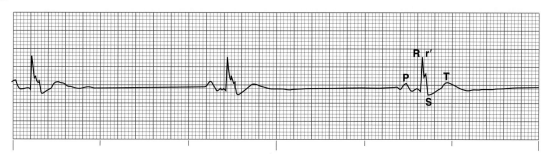

Figure 2-58

Ventricular rate/rhythm	27 beats/min; regular
Atrial rate/rhythm	27 beats/min; regular
PR interval	0.22 second
QRS duration	0.12 second
QT interval	0.52 second

64.

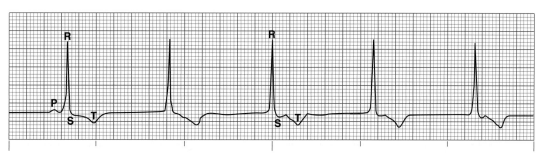

Figure 2-59

Ventricular rate/rhythm	52 beats/min; regular
Atrial rate/rhythm	None
PR interval	None
QRS duration	0.06 second
QT interval	0.44 second

65.

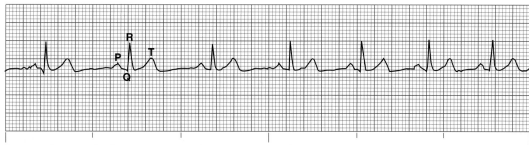

Figure 2-60

Ventricular rate/rhythm	67 to 83 beats/min; irregular
Atrial rate/rhythm	67 to 83 beats/min; irregular
PR interval	0.16 second
QRS duration	0.06 to 0.08 second
QT interval	0.32 second

66.

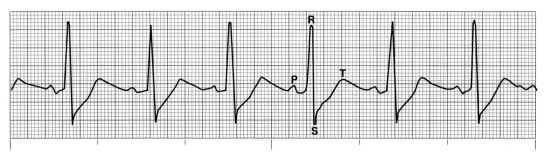

Figure **2-61**

Ventricular rate/rhythm	65 beats/min; regular
Atrial rate/rhythm	65 beats/min; regular
PR interval	0.20 second
QRS duration	0.10 second
QT interval	0.52 second

67.

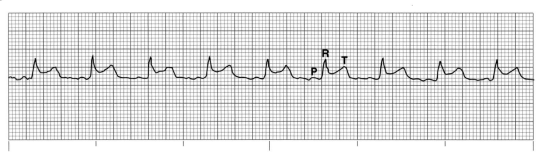

Figure **2-62**

Ventricular rate/rhythm	93 beats/min; regular
Atrial rate/rhythm	93 beats/min; regular
PR interval	0.14 second
QRS duration	0.08 second
QT interval	0.32 second

68.

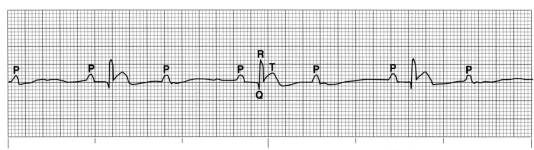

Figure **2-63**

Ventricular rate/rhythm	35 beats/min; regular
Atrial rate/rhythm	70 beats/min; regular
PR interval	0.24 to 0.26 second
QRS duration	0.08 to 0.10 second
QT interval	0.28 second

Sinus Mechanisms

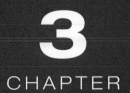

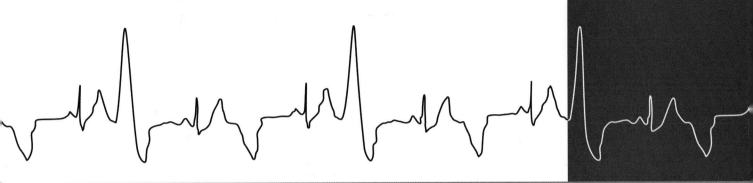

LEARNING OBJECTIVES

After reading this chapter, you should be able to:

1. Describe the electrocardiogram (ECG) characteristics of a sinus rhythm.
2. Describe the ECG characteristics, possible causes, signs and symptoms, and emergency management of sinus bradycardia.
3. Describe the ECG characteristics, possible causes, signs and symptoms, and emergency management of sinus tachycardia.
4. Describe the ECG characteristics, possible causes, signs and symptoms, and emergency management of sinus arrhythmia.
5. Describe the ECG characteristics, possible causes, signs and symptoms, and emergency management of sinoatrial block.
6. Describe the ECG characteristics, possible causes, signs and symptoms, and emergency management of sinus arrest.

KEY TERMS

Sinus arrhythmia: Dysrhythmia originating in the sinoatrial (SA) node that occurs when the SA node discharges irregularly; sinus arrhythmia is a normal phenomenon associated with the phases of breathing and changes in intrathoracic pressure

Sinus bradycardia: Dysrhythmia originating in the SA node with a ventricular response of less than 60 beats/min

Sinus rhythm: A normal heart rhythm; sometimes called a *regular sinus rhythm* (RSR) or *normal sinus rhythm* (NSR)

Sinus tachycardia: Dysrhythmia originating in the SA node with a ventricular response between 101 and 180 beats/min

INTRODUCTION

In this chapter, you will begin learning the characteristics of specific cardiac rhythms. Study these characteristics carefully and commit them to memory. Throughout this text, all ECG characteristics pertain to the adult patient unless otherwise noted.

The normal heartbeat is the result of an electrical impulse that starts in the SA node (Figure 3-1). Normally, pacemaker cells within the SA node spontaneously depolarize more rapidly than other cardiac cells. As a result, the SA node usually dominates other areas that are depolarizing at a slightly slower rate. The impulse is sent to cells at the outside edge of the SA node and then to the myocardial cells of the surrounding atrium.

A rhythm that begins in the SA node has the following characteristics:

- A positive (i.e., upright) P wave before each QRS complex
- P waves that look alike
- A constant PR interval
- A regular atrial and ventricular rhythm (usually)

An electrical impulse that begins in the SA node may be affected by the following:

- Medications
- Diseases or conditions that cause the heart rate to speed up, slow down, or beat irregularly
- Diseases or conditions that delay or block the impulse from leaving the SA node
- Diseases or conditions that prevent an impulse from being generated in the SA node

ECG Pearl

Most, but not all, rhythms that begin in the sinoatrial (SA) node are regular.

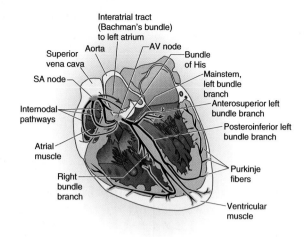

Figure 3-1   The sinoatrial (SA) node normally depolarizes faster than any other part of the heart's conduction system. As a result, the SA node is normally the heart's primary pacemaker. AV, atrioventricular.

Table **3-1**	Normal Heart Rates by Age
Age	**Beats/Min***
Infant (1 to 12 months)	100 to 160
Toddler (1 to 3 years)	90 to 150
Preschooler (4 to 5 years)	80 to 140
School-age (6 to 12 years)	70 to 120
Adolescent (13 to 18 years)	60 to 100
Adult	60 to 100

*Pulse rates for a sleeping child may be 10% lower than the low rate listed in age group.

SINUS RHYTHM

[Objective 1]

Sinus rhythm is the name given to a normal heart rhythm. Sinus rhythm is sometimes called a *regular sinus rhythm* (RSR) or *normal sinus rhythm* (NSR). Sinus rhythm reflects normal electrical activity—that is, the rhythm starts in the SA node and then heads down the normal conduction pathway through the atria, atrioventricular (AV) node and bundle, right and left bundle branches, and Purkinje fibers.

A person's heart rate varies with age (Table 3-1). In adults and adolescents, the SA node normally fires at a regular rate of 60 to 100 beats/min.

How Do I Recognize It?

Figure 3-2 shows an example of a sinus rhythm recorded simultaneously in three leads: V_1, II, and V_5. As you look as this figure from left to right, note the 10-mm calibration marker that appears at the far left of each lead. Although we will focus on lead II as we examine this rhythm strip, you will find that it is helpful to view waveforms, segments, and intervals in more than one lead.

A sinus rhythm has a regular atrial and ventricular rhythm. Find the QRS complexes on the rhythm strip. Place one point of your calipers, or make a mark on a piece of paper, on the beginning of an R wave. Place the other point of the calipers, or make a second mark on the paper, on the beginning of the R wave of the next QRS complex. Without adjusting the calipers, evaluate each succeeding R-R interval. If you are using paper, lift the paper and move it across the rhythm strip. The R-R intervals in this example are regular. Since you have already identified the R waves, determine the ventricular rate. In this rhythm strip, the ventricular rate is 80 beats/min. Remember, the built-in (i.e., intrinsic) rate for a rhythm that begins in the SA node is 60 to 100 beats/min; therefore the rate of the rhythm in our example fits within the criteria for a sinus rhythm.

Now look to the left of the QRS complexes to find the P waves on the rhythm strip. A rhythm that begins in the SA node should have a positive (i.e., upright) P wave in lead II before each QRS complex. When you look at this rhythm strip, you can see one upright P wave before each QRS complex. Every P wave looks alike. Measure the P-P interval to see if the P waves occur regularly and then determine the atrial rate. You will find that the P waves occur regularly at a rate of 80 beats/min.

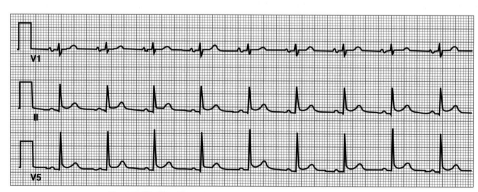

Figure 3-2   Sinus rhythm at 80 beats/min, ST-segment elevation.

Now measure the PR interval and QRS duration. In a sinus rhythm, the PR interval measures 0.12 to 0.20 second and is constant from beat to beat. In this example, the PR interval is 0.16 second. The QRS complex normally measures 0.11 second or less. If there is a delay in conduction through the bundle branches, the QRS may be wide (i.e., greater than 0.11 second). In our example, the QRS measures 0.08 second. Next, determine the QT interval by counting the number of small boxes between the beginning of the QRS complex and the end of the T wave and multiplying that number by 0.04 second. In our example, the QT interval measures about 8.5 boxes (0.34 second). This value is within normal limits.

Next, locate the TP segment and then the J point. Look 0.06 or 0.08 second to the right of the J point and assess the ST segments. You will see that the ST segments in this rhythm strip are elevated. Now interpret the rhythm, specifying the site of origin (pacemaker site) of the rhythm and the ventricular rate. Because the rhythm shown in Figure 3-2 fits the ECG criteria for a sinus rhythm, your identification should be, "Sinus rhythm at 80 beats/min with ST-segment elevation." A summary of the ECG characteristics of a sinus rhythm are shown in Table 3-2.

Table 3-2	Characteristics of Sinus Rhythm
Rhythm	R-R and P-P intervals are regular
Rate	60 to 100 beats/min
P waves	Positive (upright) in lead II; one precedes each QRS complex; P waves look alike
PR interval	0.12 to 0.20 sec and constant from beat to beat
QRS duration	0.11 sec or less unless abnormally conducted

SINUS BRADYCARDIA

[Objective 2]
If the SA node fires at a rate that is slower than normal for the patient's age, the rhythm is called **sinus bradycardia**. The rhythm starts in the SA node and then travels the normal conduction pathway, resulting in atrial and ventricular depolarization. In adults and adolescents, a sinus bradycardia has a heart rate of less than 60 beats/min. The term *severe sinus bradycardia* is sometimes used to describe a sinus bradycardia with a rate of less than 40 beats/min.

How Do I Recognize It?

Figure 3-3 is an example of sinus bradycardia. Table 3-3 lists the ECG characteristics of sinus bradycardia. You will note they are the same as the characteristics of a sinus rhythm with one exception—the rate. The rate of a sinus rhythm is 60 to 100 beats/min. The rate of a sinus bradycardia is less than 60 beats/min.

Examine this rhythm strip with the use of the same systematic format that you previously used. Begin by locating the QRS complexes on the rhythm strip. Evaluate each succeeding R-R interval. The R-R intervals in this example are regular. Now determine the ventricular rate. In this rhythm strip, the ventricular rate is 40 beats/min. Now find the P waves on the rhythm strip. Remember that a rhythm that begins in the SA node should have a positive P wave (in lead II) before each QRS complex. In our example, you can see one upright P wave before each QRS complex and every P wave looks alike. Now measure the P-to-P interval to see if the P waves occur regularly and determine the atrial rate. The P waves occur regularly at a rate of 40 beats/min. Now measure the PR interval, QRS duration, and QT interval. In this example, the PR interval is 0.16 second, the QRS complex measures 0.08 second, and the QT interval is 0.40 second. ST-segment depression is present and negative (i.e., inverted) T waves appear after each QRS complex. These findings must be noted in your final description of the rhythm. Therefore, correct identification of this rhythm would be, "Sinus bradycardia at 40 beats/min with ST-segment depression and inverted T waves."

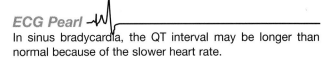

ECG Pearl
In sinus bradycardia, the QT interval may be longer than normal because of the slower heart rate.

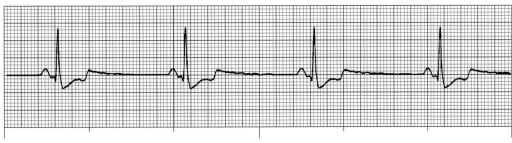

Figure 3-3   Sinus bradycardia at 40 beats/min with ST-segment depression and inverted T waves.

Table **3-3**	Characteristics of Sinus Bradycardia
Rhythm	R-R and P-P intervals are regular
Rate	Less than 60 beats/min
P waves	Positive (upright) in lead II; one precedes each QRS complex; P waves look alike
PR interval	0.12 to 0.20 sec and constant from beat to beat
QRS duration	0.11 sec or less unless abnormally conducted

What Causes It?

Sinus bradycardia occurs in adults during sleep and in well-conditioned athletes. It is also present in up to 35% of people under 25 years of age while at rest. Sinus bradycardia is common in some myocardial infarctions (MIs). Prolonged standing and stimulation of the vagus nerve can also result in slowing of the heart rate. For example, coughing, vomiting, straining to have a bowel movement, or sudden exposure of the face to cold water can result in slowing of the heart rate. In people who have a sensitive carotid sinus, slowing of the heart rate can occur when a tight collar is worn or with the impact of the stream of water on the neck while in the shower. Other causes of sinus bradycardia are shown in the box below.

CLINICAL CORRELATION

Causes of Sinus Bradycardia
- Disease of the sinoatrial (SA) node
- Hyperkalemia
- Hypokalemia
- Hypothermia
- Hypothyroidism
- Hypoxia
- Increased intracranial pressure
- Inferior myocardial infarction (MI)
- Medications such as calcium channel blockers, digitalis, beta-blockers, amiodarone, and sotalol
- Obstructive sleep apnea
- Post heart transplant
- Posterior MI
- Vagal stimulation

What Do I Do About It?

Remember that cardiac output equals stroke volume × heart rate. Therefore, a decrease in either stroke volume or heart rate may result in a decrease in cardiac output. Many patients tolerate a heart rate of 50 to 60 beats/min but become symptomatic when the rate drops below 50 beats/min. A patient with an unusually slow heart rate may complain of lightheadedness, dizziness or weakness, and fainting (i.e., syncope) can occur. Decreasing cardiac output will eventually produce hemodynamic compromise.

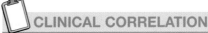

CLINICAL CORRELATION

Signs and Symptoms of Hemodynamic Compromise
- Acute changes in mental status
- Chest pain or discomfort
- Cold, clammy skin
- Fall in urine output
- Heart failure
- Low blood pressure
- Pulmonary congestion
- Shock
- Shortness of breath

If a patient presents with a bradycardia, assess how the patient is tolerating the rhythm at rest and with activity. If the patient has no symptoms, no treatment is necessary. The term *symptomatic bradycardia* is used to describe a patient who experiences signs and symptoms of hemodynamic compromise related to a slow heart rate. Treatment of a symptomatic bradycardia should include assessment of the patient's oxygen saturation level, and determining if signs of increased work of breathing are present (e.g., retractions, tachypnea, paradoxic abdominal breathing). Give supplemental oxygen if oxygenation is inadequate and assist breathing if ventilation is inadequate. Establish intravenous (IV) access and obtain a 12-lead ECG. Atropine, administered intravenously, is the drug of choice for symptomatic bradycardia. Reassess the patient's response and continue monitoring the patient.

In the setting of an MI, sinus bradycardia is often transient. A slow heart rate can be beneficial in the patient who has had an MI and who has no symptoms as a result of the slow rate. This is because the heart's demand for oxygen is less when the heart rate is slow.

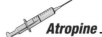

Atropine

Atropine is a vagolytic drug that is used to increase the heart rate. *Vago* refers to the vagus nerves (right and left), which are the main nerves of the parasympathetic division of the autonomic nervous system. *Lytic* refers to "lyse," which means "to interfere with." Atropine works by blocking acetylcholine at the endings of the vagus nerves. The vagus nerves innervate the heart at the sinoatrial (SA) and atrioventricular (AV) nodes. Thus, atropine is most effective for narrow-QRS bradycardias. By blocking the effects of acetylcholine, atropine allows more activity from the sympathetic division of the autonomic nervous system. As a result, the rate at which the SA node can fire is increased. Areas of the heart that are not innervated or that are minimally innervated by the vagus nerves (e.g., the ventricles) will not respond to atropine. Thus, atropine is usually ineffective for the treatment of wide-QRS bradycardias. Atropine also increases the rate at which an impulse is conducted through the AV node. It has little or no effect on the force of contraction.

SINUS TACHYCARDIA

[Objective 3]

If the SA node fires at a rate faster than normal for the patient's age, the rhythm is called **sinus tachycardia**. Sinus tachycardia begins and ends gradually. The rhythm starts in the SA node and travels the normal pathway of conduction through the heart, resulting in atrial and ventricular depolarization.

How Do I Recognize It?

A sinus tachycardia looks much like a sinus rhythm except that it is faster. At very fast rates, it may be hard to tell the difference between a P wave and T wave. Keep in mind that the QT interval normally shortens as heart rate increases.

Normal heart rates vary with age. In adults, the rate associated with sinus tachycardia is usually between 101 and 180 beats/min. Because an infant or child's heart rate can transiently increase during episodes of crying, pain, or in the presence of a fever, the term *tachycardia* is used to describe a significant and persistent increase in heart rate. In infants, a tachycardia is a heart rate of more than 200 beats/min. In a child older than 5 years, a tachycardia is a heart rate of more than 160 beats/min.

Figure 3-4 is an example of sinus tachycardia. Table 3-4 lists the ECG characteristics of sinus tachycardia. Let us examine this rhythm strip more closely. By glancing at the strip from left to right, you can see that the rate is faster than that of a sinus rhythm. Locate the QRS complexes, evaluate the R-R intervals, and then determine the ventricular rate. The R-R intervals in this example are regular and the ventricular rate is 125 beats/min. Remember that the rate range for a sinus tachycardia is between 101 and 180 beats/min; therefore, the ventricular rate fits within the parameters of a sinus tachycardia.

Look at the P waves on the rhythm strip, evaluate the P-P intervals for regularity, and then determine the atrial rate. One upright P wave appears before each QRS complex, every P wave looks alike, and the P waves occur regularly at a rate of 125 beats/min. Now measure the PR interval, QRS

Table **3-4**	Characteristics of Sinus Tachycardia
Rhythm	R-R and P-P intervals are regular
Rate	101 to 180 beats/min
P waves	Positive (upright) in lead II; one precedes each QRS complex; P waves look alike
PR interval	0.12 to 0.20 sec and constant from beat to beat
QRS duration	0.11 sec or less unless abnormally conducted

duration, and QT interval. In this example, the PR interval is 0.16 second, the QRS complex measures 0.06 second, and the QT interval is 0.32 second. Now interpret the rhythm, noting the ST-segment depression that is present. The correct interpretation is, "Sinus tachycardia at 125 beats/min with ST-segment depression."

What Causes It?

Sinus tachycardia is a normal response to the body's demand for increased oxygen, which results from many conditions (see the Clinical Correlation box below). The patient is often aware of an increase in heart rate. Some patients complain of palpitations, a racing heart, or a feeling of pounding in their chests. Sinus tachycardia is seen in some patients with acute MI, especially in those with an anterior infarction.

In a patient with coronary artery disease, sinus tachycardia can cause problems. The heart's demand for oxygen increases as the heart rate increases. As the heart rate increases, there is less time for the ventricles to fill and less blood for the ventricles to pump out with each contraction, which can lead to decreased cardiac output. Because the coronary arteries fill when the ventricles are at rest, rapid heart rates decrease the time available for coronary artery filling. This decreases the heart's blood supply. Chest discomfort can result if the supplies of blood and oxygen to the heart are inadequate. Sinus tachycardia in a patient who is having an acute MI may be an early warning signal for heart failure, cardiogenic shock, and more serious dysrhythmias.

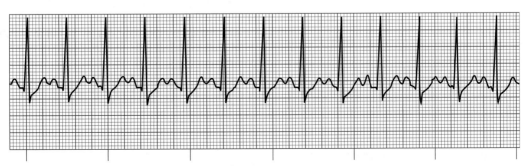

Figure 3-4 Sinus tachycardia at 125 beats/min with ST-segment depression.

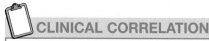

Causes of Sinus Tachycardia
- Acute myocardial infarction
- Caffeine-containing beverages
- Dehydration, hypovolemia
- Drugs such as cocaine, amphetamines, "ecstasy," cannabis
- Exercise
- Fear and anxiety
- Fever
- Heart failure
- Hyperthyroidism
- Hypoxia
- Infection
- Medications (e.g., epinephrine, atropine, dopamine)
- Nicotine
- Pain
- Pulmonary embolism
- Shock
- Sympathetic stimulation

What Do I Do About It?

Treatment for sinus tachycardia is directed at correcting the underlying cause (i.e., fluid replacement, relief of pain, removal of offending medications or substances, reducing fever, or anxiety). Sinus tachycardia in a patient experiencing an acute MI may be treated with medications to slow the heart rate and decrease myocardial oxygen demand (e.g., beta-blockers), provided there are no signs of heart failure or other contraindications.

Some dysrhythmias with very rapid ventricular rates (i.e., above 150 beats/min) require the delivery of medications or a shock to stop the rhythm. However, it is important to remember that shocking a sinus tachycardia is inappropriate; rather, treat the cause of the tachycardia.

SINUS ARRHYTHMIA

As you have seen so far, the SA node fires quite regularly most of the time. When it fires irregularly, the resulting rhythm is called **sinus arrhythmia**. Sinus arrhythmia begins in the SA node and follows the normal conduction pathway in the heart, resulting in atrial and ventricular depolarization. Sinus arrhythmia that is associated with the phases of breathing and changes in intrathoracic pressure is called *respiratory sinus arrhythmia*. Sinus arrhythmia that is not related to the ventilatory cycle is called *nonrespiratory sinus arrhythmia*.

How Do I Recognize It?

A sinus arrhythmia usually occurs at a rate of 60 to 100 beats/min. If sinus arrhythmia is associated with a slower than normal rate, it is called *sinus brady-arrhythmia*. If the rhythm is associated with a faster than normal rate, it is known as *sinus tachy-arrhythmia*.

Let's look at the rhythm strip in Figure 3-5. How does this rhythm differ from the others we have discussed so far? Without using calipers or a piece of paper, you can see that it is irregular. Recognizing that, the rhythm cannot be a sinus rhythm because a sinus rhythm is regular. Now, let us determine the atrial and ventricular rate. Because the rhythm is irregular, it is best to give a rate range. To do that we will need to find the slowest part of the rhythm and calculate that rate. We will then need to find the fastest part of the rhythm and calculate that rate. Looking from left to right, the slowest part of this rhythm strip appears to be between the first and second beats because they have the longest R-R and P-P interval. The rate between these beats is 63 beats/min. The rate between the sixth and seventh beats is 81 beats/min. This rhythm strip was obtained from a 39-year-old man who was complaining of "feeling faint." If we were able to see the patient and watch his ventilatory rate and ECG at the same time, you would see a pattern. The patient's heart rate increases gradually during inspiration (i.e., the R-R intervals shorten) and decreases with expiration (i.e., the R-R intervals lengthen). Looking closely at the rest of the rhythm strip, you can see one upright P wave before each QRS complex. The PR interval and QRS duration are within normal limits. To identify this rhythm, we will call it a sinus arrhythmia at 63 to 81 beats/min. Table 3-5 lists the characteristics of sinus arrhythmia.

What Causes It?

Respiratory sinus arrhythmia, which is the most common type of sinus arrhythmia, is a normal phenomenon that occurs with phases of breathing and changes in intrathoracic pressure. The heart rate increases with inspiration (i.e., the

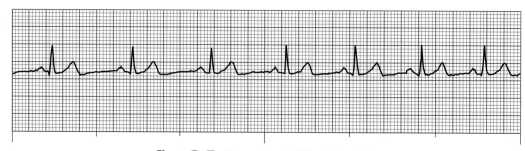

Figure 3-5   Sinus arrhythmia at 63 to 81 beats/min.

Table 3-5	Characteristics of Sinus Arrhythmia
Rhythm	Irregular and phasic with breathing; heart rate increases gradually during inspiration (R-R intervals shorten) and decreases with expiration (R-R intervals lengthen)
Rate	Usually 60 to 100 beats/min, but may be slower or faster
P waves	Positive (upright) in lead II; one precedes each QRS complex; P waves look alike
PR interval	0.12 to 0.20 sec and constant from beat to beat
QRS duration	0.11 sec or less unless abnormally conducted

R-R intervals shorten) and decreases with expiration (i.e., the R-R intervals lengthen). The changes in rhythm disappear when patients hold their breath. Sinus arrhythmia is most commonly observed in children and young adults.

Nonrespiratory sinus arrhythmia can be seen in people with normal hearts, but it is more likely to be found in older individuals and in those with heart disease. It is common after acute inferior wall MI, and it may be seen with increased intracranial pressure. Nonrespiratory sinus arrhythmia may be the result of the effects of medications (e.g., digitalis, morphine) or carotid sinus pressure.

What Do I Do About It?

Sinus arrhythmia usually does not require treatment unless it is accompanied by a slow heart rate that causes hemodynamic compromise. If hemodynamic compromise is present as a result of the slow rate, IV atropine may be indicated to treat the bradycardia.

SINOATRIAL BLOCK

With SA block, which is also called *sinus exit block*, the pacemaker cells within the SA node initiate an impulse, but it is blocked as it exits the SA node. This results in periodically absent PQRST complexes. SA block is thought to occur because of failure of the transitional cells in the SA node to conduct the impulse from the pacemaker cells to the surrounding atrium. Thus SA block is a disorder of impulse conduction.

How Do I Recognize It?

The rhythm of the SA node is not affected by SA block because impulses are generated regularly. However, because an impulse is blocked as it exits the SA node, the atria are not activated. This appears on the ECG as a single missed beat (i.e., a P wave, QRS complex, and T wave are missing). The pause caused by the missed beat is the same as, or an exact multiple of, the distance between two P-P intervals of the underlying rhythm.

Look at the example of SA block in Figure 3-6. As you quickly scan the rhythm strip from left to right, the pause between the third and fourth beats should be obvious. The atrial and ventricular rhythm is irregular because of the pause. It is also correct to say that the atrial and ventricular rhythms are regular except for the event; in this case, the pause is the event. Begin analyzing the rhythm strip by determining atrial and ventricular rate and regularity. Because there is a pause, it is best to give a rate range. In our example, the rate varies from 36 to 71 beats/min. You can see a positive P wave in front of each QRS complex. The P waves look alike. The PR interval is 0.16 second and constant from beat to beat. The QRS complex is 0.08 second and the QT interval measures 0.32 to 0.36 second, which is within normal limits. Because the P waves are upright and each P wave is associated with a QRS complex, we know that the underlying rhythm came from the SA node. So far, we can identify this rhythm as a sinus rhythm with a ventricular rate of 36 to 71 beats/min.

Now we need to figure out what caused the pause between beats 3 and 4. First, look to the left of the pause and examine the waveforms of the beat that comes before the pause. Compare these waveforms to the others in the rhythm strip. It is important to do this because sometimes waveforms "hide" on top of other waveforms and distort their shape. In our example, nothing seems to be amiss. Now use your calipers or paper and plot P waves and R waves from left to right across the strip. When you do this, make a mark on the rhythm strip where the next PQRST cycle should have occurred. You will find that exactly one PQRST cycle is missing. The P-P interval is an exact multiple of the distance between two P-P intervals of the underlying sinus rhythm.

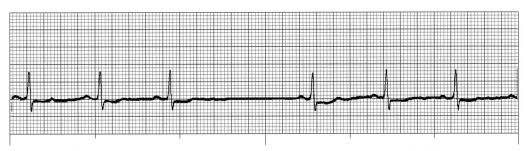

Figure 3-6   Sinus rhythm at a rate of 36 to 71 beats/min with an episode of sinoatrial (SA) block.

Table 3-6	Characteristics of Sinoatrial Block
Rhythm	Irregular as a result of the pause(s) caused by the sinoatrial (SA) block—the pause is the same as, or an exact multiple of, the distance between two other P-P intervals
Rate	Usually normal but varies because of the pause
P waves	Positive (i.e., upright) in lead II; P waves look alike; when present, one precedes each QRS complex.
PR interval	0.12 to 0.20 sec and constant from beat to beat
QRS duration	0.11 sec or less unless abnormally conducted

This occurred because impulses were generated regularly but failed to exit the SA node between beats 3 and 4. To complete our identification of this rhythm, we will explain the pause as an SA block. Putting it all together, we have a sinus rhythm at a rate of 36 to 71 beats/min with an episode of SA block. Table 3-6 lists the ECG characteristics of SA block.

What Causes It?

SA block is rather uncommon. Possible causes of SA block include hypoxia, damage or disease to the SA node from coronary artery disease, myocarditis, or acute MI; carotid sinus sensitivity, increased vagal tone on the SA node, and medications (e.g., digitalis, quinidine, procainamide, salicylates). If episodes of SA block are frequent and accompanied by a slow heart rate, the patient may show signs and symptoms of hemodynamic compromise.

What Do I Do About It?

Signs and symptoms associated with SA block depend on the number of sinus beats blocked. If the episodes of SA block are transient and there are no significant signs or symptoms, the patient is observed. If signs of hemodynamic compromise are present and are the result of medication toxicity, the offending agents should be withheld. If the episodes of SA block are frequent, IV atropine, temporary pacing, or insertion of a permanent pacemaker may be needed.

SINUS ARREST

[Objective 6]

Sinus arrest, which is also called *sinus pause* or *sinoatrial arrest*, is a disorder of impulse formation. With sinus arrest, the pacemaker cells of the SA node fail to initiate an electrical impulse for one or more beats resulting in absent PQRST complexes on the ECG.

When the SA node fails to initiate an impulse, an escape pacemaker site (e.g., the AV junction or the Purkinje fibers) should kick in and assume responsibility for pacing the heart. The term *junctional* is used to denote a beat or rhythm that originates from the AV junction. Therefore, when the SA node fails to fire and an escape pacemaker kicks in, the pause associated with a sinus arrest may be terminated by a junctional or ventricular escape beat. If an escape pacemaker site does not fire, you will see absent PQRST complexes on the ECG.

How Do I Recognize It?

Figure 3-7 shows an example of sinus arrest. Looking at the rhythm strip from left to right, you can see a period of no electrical activity between the third and fourth beats. Begin analyzing the rhythm strip by determining the atrial and ventricular rhythmicity and rate. Because the rhythmicity of this dysrhythmia occurs as the result of a specific event and the remainder of the rhythm is regular, the regularity (i.e., the rhythm) may be described as *irregular* or as *regular except for the event*. Because there is a pause, it is best to give a rate range. In our example, the rate varies from 24 to 81 beats/min. You can see a positive P wave in front of each QRS complex. The P waves look alike. The PR interval is 0.20 second and constant from beat to beat. The QRS complex is 0.10 second and the QT interval is 0.36 second. Because the P waves are upright and each P wave is associated with a QRS complex, we know that the underlying rhythm came from the SA node. Therefore the underlying rhythm is a sinus rhythm with a ventricular rate of 24 to 81 beats/min.

Now let's try to explain what caused the pause between beats 3 and 4. Look to the left of the pause and examine the waveforms of the beat that comes before the pause. Compare these waveforms to the others in the rhythm strip. There

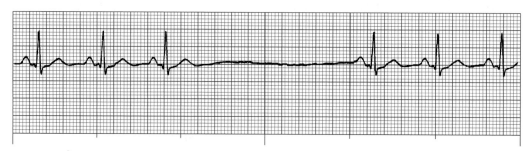

Figure 3-7   Sinus rhythm at a rate of 24 to 81 beats/min with an episode of sinus arrest.

does not appear to be any distortion of the waveforms. With the use of your calipers or paper, plot P waves and R waves from left to right across the strip. When you do this, make a mark on the rhythm strip where the next PQRST cycles should have occurred. You will find that more than one PQRST cycle is missing. Because the SA node periodically failed to produce impulses, the P-P intervals are not exact multiples of other P-P intervals. This is characteristic of a sinus arrest. To complete our identification of this rhythm strip, we must add this explanation for the pause we saw; therefore our final identification is a sinus rhythm at a rate of 24 to 81 beats/min with an episode of sinus arrest. Table 3-7 lists the ECG characteristics of sinus arrest.

Table 3-7	Characteristics of Sinus Arrest
Rhythm	Irregular; the pause is of undetermined length, more than one PQRST complex is missing, and it is not the same distance as other P-P intervals
Rate	Usually normal but varies because of the pause
P waves	Positive (i.e., upright) in lead II; P waves look alike; when present, one precedes each QRS complex
PR interval	0.12 to 0.20 sec and constant from beat to beat
QRS duration	0.11 sec or less unless abnormally conducted

What Causes It?

Causes of sinus arrest include damage to or disease of the SA node from coronary artery disease, acute MI, or rheumatic disease; carotid sinus pressure, a sudden increase in parasympathetic activity on the SA node, stimulation of the pharynx, obstructive sleep apnea, hypothermia, and reactions to medications such as beta-blockers and calcium channel blockers.

What Do I Do About It?

Signs and symptoms associated with sinus arrest depend on the number of absent sinus beats and the length of the sinus arrest because there is no cardiac output during the period of arrest. Signs of hemodynamic compromise such as weakness, lightheadedness, dizziness, or syncope may be associated with this dysrhythmia. If the episodes of sinus arrest are transient and there are no significant signs or symptoms, observe the patient. If signs and symptoms are a result of carotid sinus sensitivity and resultant vagal stimulation, remove tight clothing, if applicable. If hemodynamic compromise is present, IV atropine, temporary pacing, or both may be indicated. If the episodes of sinus arrest are frequent and prolonged (i.e., more than 3 seconds) or a result of disease of the SA node, insertion of a permanent pacemaker is generally warranted.

A summary of the characteristics of sinus mechanisms can be found in Table 3-8.

Table 3-8	Sinus Mechanisms—Summary of Characteristics					
Characteristic	Sinus Rhythm	Sinus Bradycardia	Sinus Tachycardia	Sinus Arrhythmia	Sinoatrial Block	Sinus Arrest
Rhythm	Regular	Regular	Regular	Irregular, typically phasic with breathing	Regular except for the event; pause is the same (or an exact multiple of) as the distance between two P-P intervals of underlying rhythm	Regular except for the event; pause of undetermined length—not a multiple of other P-P intervals
Rate (beats/min)	60 to 100	Less than 60	101 to 180	Usually 60 to 100	Varies	Varies
P Waves (lead II)	Positive, one precedes each QRS	Positive, one precedes each QRS	Positive, one precedes each QRS	Positive, one precedes each QRS	When present, positive, one precedes each QRS	When present, positive, one precedes each QRS
PR interval	0.12 to 0.20 sec	0.12 to 0.20 sec	0.12 to 0.20 sec	0.12 to 0.20 sec	When present, 0.12 to 0.20 sec	When present, 0.12 to 0.20 sec
QRS duration	0.11 sec or less unless abnormally conducted	0.11 sec or less unless abnormally conducted	0.11 sec or less unless abnormally conducted	0.11 sec or less unless abnormally conducted	0.11 sec or less unless abnormally conducted	0.11 sec or less unless abnormally conducted

STOP & REVIEW—CHAPTER 3

Multiple Choice

Identify the choice that best completes the statement or answers the question.

_____ 1. Sinus arrest is a disorder of:
   a. Reentry.
   b. Conductivity.
   c. Impulse formation.
   d. Impulse conduction.

_____ 2. Which of the following rhythms originates in the SA node and is commonly phasic with breathing?
   a. Sinus arrest
   b. Sinus arrhythmia
   c. Sinus tachycardia
   d. Sinus bradycardia

_____ 3. A lead II rhythm strip obtained from a 38-year-old woman with difficulty breathing reveals a regular atrial and ventricular rhythm, a ventricular rate of 120 beats/min, an upright P wave before each QRS complex, and a normal PR interval and QRS duration. This rhythm is:
   a. Sinus rhythm.
   b. Sinoatrial block.
   c. Sinus arrhythmia.
   d. Sinus tachycardia.

_____ 4. Sinoatrial block is a disorder of:
   a. Reentry.
   b. Contractility.
   c. Impulse formation.
   d. Impulse conduction.

Questions 5 through 11 pertain to the following scenario.
A 75-year-old man presents with weakness and "feeling lightheaded." His symptoms began about 30 minutes ago.

_____ 5. The patient's blood pressure is 75/40 mm Hg, pulse 44 beats/min, and ventilations 16 breaths/min. A bradycardia is present when the heart rate is less than:
   a. 60 beats/min.
   b. 75 beats/min.
   c. 85 beats/min.
   d. 100 beats/min.

_____ 6. You prepare to apply electrodes and lead wires to the patient for continuous ECG monitoring in lead II. Lead II views the:
   a. Lateral surface of the left ventricle.
   b. Inferior surface of the left ventricle.
   c. Anterior surface of the left ventricle.
   d. Posterior surface of the right ventricle.

_____ 7. You are examining the waveforms on this patient's ECG. What is the name given to the first negative deflection observed after the P wave?
   a. Q wave
   b. R wave
   c. S wave
   d. T wave

_____ 8. As you measure the intervals on this patient's rhythm strip, you recall that the normal duration of the PR interval is _____ second.
   a. 0.04 to 0.10
   b. 0.06 to 0.14
   c. 0.12 to 0.20
   d. 0.16 to 0.24

_____ 9. Analysis of the patient's ECG reveals ST-segment depression in lead II. Although this ECG finding must be noted in additional leads viewing the same area of the heart to be considered clinically significant, the presence of ST-segment depression suggests:
   a. Myocardial injury.
   b. Myocardial ischemia.
   c. Death of a portion of the left ventricular tissue.
   d. Death of a portion of the cardiac conduction system.

_____ 10. You interpret the patient's cardiac rhythm to be a sinus bradycardia. A coworker applied a pulse oximeter, which revealed an oxygen saturation level of 92% on room air. Supplemental oxygen is now being administered. The patient reports that he continues to feel weak and lightheaded. A second set of vital signs have been obtained and are essentially unchanged. Which of the following statements is true regarding this patient situation?
   a. The patient is asymptomatic. No treatment is necessary.
   b. The patient is showing signs of hemodynamic compromise. An IV should be established and a 12-lead ECG obtained.
   c. The patient's complaints of weakness and lightheadedness warrant an IV start but no further interventions.
   d. The patient is not complaining of chest pain or discomfort, therefore no additional interventions are necessary at this time.

_____ 11. The patient's symptoms persist and his vital signs are essentially unchanged. The cardiac monitor shows a sinus bradycardia with ST-segment depression. You should prepare to administer:
   a. Atropine.
   b. Atenolol.
   c. Adenosine.
   d. Amiodarone.

Matching

Match the key terms with their definitions by placing the letter of each correct answer in the space provided.

a. Inferior MI, prolonged standing
b. AV junction
c. Symptomatic bradycardia
d. Sinus tachycardia
e. Palpitations, racing heart, pounding in the chest
f. SA block
g. Exercise, fever, pain, dehydration

h. Sinus arrhythmia
i. Smooth, rounded, upright
j. Sinus arrest
k. Atropine
l. Damage or disease to the SA node from acute MI

_____12. Possible causes of sinus tachycardia

_____13. Appearance of P waves that originate from the SA node

_____14. Dysrhythmia with a pause that is the same as (or an exact multiple of) the distance between two other P-P intervals

_____15. If the SA node fails to generate an impulse, the next (escape) pacemaker that should generate an impulse

_____16. Common dysrhythmia associated with changes in intrathoracic pressure

_____17. Possible causes of sinoatrial block

_____18. Dysrhythmia with a pause of undetermined length that is not the same distance as other P-P intervals

_____19. Examples of symptoms that may be associated with a sinus tachycardia

_____20. Vagolytic medication used to increase heart rate

_____21. Signs and symptoms of hemodynamic compromise related to a slow heart rate

_____22. Possible causes of sinus bradycardia

_____23. Dysrhythmia that originates from the SA node and has a ventricular rate of 101 to 180 beats/min

Short Answer

24. Fill in the blank areas in the table below to help you to recall the primary differences among sinus bradycardia, sinus tachycardia, and sinus arrhythmia.

ECG Finding	Sinus Bradycardia	Sinus Tachycardia	Sinus Arrhythmia
Rhythm			
Rate (beats/min)			
P waves (lead II)	Positive, one precedes each QRS	Positive, one precedes each QRS	Positive, one precedes each QRS
PR interval	0.12 to 0.20 sec	0.12 to 0.20 sec	0.12 to 0.20 sec
QRS duration	0.11 sec or less unless abnormally conducted	0.11 sec or less unless abnormally conducted	0.11 sec or less unless abnormally conducted

25. Fill in the blank areas in the table below to help you to recall the differences among sinus rhythm, sinoatrial block, and sinus arrest.

ECG Finding	Sinus Rhythm	Sinoatrial Block	Sinus Arrest
Rhythm			
Rate (beats/min)			
P waves (lead II)	Positive, one precedes each QRS	When present, positive, one precedes each QRS	When present, positive, one precedes each QRS
PR interval	0.12 to 0.20 sec	When present, 0.12 to 0.20 sec	When present, 0.12 to 0.20 sec
QRS duration	0.11 sec or less unless abnormally conducted	0.11 sec or less unless abnormally conducted	0.11 sec or less unless abnormally conducted

For each of the following rhythm strips, determine the atrial and ventricular rate and rhythm, measure the PR interval, QRS duration, and QT interval, and then identify the rhythm.

26. This rhythm strip is from a 19-year-old woman complaining of a sudden onset of fever, weakness, and chills.

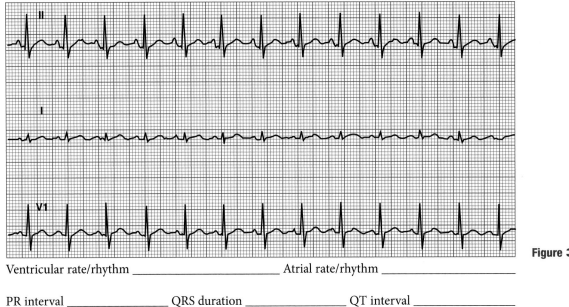

Figure 3-8

Ventricular rate/rhythm _____ Atrial rate/rhythm _____

PR interval _____ QRS duration _____ QT interval _____

Identification _____

27. This rhythm strip (lead II) is from a 33-year-old woman complaining of abdominal pain.

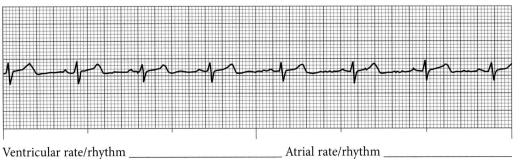

Figure 3-9

Ventricular rate/rhythm _____ Atrial rate/rhythm _____

PR interval _____ QRS duration _____ QT interval _____

Identification _____

28. This rhythm strip is from a 37-year-old asymptomatic man.

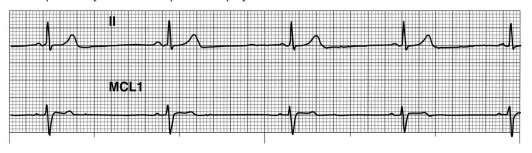

Figure 3-10

Ventricular rate/rhythm _____ Atrial rate/rhythm _____

PR interval _____ QRS duration _____ QT interval _____

Identification _____

29. This rhythm strip (lead II) is from a 50-year-old man complaining of chest pressure. His blood pressure is 70/50 mm Hg.

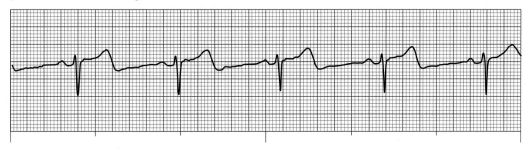

Figure 3-11

Ventricular rate/rhythm _____ Atrial rate/rhythm _____

PR interval _____ QRS duration _____ QT interval _____

Identification _____

30. Identify the rhythm (lead II).

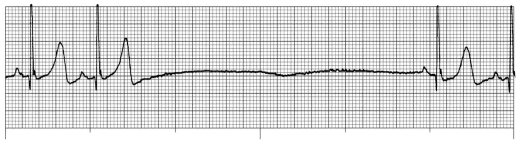

Figure 3-12

Ventricular rate/rhythm _____ Atrial rate/rhythm _____

PR interval _____ QRS duration _____ QT interval _____

Identification _____

31. This rhythm strip is from a 6-year-old girl complaining of abdominal pain. Her blood pressure is 100/60 mm Hg.

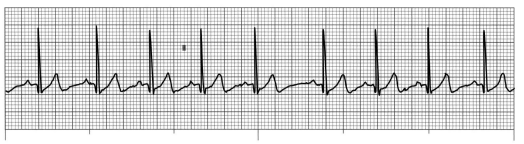

Figure **3-13**

Ventricular rate/rhythm _____ Atrial rate/rhythm _____

PR interval _____ QRS duration _____ QT interval_____

Identification _____

32. Identify the rhythm (lead II).

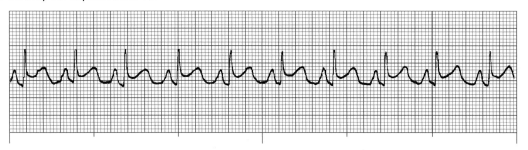

Figure **3-14**

Ventricular rate/rhythm _____ Atrial rate/rhythm _____

PR interval _____ QRS duration _____ QT interval _____

Identification _____

33. This rhythm strip is from a 73-year-old man complaining of chest pain. He has a history of hypertension and lung disease. Medications include aspirin, albuterol, and benazepril (Lotensin).

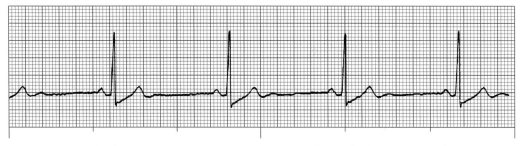

Figure **3-15**

Ventricular rate/rhythm _____ Atrial rate/rhythm _____

PR interval _____ QRS duration _____ QT interval _____

Identification _____

34. This rhythm strip is from a 61-year-old woman with an altered level of responsiveness. Her blood pressure is 112/62 mm Hg and her blood sugar is 42 mg/dL.

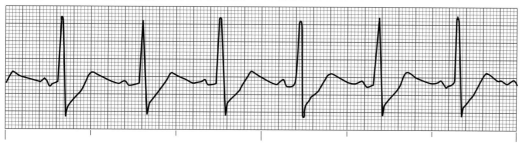

Figure 3-16

Ventricular rate/rhythm _____ Atrial rate/rhythm _____

PR interval _____ QRS duration _____ QT interval _____

Identification _____

35. This rhythm strip is from a 72-year-old man presenting with left-sided weakness. He has a history of a brain tumor.

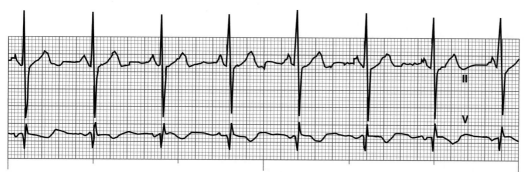

Figure 3-17

Ventricular rate/rhythm _____ Atrial rate/rhythm _____

PR interval _____ QRS duration _____ QT interval _____

Identification _____

36. This rhythm strip is from a 40-year-old man complaining of back pain after jumping from a burning second floor balcony. His blood pressure is 128/84 mm Hg.

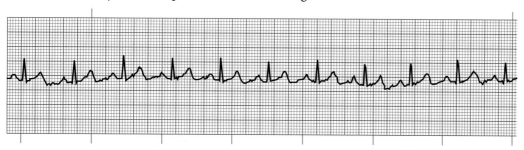

Figure 3-18

Ventricular rate/rhythm _____ Atrial rate/rhythm _____

PR interval _____ QRS duration _____ QT interval _____

Identification _____

37. This rhythm strip (lead II) is from a 90-year-old woman with difficulty breathing.

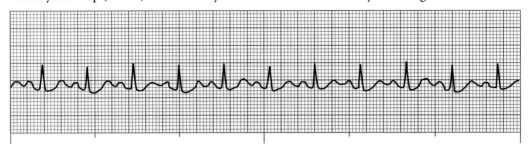

Figure **3-19**

Ventricular rate/rhythm _____ Atrial rate/rhythm _____

PR interval _____ QRS duration _____ QT interval _____

Identification _____

38. Identify the rhythm (lead II).

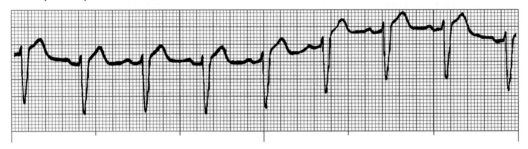

Figure **3-20**

Ventricular rate/rhythm _____ Atrial rate/rhythm _____

PR interval _____ QRS duration _____ QT interval _____

Identification _____

39. Identify the rhythm (top = lead II, middle = lead I, bottom = lead III).

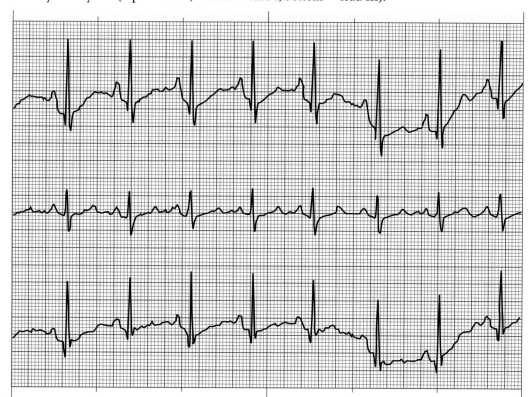

Figure 3-21

Ventricular rate/rhythm _____ Atrial rate/rhythm _____

PR interval _____ QRS duration _____ QT interval _____

Identification _____

40. This rhythm strip (lead II) is from a 44-year-old construction worker with a sudden onset of chest pressure.

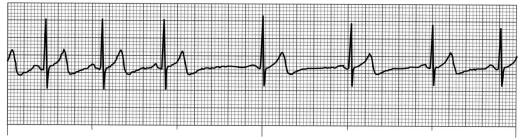

Figure 3-22

Ventricular rate/rhythm _____ Atrial rate/rhythm _____

PR interval _____ QRS duration _____ QT interval _____

Identification _____

41. This rhythm strip (lead II) is from a 29-year-old woman with a kidney stone.

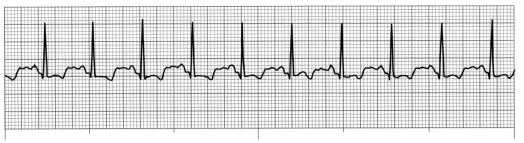

Figure **3-23**

Ventricular rate/rhythm _____ Atrial rate/rhythm _____

PR interval _____ QRS duration _____ QT interval _____

Identification _____

42. Identify the rhythm.

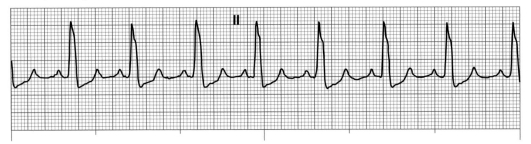

Figure **3-24**

Ventricular rate/rhythm _____ Atrial rate/rhythm _____

PR interval _____ QRS duration _____ QT interval _____

Identification _____

43. These rhythm strips are from a 44-year-old man complaining of dizziness secondary to cocaine use.

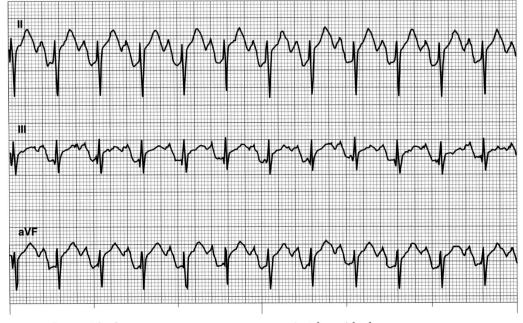

Figure **3-25**

Ventricular rate/rhythm _____ Atrial rate/rhythm _____

PR interval _____ QRS duration _____ QT interval _____

Identification _____

44. This rhythm strip (lead II) is from a 35-year-old woman who attempted suicide. Her blood pressure is 118/80, ventilations 16 breaths/min.

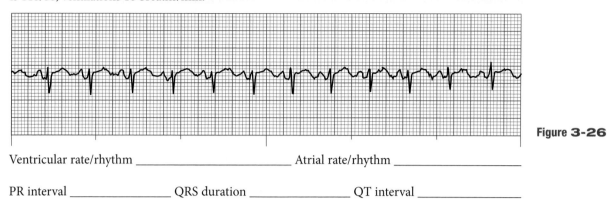

Figure 3-26

Ventricular rate/rhythm _____ Atrial rate/rhythm _____

PR interval _____ QRS duration _____ QT interval _____

Identification _____

45. Identify the rhythm.

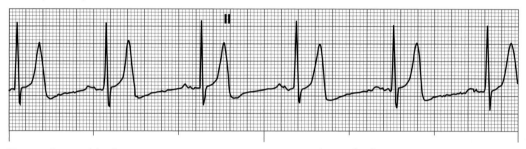

Figure 3-27

Ventricular rate/rhythm _____ Atrial rate/rhythm _____

PR interval _____ QRS duration _____ QT interval _____

Identification _____

46. Identify the rhythm (lead II).

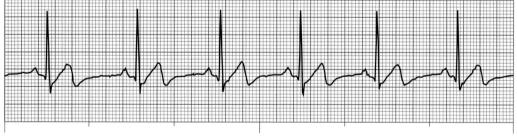

Figure 3-28

Ventricular rate/rhythm _____ Atrial rate/rhythm _____

PR interval _____ QRS duration _____ QT interval _____

Identification _____

47. These rhythm strips are from a 44-year-old woman with chest pain.

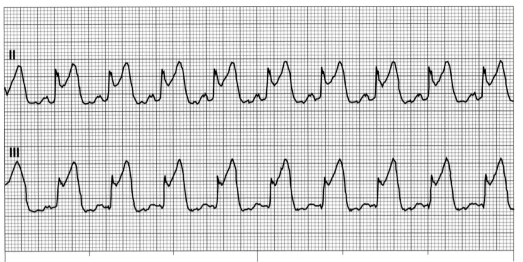

Figure 3-29

Ventricular rate/rhythm _____ Atrial rate/rhythm _____

PR interval _____ QRS duration _____ QT interval _____

Identification _____

48. This rhythm strip is from a 27-year-old man with a stab wound to his mid-abdomen. His blood pressure is 126/68 mm Hg.

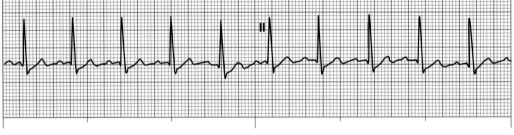

Figure 3-30

Ventricular rate/rhythm _____ Atrial rate/rhythm _____

PR interval _____ QRS duration _____ QT interval _____

Identification Identification _____

STOP & REVIEW ANSWERS

Multiple Choice

1. ANS: C

Sinus arrest is a disorder of impulse formation. In sinus arrest, the pacemaker cells of the sinoatrial (SA) node fail to initiate an electrical impulse for one or more beats resulting in absent PQRST complexes on the ECG.

OBJ: Describe the ECG characteristics, possible causes, signs and symptoms, and emergency management of sinus arrest.

2. ANS: B

Sinus arrhythmia that is associated with the phases of breathing and changes in intrathoracic pressure is called *respiratory sinus arrhythmia*. Sinus arrhythmia that is not related to the ventilatory cycle is called *nonrespiratory sinus arrhythmia*.

OBJ: Describe the ECG characteristics, possible causes, signs and symptoms, and emergency management of sinus arrhythmia.

3. ANS: D

A sinus tachycardia is differentiated from other rhythms that originate in the SA node by its rate (101 to 180 beats/min).

OBJ: Describe the ECG characteristics, possible causes, signs and symptoms, and emergency management of sinus tachycardia.

4. ANS: D

In SA block, the pacemaker cells within the SA node initiate an impulse, but it is blocked as it exits the SA node. This results in periodically absent PQRST complexes. SA block is thought to occur because of failure of the transitional cells in the SA node to conduct the impulse from the pacemaker cells to the surrounding atrium. Thus SA block is a disorder of impulse conduction.

OBJ: Describe the ECG characteristics, possible causes, signs and symptoms, and emergency management of sinoatrial block.

5. ANS: A

In adults, a bradycardia exists if the rate is less than 60 beats per minute (brady = slow).

OBJ: Describe the ECG characteristics, possible causes, signs and symptoms, and emergency management of sinus bradycardia.

6. ANS: B

Lead II views the inferior surface of the left ventricle.

OBJ: Relate the cardiac surfaces or areas represented by the ECG leads.

Matching

12. ANS: G

13. ANS: I

14. ANS: F

15. ANS: B

16. ANS: H

17. ANS: L

7. ANS: A

A QRS complex normally follows each P wave. The QRS complex begins as a downward deflection, the *Q wave,* and represents depolarization of the interventricular septum.

OBJ: Define and describe the significance of each of the following as they relate to cardiac electrical activity: P wave, QRS complex, T wave, U wave, PR segment, TP segment, ST segment, PR interval, QRS duration, and QT interval.

8. ANS: C

The PR interval changes with heart rate but normally measures 0.12 to 0.20 second in adults. As the heart rate increases, the duration of the PR interval shortens. A PR interval is considered *short* if it is less than 0.12 second and *long* if it is more than 0.20 second.

9. ANS: B

ST-segment depression of more than 0.5 mm in leads V_2 and V_3 and more than 1 mm in all other leads is suggestive of myocardial ischemia.

OBJ: Recognize the changes on the ECG that may reflect evidence of myocardial ischemia and injury.

10. ANS: B

The term *symptomatic bradycardia* is used to describe a patient who experiences signs and symptoms of hemodynamic compromise related to a slow heart rate. Because this patient is complaining of weakness, light-headedness, and is hypotensive, he is clearly symptomatic with his slow heart rate. Treatment of a symptomatic bradycardia should include application of a pulse oximeter and administration of supplemental oxygen if indicated, which have already been done. Next, establish intravenous (IV) access and obtain a 12-lead ECG.

OBJ: Describe the ECG characteristics, possible causes, signs and symptoms, and emergency management of sinus bradycardia.

11. ANS: A

Atropine, administered intravenously, is the drug of choice for symptomatic bradycardia. Reassess the patient's response to the therapeutic interventions provided and continue monitoring the patient. Adenosine is used to slow the ventricular rate. Atenolol, a beta-blocker, would further slow the heart rate. Although amiodarone is an antiarrhythmic used to treat many atrial and ventricular dysrhythmias, it is not used to treat a sinus bradycardia.

18. ANS: J

19. ANS: E

20. ANS: K

21. ANS: C

22. ANS: A

23. ANS: D

Short Answer

24. ANS:

ECG Finding	Sinus Bradycardia	Sinus Tachycardia	Sinus Arrhythmia
Rhythm	**Regular**	**Regular**	**Irregular, typically phasic with breathing**
Rate (beats/min)	**Slower than 60**	**101 to 180**	**Usually 60 to 100**
P waves (lead II)	Positive, one precedes each QRS	Positive, one precedes each QRS	Positive, one precedes each QRS
PR interval	0.12 to 0.20 sec	0.12 to 0.20 sec	0.12 to 0.20 sec
QRS duration	0.11 sec or less unless abnormally conducted	0.11 sec or less unless abnormally conducted	0.11 sec or less unless abnormally conducted

OBJ: Describe the ECG characteristics, possible causes, signs and symptoms, and emergency management of sinus brady-cardia. Describe the ECG characteristics, possible causes, signs and symptoms, and emergency management of sinus tachycardia. Describe the ECG characteristics, possible causes, signs and symptoms, and emergency management of sinus arrhythmia.

25. ANS:

ECG Finding	Sinus Rhythm	Sinoatrial Block	Sinus Arrest
Rhythm	**Regular**	**Regular except for the event; pause is the same (or an exact multiple of) as the distance between two P-P intervals of underlying rhythm**	**Regular except for the event; pause of undetermined length—not a multiple of other P-P intervals**
Rate (beats/min)	**60 to 100**	**Varies**	**Varies**
P waves (lead II)	Positive, one precedes each QRS	When present, positive, one precedes each QRS	When present, positive, one precedes each QRS
PR interval	0.12 to 0.20 sec	When present, 0.12 to 0.20 sec	When present, 0.12 to 0.20 sec
QRS duration	0.11 sec or less unless abnormally conducted	0.11 sec or less unless abnormally conducted	0.11 sec or less unless abnormally conducted

OBJ: Describe the ECG characteristics, possible causes, signs and symptoms, and emergency management of sinoatrial block. Describe the ECG characteristics, possible causes, signs and symptoms, and emergency management of sinus arrest.

26. Figure 3-8 answer

Ventricular rate/rhythm	120 beats/min; regular
Atrial rate/rhythm	120 beats/min; regular
PR interval	0.12 to 0.14 sec
QRS duration	0.08 sec
QT interval	0.28 sec
Identification	Sinus tachycardia at 120 beats/min

27. Figure 3-9 answer

Ventricular rate/rhythm	71 beats/min; regular
Atrial rate/rhythm	71 beats/min; regular
PR interval	0.12 sec
QRS duration	0.08 sec
QT interval	0.36 sec
Identification	Sinus rhythm at 71 beats/min

28. Figure 3-10 answer

Ventricular rate/rhythm	37 beats/min; regular
Atrial rate/rhythm	37 beats/min; regular
PR interval	0.16 sec
QRS duration	0.08 to 0.10 sec
QT interval	0.36 sec
Identification	Sinus bradycardia at 37 beats/min

29. Figure 3-11 answer

Ventricular rate/rhythm	52 beats/min; regular
Atrial rate/rhythm	52 beats/min; regular
PR interval	0.18 to 0.20 sec
QRS duration	0.08 to 0.10 sec
QT interval	0.44 sec
Identification	Sinus bradycardia at 52 beats/min with ST-segment elevation

30. **Figure 3-12 answer**
Ventricular rate/rhythm — 0 to 75 beats/min; irregular
Atrial rate/rhythm — 0 to 75 beats/min; irregular
PR interval — 0.16 sec
QRS duration — 0.08 sec
QT interval — 0.44 sec
Identification — Sinus rhythm at about 75 beats/min with an episode of sinus arrest; tall T waves

31. **Figure 3-13 answer**
Ventricular rate/rhythm — 75 to 100 beats/min; irregular
Atrial rate/rhythm — 75 to 100 beats/min; irregular
PR interval — 0.14 to 0.16 sec
QRS duration — 0.08 sec
QT interval — 0.32 sec
Identification — Sinus arrhythmia at 75 to 100 beats/min

32. **Figure 3-14 answer**
Ventricular rate/rhythm — 98 beats/min; regular
Atrial rate/rhythm — 98 beats/min; regular
PR interval — 0.16 sec
QRS duration — 0.04 to 0.06 sec
QT interval — 0.32 sec
Identification — Sinus rhythm at 98 beats/min; ST-segment elevation

33. **Figure 3-15 answer**
Ventricular rate/rhythm — 44 beats/min; regular
Atrial rate/rhythm — 44 beats/min; regular
PR interval — 0.16 sec
QRS duration — 0.06 sec
QT interval — 0.44 sec
Identification — Sinus bradycardia at 44 beats/min, ST-segment depression; note the upright U waves following each T wave.

34. **Figure 3-16 answer**
Ventricular rate/rhythm — 65 beats/min; regular
Atrial rate/rhythm — 65 beats/min; regular
PR interval — 0.20 sec
QRS duration — 0.10 sec
QT interval — 0.64 sec (prolonged)
Identification — Sinus rhythm at 65 beats/min with ST-segment depression; prolonged QT interval

35. **Figure 3-17 answer**
Ventricular rate/rhythm — 75 beats/min; regular
Atrial rate/rhythm — 75 beats/min; regular
PR interval — 0.12 sec
QRS duration — 0.08 sec
QT interval — 0.36 sec
Identification — Sinus rhythm at 75 beats/min

36. **Figure 3-18 answer**
Ventricular rate/rhythm — 86 beats/min; regular
Atrial rate/rhythm — 86 beats/min; regular
PR interval — 0.16 sec
QRS duration — 0.06 sec
QT interval — 0.32 sec
Identification — Sinus rhythm at 86 beats/min

37. **Figure 3-19 answer**
Ventricular rate/rhythm — 111 beats/min; regular
Atrial rate/rhythm — 111 beats/min; regular
PR interval — 0.16 sec
QRS duration — 0.04 to 06 sec
QT interval — 0.34 sec
Identification — Sinus tachycardia at 111 beats/min

38. **Figure 3-20 answer**
Ventricular rate/rhythm — 83 beats/min; regular
Atrial rate/rhythm — 83 beats/min; regular
PR interval — 0.18 sec
QRS duration — 0.12 sec
QT interval — 0.32 sec
Identification — Sinus rhythm at 83 beats/min with a wide QRS

39. **Figure 3-21 answer**
Ventricular rate/rhythm — 79 beats/min; regular
Atrial rate/rhythm — 79 beats/min; regular
PR interval — 0.16 sec
QRS duration — 0.06 sec
QT interval — 0.40 sec
Identification — Sinus rhythm at 79 beats/min

40. **Figure 3-22 answer**
Ventricular rate/rhythm — 52 to 94 beats/min; irregular
Atrial rate/rhythm — 52 to 94 beats/min; irregular
PR interval — 0.12 sec
QRS duration — 0.08 sec
QT interval — 0.32 sec
Identification — Sinus arrhythmia at 52 to 94 beats/min with ST-segment elevation

41. **Figure 3-23 answer**

Ventricular rate/rhythm	103 beats/min; regular
Atrial rate/rhythm	103 beats/min; regular
PR interval	0.14 sec
QRS duration	0.08 sec
QT interval	0.32 sec
Identification	Sinus tachycardia at 103 beats/min; inverted T waves

42. **Figure 3-24 answer**

Ventricular rate/rhythm	71 beats/min; regular
Atrial rate/rhythm	71 beats/min; regular
PR interval	0.16 to 0.20 sec
QRS duration	0.12 to 0.14 sec
QT interval	0.40 sec
Identification	Sinus rhythm at 71 beats/min with a wide QRS and ST-segment depression

43. **Figure 3-25 answer**

Ventricular rate/rhythm	115 beats/min; regular
Atrial rate/rhythm	115 beats/min; regular
PR interval	0.20 sec
QRS duration	0.08 sec
QT interval	0.32 sec
Identification	Sinus tachycardia at 115 beats/min with ST-segment elevation

44. **Figure 3-26 answer**

Ventricular rate/rhythm	130 beats/min; regular
Atrial rate/rhythm	130 beats/min; regular
PR interval	0.16 sec
QRS duration	0.08 sec
QT interval	0.28 to 0.32 sec
Identification	Sinus tachycardia at 130 beats/min with ST-segment elevation

45. **Figure 3-27 answer**

Ventricular rate/rhythm	55 beats/min; regular
Atrial rate/rhythm	55 beats/min; regular
PR interval	0.20 sec
QRS duration	0.08 sec
QT interval	0.38 sec
Identification	Sinus bradycardia at 55 beats/min with tall T waves

46. **Figure 3-28 answer**

Ventricular rate/rhythm	54 to 65 beats/min; irregular
Atrial rate/rhythm	54 to 65 beats/min; irregular
PR interval	0.18 sec
QRS duration	0.08 sec
QT interval	0.36 sec
Identification	Sinus arrhythmia at 54 to 65 beats/min

47. **Figure 3-29 answer**

Ventricular rate/rhythm	94 beats/min; regular
Atrial rate/rhythm	94 beats/min; regular
PR interval	0.16 sec
QRS duration	0.08 sec
QT interval	0.28 sec
Identification	Sinus rhythm at 94 beats/min with ST-segment elevation

48. **Figure 3-30 answer**

Ventricular rate/rhythm	98 beats/min; regular
Atrial rate/rhythm	98 beats/min; regular
PR interval	0.16 sec
QRS duration	0.08 sec
QT interval	0.32 sec
Identification	Sinus rhythm at 98 beats/min

Atrial Rhythms

CHAPTER

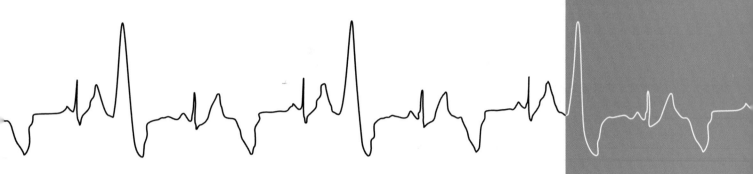

LEARNING OBJECTIVES

After reading this chapter, you should be able to:

1. Explain the concepts of altered automaticity, triggered activity, and reentry.
2. Explain the terms *bigeminy*, *trigeminy*, *quadrigeminy*, and *run* when used to describe premature complexes.
3. Describe the electrocardiogram (ECG) characteristics, possible causes, signs and symptoms, and initial emergency care for premature atrial complexes (PACs).
4. Explain the difference between a compensatory and noncompensatory pause.
5. Explain the terms *wandering atrial pacemaker* and *multifocal atrial tachycardia*.
6. Describe the ECG characteristics, possible causes, signs and symptoms, and initial emergency care for wandering atrial pacemaker (multiformed atrial rhythm).
7. Describe the ECG characteristics, possible causes, signs and symptoms, and initial emergency care for multifocal atrial tachycardia (MAT).
8. List four examples of vagal maneuvers.
9. Describe the ECG characteristics, possible causes, signs and symptoms, and initial emergency care for atrial tachycardia (AT).
10. Explain the terms *paroxysmal atrial tachycardia* (PAT) and *paroxysmal supraventricular tachycardia* (PSVT).
11. Discuss the indications and procedure for synchronized cardioversion.
12. Describe the ECG characteristics, possible causes, signs and symptoms, and initial emergency care for atrioventricular nodal reentrant tachycardia (AVNRT).
13. Describe the ECG characteristics, possible causes, signs and symptoms, and initial emergency care for atrioventricular reentrant tachycardia (AVRT).
14. Describe the ECG characteristics, possible causes, signs and symptoms, and initial emergency care for atrial flutter.
15. Describe the ECG characteristics, possible causes, signs and symptoms, and initial emergency care for atrial fibrillation (AFib).

KEY TERMS

Accessory pathway: An extra bundle of working myocardial tissue that forms a connection between the atria and ventricles outside the normal conduction system

Altered automaticity: A disorder of impulse formation in which cardiac cells fire and initiate impulses before a normal sinoatrial (SA) node impulse

Atrial kick: Blood pushed into the ventricles because of atrial contraction

Atrial tachycardia: Three or more sequential PACs occurring at a rate of more than 100 beats/min

Bigeminy: Dysrhythmia in which every other beat is a premature ectopic beat

Blocked premature atrial complex: PAC not followed by a QRS complex

Bruit: Blowing or swishing sound

Burst: Three or more sequential ectopic beats; also referred to as a salvo or run

Bypass tract: Term used when one end of an accessory pathway is attached to normal conductive tissue

Carotid sinus pressure: Type of vagal maneuver in which pressure is applied to the carotid sinus for a brief period to slow conduction through the atrioventricular (AV) node

Compensatory pause: Pause for which the normal beat after a premature complex occurs when expected; also called a *complete pause*

Couplet: Two consecutive premature complexes

Delta wave: Slurring of the beginning portion of the QRS complex, caused by pre-excitation

f waves: Fibrillation waves; irregularly shaped atrial waves associated with atrial fibrillation; occurring at a rate of 400 to 600 beats/min

F waves: Flutter waves; atrial waves associated with atrial flutter; usually shaped like the teeth of a saw or a picket fence

Focal atrial tachycardia: AT that begins in a small area (focus) within the heart

Multiformed atrial rhythm: Dysrhythmia that occurs because of impulses originating from various sites, including the SA node, the atria, and/or the AV junction; requires at least three different P waves, seen in the same lead, for proper diagnosis

Nonconducted PAC (blocked PAC): PAC that is not followed by a QRS complex

Noncompensatory pause: A pause that often follows a premature atrial complex that represents the delay during which the SA node resets its rhythm for the next beat; the pause is noncompensatory if the normal beat following the premature complex occurs before it was expected (i.e., the period between the complex before and after the premature beat is less than two normal R-R intervals).

Paired beats: Two consecutive complexes

Palpitations: An unpleasant awareness of one's heartbeat

Paroxysmal atrial tachycardia (PAT): AT that starts or ends suddenly

Paroxysmal supraventricular tachycardia (PSVT): A regular, narrow-QRS tachycardia that starts or ends suddenly; also called paroxysmal atrial tachycardia (PAT)

Preexcitation: Term used to describe rhythms that originate from above the ventricles but in which the impulse travels by a pathway other than the AV node and bundle of His; thus the supraventricular impulse excites the ventricles earlier than normal.

Premature complex: Early beat occurring before the next expected beat; can be atrial, junctional, or ventricular

Quadrigeminy: Dysrhythmia in which every fourth beat is a premature ectopic beat

Supraventricular: Originating from a site above the bifurcation of the bundle of His, such as the SA node, atria, or AV junction

Trigeminy: Dysrhythmia in which every third beat is a premature ectopic beat

Vagal maneuver: Methods used to stimulate the vagus nerve in an attempt to slow conduction through the AV node, resulting in slowing of the heart rate

Wandering atrial pacemaker (multiformed atrial rhythm): Cardiac dysrhythmia that occurs because of impulses originating from various sites, including the sinoatrial node, the atria, and/or the AV junction; requires at least three different P waves, seen in the same lead, for proper diagnosis.

Wolff-Parkinson-White syndrome: Type of preexcitation syndrome, characterized by a slurred upstroke of the QRS complex (delta wave) and wide QRS

INTRODUCTION

The atria are thin-walled, low-pressure chambers that receive blood from the systemic circulation and lungs. There is normally a continuous flow of blood from the superior and inferior vena cavae into the atria. Approximately 70% of this blood flows directly through the atria and into the ventricles before the atria contract. When the atria contract, an additional 30% is added to filling of the ventricles. This additional contribution of blood because of atrial contraction is called **atrial kick**.

P waves reflect atrial depolarization. A rhythm that begins in the SA node has one positive (i.e., upright) P wave before each QRS complex. A rhythm that begins in the atria will have a positive P wave that is shaped differently than P waves that begin in the SA node. This difference in P wave configuration occurs because the impulse begins in the atria and follows a different conduction pathway to the AV node.

ATRIAL DYSRHYTHMIAS: MECHANISMS

[Objective 1]
Atrial dysrhythmias reflect abnormal electrical impulse formation and conduction in the atria. They result from altered automaticity, triggered activity, or reentry. Altered automaticity and triggered activity are disorders in impulse *formation*. Reentry is a disorder in impulse *conduction*. Dysrhythmias that result from disorders of impulse formation are often referred to as *automatic*. Dysrhythmias that result from a disorder in impulse conduction are referred to as *reentrant*.

Altered Automaticity

Altered automaticity occurs in normal pacemaker cells and in myocardial working cells that do not normally function

as pacemaker sites. In altered automaticity, these cells fire and initiate impulses before a normal SA node impulse. If the rapid firing rate occurs for more than 50% of the day, it is said to be *incessant*. The rapid firing rate may also occur periodically. In these cases it is said to be *episodic*. Atrial dysrhythmias associated with altered automaticity include PACs and AFib.

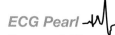
ECG Pearl

Causes of Altered Automaticity
- Drug toxicity
- Hypocalcemia
- Imbalance of electrolytes across the cardiac cell membrane
- Ischemia

Triggered Activity

Triggered activity results from abnormal electrical impulses that sometimes occur during repolarization (i.e., afterdepolarizations), when cells are normally quiet. Triggered activity occurs when escape pacemaker and myocardial working cells fire more than once after stimulation by a single impulse. Triggered activity can result in atrial or ventricular beats that occur alone, in pairs, in "runs" (i.e., three or more beats), or as a sustained ectopic rhythm.

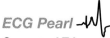
ECG Pearl

Causes of Triggered Activity
- Catecholamine increase
- Hypomagnesemia
- Hypoxia
- Medications that prolong repolarization (e.g., quinidine)
- Myocardial ischemia and injury

Reentry

Reentry, which is also called *reactivation*, is a condition in which an impulse returns to stimulate tissue that was previously depolarized. You will recall from Chapter 2 that reentry requires the following three conditions (Figure 4-1):

- A potential conduction circuit or circular conduction pathway
- A block within part of the circuit
- Delayed conduction within the remainder of the circuit

Normally, an impulse spreads through the heart only once after it is initiated by pacemaker cells. In reentry, an electrical impulse is delayed, blocked, or both in one or more areas of the conduction system while being conducted normally through the rest of the system. This results in the delayed electrical impulse entering cardiac cells that have just been depolarized by the normally conducted impulse. If the delayed impulse stimulates a relatively refractory area, the impulse can cause those cells to fire. This can produce a single early (i.e., premature) beat or repetitive electrical impulses, resulting in short periods of rapid rhythms (i.e., tachydysrhythmias).

Macroreentry circuits and microreentry circuits are two main types of reentry circuits. If the reentry circuit involves conduction through a large area of the heart, such as the entire right or left atrium, it is called a *macroreentry circuit*. A reentry circuit involving conduction within a small area is called a *microreentry circuit*. Atrial rhythms associated with reentry include atrial flutter, AVNRT, and AVRT. Common causes of reentry include hyperkalemia, myocardial ischemia, and some antiarrhythmic medications.

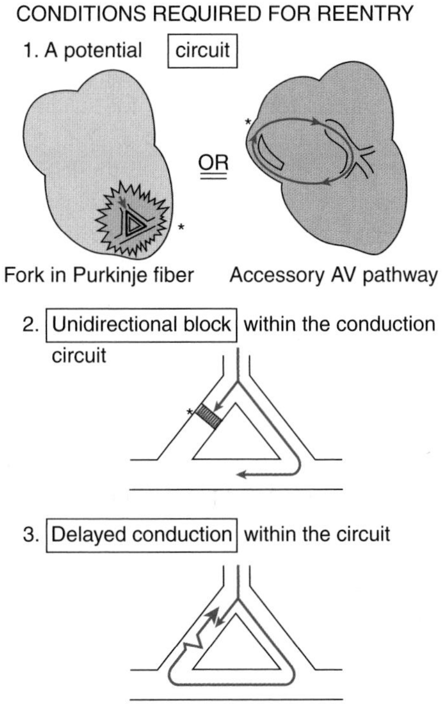

CONDITIONS REQUIRED FOR REENTRY

Figure 4-1 Reentry requires (1) a potential conduction circuit or circular conduction pathway, (2) a block within part of the circuit, and (3) delayed conduction with the remainder of the circuit. AV, atrioventricular.

Most atrial dysrhythmias are not life-threatening, but some may be associated with extremely fast ventricular rates. Increases in heart rate shorten all phases of the cardiac cycle, but the most important is a decrease in the length of time spent in diastole. Remember that as the heart rate increases, there is less time for the ventricles to fill and less blood for the ventricles to pump out with each contraction. Thus an excessively fast heart rate can lead to decreased cardiac output. Examples of factors that influence heart rate include hormone levels (e.g., thyroxin, epinephrine, norepinephrine), medications, stress, anxiety, fear, and body temperature.

PREMATURE ATRIAL COMPLEXES

[Objective 2]
Premature beats appear early, that is, they occur before the next expected beat. Premature beats are identified by their site of origin:

- Premature atrial complexes (PACs)
- Premature junctional complexes (PJCs)
- Premature ventricular complexes (PVCs)

The term *complex* is used instead of *contraction* to correctly identify an early beat because the ECG depicts electrical activity, not mechanical function of the heart. Some practitioners prefer the term *conduction* instead of complex.

Premature beats may occur in patterns:

- Paired beats (**couplet**): Two premature beats in a row
- "Runs" or "**bursts**": Three or more premature beats in a row
- **Bigeminy**: Every other beat is a premature beat
- **Trigeminy**: Every third beat is a premature beat
- **Quadrigeminy**: Every fourth beat is a premature beat

How Do I Recognize It?

[Objective 3]
A PAC occurs when an irritable site (i.e., focus) within the atria fires before the next SA node impulse is expected to fire. This interrupts the sinus rhythm. If the irritable site is close to the SA node, the atrial P wave will look very similar to the P waves initiated by the SA node. The P wave of a PAC may be biphasic (i.e., partly positive, partly negative), flattened, notched, pointed, or lost in the preceding T wave.

ECG Pearl

A premature atrial complex (PAC) has a positive P wave before the QRS complex. Sometimes the P waves are clearly seen and sometimes they are not. If the P wave of an early beat isn't obvious, look for it in the T wave of the preceding beat. The T wave of the preceding beat may be of higher amplitude than other T waves or have an extra "hump," which suggests the presence of a hidden P wave.

When compared with the P-P intervals of the underlying rhythm, a PAC is premature—occurring before the next expected sinus P wave. PACs are identified by the following:

- Early (premature) P waves
- Positive (upright) P waves (in lead II) that differ in shape from sinus P waves
- Early P waves that may or may not be followed by a QRS complex

Look closely at the rhythm strip in Figure 4-2. Begin by locating the QRS complexes on the rhythm strip. Evaluate each succeeding R-R interval. The R-R intervals in this example occur regularly except for three beats. Determine the ventricular rate between the regular R-R intervals. The ventricular rate between the regular R-R intervals is 111 beats/min.

Now find the P waves on the rhythm strip. Remember that P waves that begin in the SA node are normally smooth and rounded. Atrial P waves will look different. Using a pen or pencil, mark an "S," for SA node, above each normal looking P wave. Mark an "A," for atrial, above those P waves that look different. When you are finished, you should have an "A" marked over the P waves in beats 2, 7, and 10. The rest of the P waves should be marked with an "S."

Notice that the waveforms marked with an "S" above them occur regularly except when they are interrupted by the three atrial beats. Using the sinus beats as your guide, determine the atrial rate. The atrial rate between the regular P-P intervals is 111 beats/min. Based on the rate (i.e., faster than 100 beats/min) and an upright P wave before each QRS, we know that the underlying rhythm is a sinus tachycardia. With the use of your calipers or a piece of paper, find two sinus beats that appear next to each other, such as beats 4 and 5. Now move your calipers or paper to the right. If beat 6 occurred on time, it will line up with your calipers or paper. It is on time. Now move your calipers to the right again. The right point of your calipers shows where the next sinus beat should have occurred. You can see that beat 7 occurred earlier than expected. This is a premature beat. When you continue this process you will find that beat 10 is also early. Working backward and without adjusting your calipers, if you place the left point of your calipers on beat 1 in the rhythm strip, you will see that beat 2 is also early. So far we can identify this rhythm as a sinus tachycardia at 111 beats/min with three premature beats.

Next, measure the PR interval, QRS duration, and QT interval. The PR interval is 0.16 sec and the QRS is 0.08 sec in duration. Because it is difficult to clearly identify T waves in this rhythm strip, accurate determination of the QT interval is not possible.

Because premature beats can start from more than one area of the heart, we must identify where the premature beats came from. To do this, we must examine the premature beats more closely. Look carefully at beats 2, 7, and 10. The QRS complexes look the same as those of the underlying rhythm. This is because the impulse is conducted normally through the AV node and bundle, right and left bundle branches, and Purkinje fibers. Now look to the left of the QRS complex in each of these early beats and look at the P waves. Each P wave is positive (i.e., upright) but looks different from the P waves of the sinus beats. This is an important finding and one that tells you that the P waves came from the atria. The early beats are premature atrial complexes. A PAC is not an entire rhythm—it is a single beat; therefore you must identify the underlying rhythm and the ectopic beat(s). To complete our identification of this rhythm, we have a sinus tachycardia at 111 beats/min with three premature atrial complexes. The ECG characteristics of PACs are shown in Table 4-1.

Noncompensatory versus Compensatory Pause

[Objective 4]

A **noncompensatory** (i.e., incomplete) **pause** often follows a PAC. This represents the delay during which the SA node resets its rhythm for the next beat. A **compensatory** (i.e., complete) **pause** often follows PVCs. To find out whether or not the pause following a premature complex is compensatory or noncompensatory, measure the distance between the R-R intervals of three normal beats. Then compare that measurement to the distance between the R-R intervals of three beats, one of which includes the premature complex. The pause is *noncompensatory* if the period between the complex before and after a premature beat is less than two normal R-R intervals (Figure 4-3). The pause is *compensatory* if the period between the complex before and after a premature beat is the same as two normal R-R intervals (Figure 4-4).

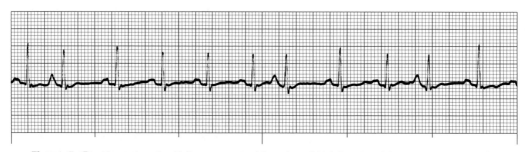

Figure 4-2   Sinus tachycardia with three premature atrial complexes (PACs). From the left, beats 2, 7, and 10 are PACs.

Table 4-1	Characteristics of Premature Atrial Complexes
Rhythm	Regular with premature beats
Rate	Usually within normal range, but depends on underlying rhythm
P waves	Premature (occurring earlier than the next expected sinus P wave), positive (upright) in lead II, one before each QRS complex, often differ in shape from sinus P waves—may be flattened, notched, pointed, biphasic, or lost in the preceding T wave
PR interval	May be normal or prolonged depending on the prematurity of the beat
QRS duration	Usually 0.11 sec or less but may be wide (aberrant) or absent, depending on the prematurity of the beat; the QRS of the premature atrial complex (PAC) is similar in shape to those of the underlying rhythm unless the PAC is abnormally conducted

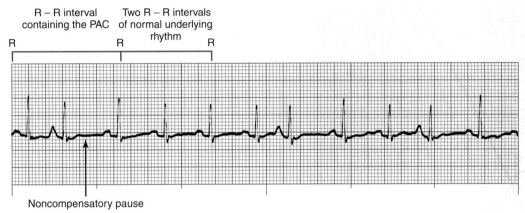

Figure 4-3   A noncompensatory pause is present if the period between the complex before and after a premature beat is less than two normal R-R intervals. PAC, premature atrial complex.

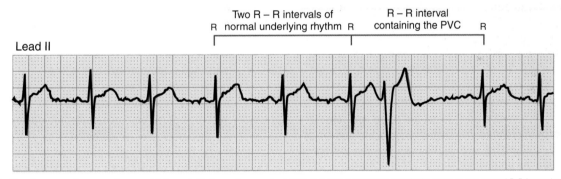

Figure 4-4   A compensatory pause is present if the period between the complex before and after a premature beat is the same as two normal R-R intervals; PVC, premature ventricular complex.

Aberrantly Conducted Premature Atrial Complexes

If a PAC occurs very early, the right bundle branch can be slow to respond to the impulse (i.e., refractory). The impulse travels down the left bundle branch with no problem. Stimulation of the left bundle branch subsequently results in stimulation of the right bundle branch. The QRS will appear wide (i.e., greater than 0.11 sec) because of this delay in ventricular depolarization. PACs associated with a wide QRS complex are called *aberrantly conducted PACs*. This indicates that conduction through the ventricles is abnormal. Figure 4-5 shows a rhythm

strip with two PACs. The first PAC (arrow) was conducted abnormally, producing a wide QRS complex. The second PAC (arrow) was conducted normally. Compare the T waves before each PAC with those of the underlying sinus bradycardia.

Nonconducted Premature Atrial Complexes

Sometimes, when a PAC occurs very early and close to the T wave of the preceding beat, only a P wave may be seen with no QRS after it, appearing as a pause (Figure 4-6). This type of PAC is called a ***nonconducted*** or ***blocked*** PAC because the

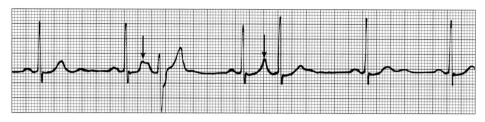

Aberrantly conducted PAC   PAC conducted normally

Figure 4-5   Premature atrial complexes (PACs) with and without abnormal conduction (aberrancy).

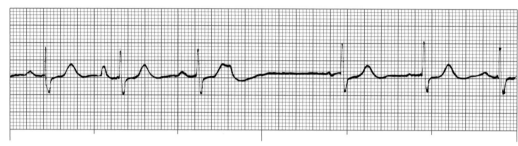

Figure 4-6   Sinus rhythm with a nonconducted (blocked) premature atrial complex (PAC). Note the distorted T wave of the third QRS complex from the left.

P wave occurred too early to be conducted. Nonconducted PACs occur because the AV junction is still refractory to stimulation and unable to conduct the impulse to the ventricles (thus no QRS complex). Look for the early P wave in the T wave of the preceding beat.

What Causes Them?

[Objective 3]

PACs may be the result of altered automaticity or reentry. PACs are very common and can occur at any age. They are very frequent in older adults. Their presence does not necessarily imply underlying cardiac disease. Possible causes of PACs include the following:

- Acute coronary syndromes
- Atrial enlargement
- Digitalis toxicity
- Electrolyte imbalance
- Emotional stress
- Heart failure
- Hyperthyroidism
- Mental and physical fatigue
- Stimulants: caffeine, tobacco, cocaine
- Sympathomimetic medications, such as epinephrine
- Valvular heart disease

What Do I Do About Them?

[Objective 3]

PACs usually do not require treatment if they are infrequent. The patient may complain of a "skipped beat" or occasional "**palpitations**" if PACs are frequent or may be unaware of their occurrence. In susceptible individuals, frequent PACs may induce episodes of AFib or PSVT. Frequent PACs are treated by correcting the underlying cause:

- Correcting electrolyte imbalances
- Reducing stress
- Reducing or eliminating stimulants
- Treating heart failure

If the patient is symptomatic, frequent PACs may be treated with beta-blockers, such as atenolol or metoprolol.

WANDERING ATRIAL PACEMAKER

How Do I Recognize It?

[Objectives 5, 6]

Multiformed atrial rhythm is an updated term for the rhythm formerly known as **wandering atrial pacemaker**. With this rhythm, the size, shape, and direction of the P waves vary, sometimes from beat to beat. The difference in the look of the P waves is a result of the gradual shifting of the dominant pacemaker among the SA node, the atria, and the AV junction (Figure 4-7). Wandering atrial pacemaker is associated with a normal or slow rate and irregular P-P, R-R, and PR intervals because of the different sites of impulse formation. The QRS duration is normally 0.11 second or less because conduction through the ventricles is usually normal. The ECG characteristics of wandering atrial pacemaker are shown in Table 4-2.

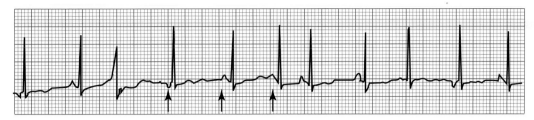

Figure 4-7   Wandering atrial pacemaker. Note the differences in the shapes of the P waves.

Table 4-2	Characteristics of Wandering Atrial Pacemaker
Rhythm	Usually irregular as the pacemaker site shifts from the SA node to ectopic atrial locations or AV junction
Rate	Usually 60 to 100 beats/min, but may be slower; if the rate is faster than 100 beats/min, the rhythm is termed *multifocal* (or *chaotic*) *atrial tachycardia*
P waves	Size, shape, and direction may change from beat to beat; may be upright, inverted, biphasic, rounded, flat, pointed, notched, or buried in the QRS complex
PR interval	Varies as the pacemaker site shifts from the SA node to ectopic atrial locations or AV junction
QRS duration	0.11 sec or less unless abnormally conducted

AV, atrioventricular; SA, sinoatrial.

ECG Pearl

At least three different P wave configurations, seen in the same lead, are required for a diagnosis of wandering atrial pacemaker or multifocal atrial tachycardia.

What Causes It?

Wandering atrial pacemaker may be observed in normal, healthy hearts (particularly in athletes) and during sleep. It may also occur with some types of underlying heart disease and with digitalis toxicity. This dysrhythmia usually produces no signs and symptoms unless it is associated with a slow rate.

What Do I Do About It?

Wandering atrial pacemaker is usually a transient rhythm that resolves on its own when the firing rate of the SA node increases and the sinus resumes pacing responsibility. If the rhythm occurs because of digitalis toxicity, the drug should be withheld.

MULTIFOCAL ATRIAL TACHYCARDIA

How Do I Recognize It?

[Objective 7]

When the wandering atrial pacemaker rhythm is associated with a ventricular rate of more than 100 beats/min, the dysrhythmia is called multifocal atrial tachycardia (MAT) or *chaotic atrial tachycardia* (Figure 4-8). In MAT, multiple ectopic sites stimulate the atria. MAT may be confused with AFib because both rhythms are irregular; however, P waves, although varying in size, shape, and direction, are clearly visible in MAT. The ECG characteristics of MAT are shown in Table 4-3.

What Causes It?

MAT is most often seen in patients with severe chronic obstructive pulmonary disease (COPD), but it is also seen in the setting of acute coronary syndromes, hypokalemia, or hypomagnesemia; and it may be a precursor of AFib.[1]

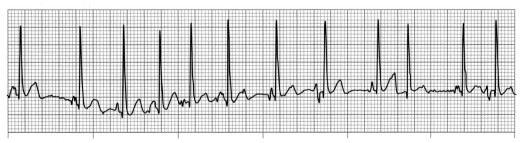

Figure 4-8   Multifocal atrial tachycardia (MAT), also known as chaotic atrial tachycardia.

Table **4-3**	Characteristics of Multifocal Atrial Tachycardia
Rhythm	Usually irregular as the pacemaker site shifts from the SA node to ectopic atrial locations or AV junction
Rate	Faster than 100 beats/min
P waves	Size, shape, and direction may change from beat to beat; may be upright, inverted, biphasic, rounded, flat, pointed, notched, or buried in the QRS complex
PR interval	Varies as the pacemaker site shifts from the SA node to ectopic atrial locations or AV junction
QRS duration	0.11 sec or less unless abnormally conducted

AV, atrioventricular; SA, sinoatrial.

What Do I Do About It?

The treatment of MAT is directed at the underlying cause. If you know the rhythm is MAT and the patient is symptomatic, it is best to consult a cardiologist before starting treatment. If the patient is stable but symptomatic and you are uncertain that the rhythm is MAT, you can try a vagal maneuver. **Vagal maneuvers** are discussed below. If vagal maneuvers are ineffective, intravenous (IV) adenosine can be tried. Remember that MAT is the result of the random and chaotic firing of multiple sites in the atria; MAT does not involve reentry through the AV node. Therefore, it is unlikely that vagal maneuvers or giving adenosine will terminate the rhythm; however, they may momentarily slow the rate enough so that you can look at the P waves and determine the specific type of tachycardia. By determining the type of tachycardia, treatment specific to that rhythm can be given.

Adenosine

- Adenosine slows the rate of the sinoatrial (SA) node, slows conduction time through the atrioventricular (AV) node, can interrupt reentry pathways that involve the AV node, and can restore sinus rhythm in supraventricular tachycardia (SVT). Reentry circuits are the underlying mechanism for many episodes of SVT. Adenosine acts at specific receptors to cause a temporary block of conduction through the AV node, interrupting these reentry circuits.
- Adenosine has an onset of action of 10 to 40 sec and duration of 1 to 2 min. Because of its short half-life (i.e., 10 seconds), and to boost delivery of the drug to its site of action in the heart, select the injection port on the intravenous (IV) tubing that is nearest the patient. Administer the drug using a two-syringe technique. Prepare one syringe with the drug, and the other with a 20-mL normal saline flush. Insert both syringes into the injection port in the IV tubing. Administer the medication IV as rapidly as possible (i.e., over a period of seconds) and *immediately* follow with the saline flush. If the patient has a central line in place, the dosages of adenosine should be reduced to avoid prolonged bradycardia or severe adverse effects.
- Adenosine may cause facial flushing because the drug causes mild dilation of blood vessels in the skin. Coughing, dyspnea, and bronchospasm may occur because it is a mild bronchoconstrictor. Adenosine should be avoided in patients with severe asthma.
- A 12-lead ECG recording is desirable when adenosine is used.

Vagal Maneuvers
[Objective 8]

Vagal maneuvers are methods that are used to stimulate baroreceptors located in the internal carotid arteries and the aortic arch. The stimulation of these receptors results in reflex stimulation of the vagus nerve and the release of acetylcholine. Acetylcholine slows conduction through the AV node, thereby resulting in the slowing of the heart rate. Although there is some overlap of the right and left vagus nerves, it is thought that the right vagus nerve has more fibers to the SA node and atrial muscle and the left vagus more fibers to the AV node and some ventricular muscle.

Examples of vagal maneuvers include the following:

- Coughing
- Squatting
- Breath-holding
- Carotid sinus massage, which is also called *carotid sinus pressure*. This procedure is performed with the patient's neck extended. Firm pressure is applied just underneath the angle of the jaw for up to 10 seconds (Figure 4-9). Carotid sinus pressure should be avoided in older adults and in patients who have a history of stroke, known carotid artery stenosis, or a carotid artery **bruit** on auscultation.[2] Simultaneous, bilateral carotid pressure should *never* be performed.
- Application of a cold stimulus to the face (e.g., a washcloth soaked in iced water, a cold pack, or crushed ice

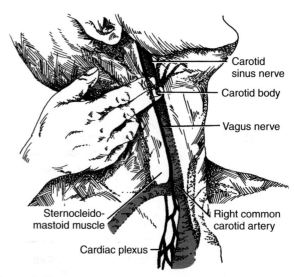

Figure 4-9   Carotid sinus massage. The carotid sinus (carotid body) is located at the bifurcation of the carotid artery at the angle of the jaw.

mixed with water in a plastic bag or glove): This is done for up to 10 seconds. This technique is often effective for infants and young children. When using this method, do not obstruct the patient's mouth or nose or apply pressure to the eyes.

- Valsalva maneuver: Instruct the patient to blow through an occluded straw or take a deep breath and bear down as if having a bowel movement for up to 10 seconds. This strains the abdominal muscles and increases intra-thoracic pressure.
- Gagging: Use a tongue depressor or a culturette swab to briefly touch the back of the throat.
- The procedure for performing carotid sinus massage is shown in Skill 4-1.

SKILL 4-1   Carotid Sinus Massage

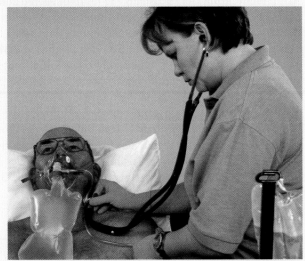

Step 1. Before performing this procedure, take appropriate standard precautions. Make sure that suction, a defibrillator, and emergency medications are available and that you have a physician's order to perform the procedure. Place the patient on oxygen, assess the patient's vital signs, establish intravenous (IV) access, and apply ECG electrodes. Explain the procedure to the patient. Gently palpate each carotid artery separately to assess pulse quality. If the pulses are markedly unequal, consult a physician before performing the procedure. Check for carotid bruits by listening to each carotid artery with a stethoscope. A bruit is a blowing or rushing sound that is created by the turbulence within the vessel. If a bruit is heard, do not perform this procedure

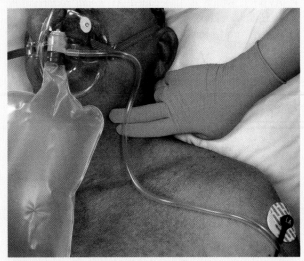

Step 2. If no bruit is heard and no contraindications are present, turn the patient's head to one side. Press "Print" or "Record" on the cardiac monitor to run a continuous ECG strip during the procedure. With two fingers, locate the carotid pulse just underneath the angle of the jaw. With firm pressure, press the carotid artery toward the cervical vertebrae. Begin an up-and-down motion, and perform this for no longer than 10 seconds. *Never* massage both carotid arteries at the same time. Visually monitor the patient and the ECG throughout the procedure. Note the onset and end of the vagal maneuver on the rhythm strip.

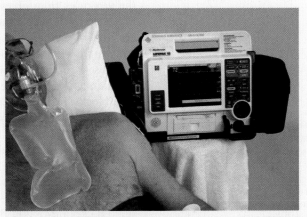

Step 3. After the procedure, reassess the patient's vital signs and the ECG rhythm.

SUPRAVENTRICULAR TACHYCARDIA

Supraventricular arrhythmias begin above the bifurcation of the bundle of His. This means that supraventricular arrhythmias include rhythms that begin in the SA node, atrial tissue, or the AV junction. The term *supraventricular tachycardia* (SVT) includes three main types of fast rhythms, which are shown in Figure 4-10.

- AT: During AT, an irritable site in the atria fires automatically at a rapid rate.
- AVNRT, which is also called *AV nodal reciprocating tachycardia*: During AVNRT, fast and slow pathways in the AV node form an electrical circuit or loop. The impulse moves in a repeating loop around the AV nodal (junctional) area.
- AVRT, which is also called *AV reciprocating tachycardia*: During AVRT, the impulse begins above the ventricles but travels by means of a pathway other than the AV node and bundle of His.

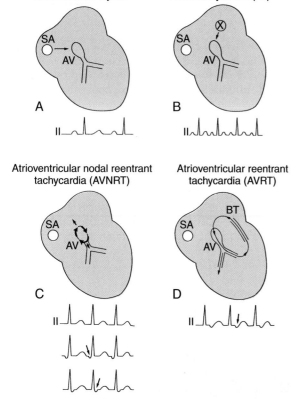

Figure 4-10   Types of supraventricular tachycardias. **A,** Normal sinus rhythm is shown here as a reference. **B,** With atrial tachycardia (AT), a focus (X) outside the sinoatrial (SA) node fires off automatically at a rapid rate. **C,** With atrioventricular (AV) nodal reentrant tachycardia (AVNRT), the cardiac stimulus originates as a wave of excitation that spins around the AV junctional area. As a result, P waves may be buried in the QRS or appear immediately before or just after the QRS complex (arrows) because of nearly simultaneous activation of the atria and ventricles. **D,** A similar type of reentrant (circus movement) mechanism in Wolff-Parkinson-White syndrome. This mechanism is referred to as atrioventricular reentrant tachycardia (AVRT). Note the P wave in lead II somewhat after the QRS complex. BT, bypass tract.

ECG Pearl —

It is important to look closely for P waves in all dysrhythmias, but is very important when trying to figure out the origin of a tachycardia. If P waves are not visible in one lead, try looking in another before finalizing your rhythm diagnosis.

Atrial Tachycardia

How Do I Recognize It?
[Objectives 9, 10]

Atrial tachycardia (AT) is usually the result of altered automaticity or triggered activity. An irritable site in the atria fires at a rate of 150 to 250 times per minute (Figure 4-11). This rapid atrial rate overrides the SA node and becomes the pacemaker. Conduction of the atrial impulse to the ventricles is often 1:1. This means that every atrial impulse is conducted through the AV node to the ventricles. This results in a P wave preceding each QRS complex. Although the P waves appear upright, they tend to look different from those seen when the impulse is initiated from the SA node. Because conducted impulses travel through the ventricles in the usual manner, the QRS complexes appear normal. The ECG characteristics of AT are shown in Table 4-4.

ECG Pearl —

Atrial tachycardia is often precipitated by a premature atrial complex (PAC). When three or more PACs occur in a row at a rate of more than 100 beats/min, atrial tachycardia is present.

The term *paroxysmal* is used to describe a rhythm that starts or ends suddenly. AT that starts or ends suddenly is called **paroxysmal supraventricular tachycardia (PSVT)**, once called **paroxysmal atrial tachycardia (PAT)** (Figure 4-12). PSVT may last for minutes, hours, or days. If the onset or end of PSVT is not observed on the ECG, the dysrhythmia is simply called *SVT*.

With very rapid atrial rates, the AV node begins to filter some of the impulses coming to it. By doing so, it protects the ventricles from excessively rapid rates. When the AV node selectively filters conduction of some of these impulses, the rhythm is called *paroxysmal supraventricular (or atrial) tachycardia with block*. PSVT with block is often associated with disease of the AV node, medications that slow conduction through the AV node, or digitalis toxicity. When PSVT with block exists, more than one P wave is present before each QRS. When the AV node blocks every other atrial impulse from traveling to the ventricles the rhythm is called *PSVT with 2:1 block* (Figure 4-13).

There is more than one type of AT. MAT has already been discussed.

- AT that begins in a small area (focus) within the heart is called *focal AT*. There are several types of focal AT. **Focal atrial tachycardia** may be caused by an automatic, triggered, or reentrant mechanism. A patient

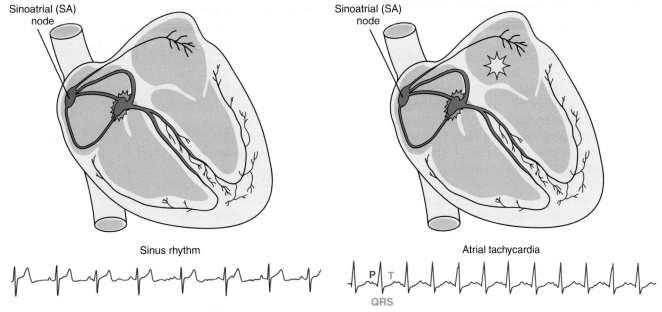

Figure 4-11   Atrial tachycardia. AV, atrioventricular; SA, sinoatrial.

Table 4-4	Characteristics of Atrial Tachycardia
Rhythm	Regular
Rate	150 to 250 beats/min
P waves	One P wave precedes each QRS complex in lead II; these P waves differ in shape from sinus P waves; an isoelectric baseline is usually present between P waves; if the atrial rhythm originates in the low portion of the atrium, P waves will be negative in lead II; with rapid rates, it may be difficult to distinguish P waves from T waves.
PR interval	May be shorter or longer than normal; may be difficult to measure because P waves may be hidden in the T waves of preceding beats
QRS duration	0.11 sec or less unless abnormally conducted

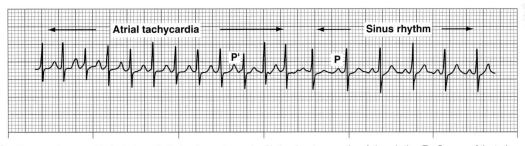

Figure 4-12   Paroxysmal supraventricular tachycardia that ends spontaneously with the abrupt resumption of sinus rhythm. The P waves of the tachycardia (rate: about 150 beats/min) are superimposed on the preceding T waves.

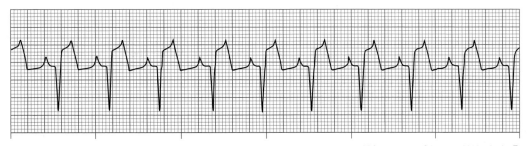

Figure 4-13   Paroxysmal supraventricular tachycardia with 2:1 block. P waves are clearly seen before the QRS complexes. Others are hidden in the T waves. Atrial rate is 180 beats/min. Ventricular rate is 90 beats/min.

with focal AT often presents with paroxysmal AT. The atrial rate is usually between 100 and 250 beats/min; it rarely reaches 300 beats/min.

- *Automatic* AT, which is also called *ectopic AT*, is another type of AT in which a small cluster of cells with altered automaticity fire. The impulse is spread from the cluster of cells to the surrounding atrium and then to the ventricles via the AV node. This type of AT often involves a "warm-up period." This means that there is a progressive shortening of the P-P interval for the first few beats of the arrhythmia. Automatic AT gradually slows down as it ends, which has been called the "cool-down period." The atrial rate is usually between 100 and 250 beats/min. P waves look different from sinus P waves, but they are still related to the QRS complex. Vagal maneuvers do not usually stop the tachycardia, but they may slow the ventricular rate.

CLINICAL CORRELATION

Although correct use of the term *paroxysmal* requires observing the onset or cessation of the dysrhythmia and identification of the underlying rhythm that preceded it, some practitioners use the term to describe the sudden onset or cessation of a patient's *symptoms* associated with the dysrhythmia.

What Causes It?

AT can occur in persons with normal hearts or in patients with organic heart disease. AT that is associated with automaticity or reentry is often related to an acute event such as the following:

- Acute illness with excessive catecholamine release
- Digitalis toxicity
- Electrolyte imbalance
- Heart disease including coronary artery disease, valvular disease, cardiomyopathies, and congenital heart disease
- Infection
- Pulmonary embolism
- Stimulant use (e.g., caffeine, albuterol, theophylline, cocaine)

Did You Know?

Some supraventricular tachycardias (SVTs) need the atrioventricular (AV) node to sustain the rhythm and some do not. For example, atrioventricular nodal reentrant tachycardia (AVNRT) and atrioventricular reentrant tachycardia (AVRT) require the AV node as part of the reentry circuit to continue the tachycardia. Other SVTs use the AV node only to conduct the rhythm to the ventricles. For example, atrial tachycardia, atrial flutter, and atrial fibrillation arise from a site (or sites) within the atria; they do not need the AV node to sustain the rhythm.

What Do I Do About It?
[Objective 9]

Assessment findings and symptoms associated with AT vary widely and may include the following:

- Acute changes in mental status
- Asymptomatic
- Dizziness or lightheadedness
- Dyspnea
- Fatigue
- Fluttering sensation in the chest
- Hypotension
- Ischemic chest discomfort
- Palpitations
- Signs of shock
- Syncope or near-syncope

When taking the patient's history, try to find out how often the episodes occur, how long they last, and possible triggers. If the patient complains of palpitations, find out if they are regular or irregular. Palpitations that occur regularly with a sudden onset and end usually are the result of AVNRT or AVRT. Irregular palpitations may be the result of premature complexes, AFib, or MAT. Tachycardias may cause syncope because the rapid ventricular rate decreases cardiac output and blood flow to the brain. Syncope is most likely to occur just after the onset of a rapid AT or when the rhythm stops abruptly. Predisposed persons may experience angina or heart failure. ▶

CLINICAL CORRELATION

The signs and symptoms experienced by a patient with a tachycardia depend on the ventricular rate, how long the tachycardia lasts, the patient's general health, and the presence of underlying heart disease. The faster the heart rate, the more likely the patient is to have signs and symptoms resulting from the rapid rate.

If episodes of AT are short, the patient may be asymptomatic. A rhythm that lasts from three beats up to 30 seconds is a *nonsustained rhythm*. A *sustained rhythm* is one that lasts more than 30 seconds. If AT is sustained and the patient is symptomatic as a result of the rapid rate, treatment should include applying a pulse oximeter and administering oxygen (if indicated), obtaining the patient's vital signs, and establishing IV access. A 12-lead ECG should be obtained. If the patient is not hypotensive, vagal maneuvers may be tried. Although AT will rarely stop with vagal maneuvers, they are used to try to stop the rhythm or slow conduction through the AV node. If vagal maneuvers fail, antiarrhythmic medications should be tried. Adenosine is the drug of choice, except for patients with severe asthma. If needed, calcium channel blockers or beta-blockers may be used to slow the ventricular rate. If AT is sustained and causing persistent signs of hemodynamic compromise, synchronized cardioversion should be performed. Synchronized cardioversion seldom stops automatic ATs, but may be successful for ATs that are the result of reentry or triggered automaticity. Synchronized cardioversion is discussed in the next section of this chapter.

PSVT with AV block often occurs because of excess digitalis. In these cases, the patient's ventricular rate is not excessively fast. The drug should be withheld and serum digoxin levels obtained. Long-term medication therapy may include the use of calcium channel blockers or beta-blockers.

When AT is difficult to control and causes serious signs and symptoms, radiofrequency catheter ablation may be necessary. When catheter ablation is performed, electrophysiologic studies are done to locate the abnormal pathways and reentry circuits in the heart. Once localized, a special ablation catheter is placed at the site of the abnormal pathway. Low-energy, high-frequency current is delivered through this catheter. With each burst of energy from the catheter, an area of tissue is destroyed (ablated). The energy is applied in various areas until the unwanted pathway is no longer functional and the circuit is broken. ATs occasionally can recur at a different site following a successful ablation.

Synchronized Cardioversion
[Objective 11]
Synchronized cardioversion is the delivery of a shock to the heart by means of a defibrillator to terminate a rapid dysrhythmia. A synchronized shock means the shock is timed to avoid the relative refractory period of the cardiac cycle. On the ECG, this period occurs during the peak of the T wave to approximately the end of the T wave. When the "sync" control is pressed, the machine searches for the highest (i.e., the R wave deflection) or deepest (i.e., the QS deflection) part of the QRS complex. When a QRS complex is detected, the monitor places a "flag" or "sync marker" on that complex that may appear as an oval, square, line, or highlighted triangle on the ECG display, depending on the machine used. When the shock controls are pressed while the defibrillator is charged in "sync" mode, the machine will discharge energy only if both discharge buttons are pushed and the monitor tells the defibrillator that a QRS complex has been detected.

Indications
Because the machine must be able to detect a QRS complex in order to "sync," synchronized cardioversion is used to treat rhythms that have a clearly identifiable QRS complex and a rapid ventricular rate in patients who show signs of hemodynamic compromise. Examples of rhythms treated with cardioversion include narrow-QRS tachycardias, AFib, atrial flutter, and monomorphic ventricular tachycardia.

Procedure
Before performing synchronized cardioversion, take appropriate standard precautions and verify that the procedure is indicated (Figure 4-14). Identify the rhythm on the cardiac monitor. Print an ECG strip to document the patient's rhythm. Assess the patient for serious signs and symptoms from the

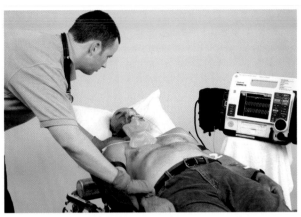
Figure 4-14 Before performing synchronized cardioversion, take appropriate standard precautions and verify that the procedure is indicated.

tachycardia. Make sure suction and emergency medications are available. Give supplemental oxygen, if indicated, and start an IV. If the patient is awake, explain the procedure.

Remove clothing from the patient's upper body (Figure 4-15). With gloves, remove nitroglycerin paste or transdermal patches from the patient's chest if present and quickly wipe away any medication residue. If present, remove excessive hair from the sites where the paddles or electrodes will be placed. Clip or shave hair if necessary and if time permits. Avoid cutting the skin. Do not apply alcohol, tincture of benzoin, or antiperspirant to the skin.

Turn the power on to the defibrillator. If using standard paddles, you must use defibrillation gel or defibrillation gel pads between the paddle electrode surface and the patient's skin. Place pregelled defibrillation pads on the patient's chest at this time. If using combination pads, place them in proper position on the patient's bare chest.

Press the "sync" control on the defibrillator (Figure 4-16). Select a lead with an optimum QRS complex amplitude (positive or negative) and no artifact. Make sure the machine is marking or flagging each QRS complex and no artifact is

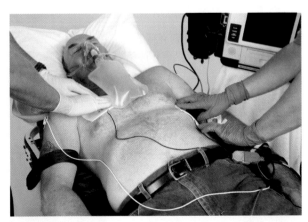
Figure 4-15 Remove clothing, transdermal patches, and medication residue from the patient's upper body. Place pregelled defibrillation pads (if using handheld paddles) on the patient's chest at this time. If using multipurpose adhesive electrodes, place them in proper position on the patient's bare chest according to the defibrillator manufacturer's instructions.

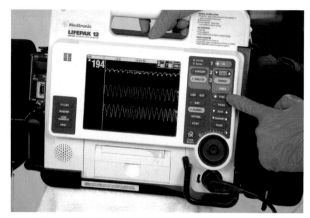

Figure 4-16   Press the "sync" control on the defibrillator.

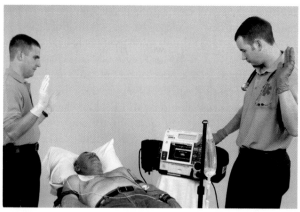

Figure 4-18   Charge the defibrillator, call "Clear!" and look around you.

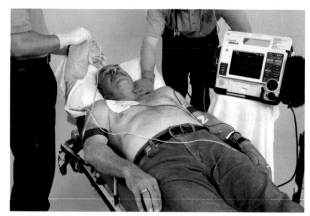

Figure 4-19   Reassess the rhythm and the patient.

present. The sense marker should appear near the middle of each QRS complex. If sense markers do not appear or are seen in the wrong place (such as on a T wave), adjust the ECG size or select another lead.

If the patient is awake and time permits, administer sedation per local protocol or physician orders unless contraindicated. Make sure the machine is in "sync" mode and then select the appropriate energy level on the defibrillator (Figure 4-17).

Charge the defibrillator and recheck the ECG rhythm. If using standard paddles, place the paddles on the pregelled defibrillator pads on the patient's chest and apply firm pressure. If the rhythm is unchanged, call "Clear!" and look around you (Figure 4-18). Make sure everyone is clear of the patient, bed, and any equipment connected to the patient. Make sure oxygen is not flowing over the patient's chest. If the area is clear, press and hold the shock control(s) until the shock is delivered. A slight delay may occur while the machine detects the next QRS complex. Release the shock control after the shock has been delivered. Reassess the rhythm and the patient (Figure 4-19).

Atrioventricular Nodal Reentrant Tachycardia

[Objectives 10, 12]

AVNRT is the most common type of SVT. It is caused by re-entry in the area of the AV node. Although AVNRT begins in the area of the AV node and could be discussed in Chapter 5 with junctional rhythms, it is discussed here because it was once thought to be a type of PAT.

In the normal AV node, there is only one pathway through which an electrical impulse is conducted from the SA node to the ventricles. Patients with AVNRT have two conduction pathways within the AV node that conduct impulses at different speeds and that recover at different rates. The fast pathway conducts impulses rapidly but has a long refractory period (i.e., slow recovery time). The slow pathway conducts impulses slowly but has a short refractory period (i.e., fast recovery time) (Figure 4-20). Under the right conditions, the fast and slow pathways can form an electrical circuit or loop. As one side of the loop is recovering, the other is firing.

AVNRT is usually caused by a PAC that is spread by the electrical circuit. This allows the impulse to spin around in a circle indefinitely, and to reenter the normal electrical

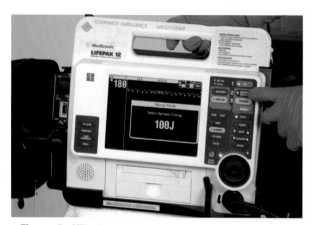

Figure 4-17   Select the appropriate energy level on the defibrillator.

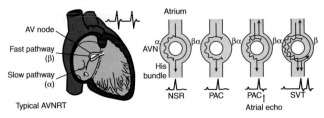

Figure 4-20   Schematic for supraventricular tachycardia (SVT) caused by atrioventricular (AV) nodal reentry. AVN, atrioventricular node; AVNRT, atrioventricular nodal reentrant tachycardia; NSR, normal sinus rhythm; PAC, premature atrial complex.

pathway with each pass around the circuit. The result is a very rapid and regular ventricular rhythm that ranges from 150 to 250 beats/min.

Look at the example of AVNRT in Figure 4-21. You can see narrow-QRS complexes that occur at a regular rate of 168 beats/min. P waves are not clearly seen. Because AVNRT begins in the area of the AV node, the impulse spreads to the atria and ventricles at almost the same time. This results in P waves that are usually hidden in the QRS complex. If the ventricles are stimulated first and then the atria, a negative (inverted) P wave will appear after the QRS in leads II, III, and aVF. When the atria are depolarized after the ventricles, the P wave typically distorts the end of the QRS complex. Since P waves are not seen before the QRS complex, the PR interval is not measurable. In our example of AVNRT, you can see ST-segment depression. ST-segment changes

(usually depression) are common in patients with SVTs. In most patients, these ST-segment changes are thought to be the result of repolarization changes. However, in older adults and those with a high likelihood of ischemic heart disease, ST-segment changes may represent ECG changes consistent with an acute coronary syndrome. The patient should be watched closely. Appropriate laboratory tests and a 12-lead ECG should be obtained to rule out infarction as needed. The ECG characteristics of AVNRT are summarized in Table 4-5. To review an animation on this topic, go to the Evolve site.

What Causes It?

AVNRT can occur at any age. Whether a person is born with a tendency to have AVNRT or whether it develops later in life for an unknown reason has not been clearly determined. AVNRT is common in individuals with no structural heart disease but can be triggered by hypoxia, stress, anxiety, caffeine, smoking, sleep deprivation, and many medications. In adults, AVNRT frequently presents in the third or fourth decade of life, occurring more often in women than in men. AVNRT also occurs in persons with COPD, coronary artery disease, valvular heart disease, heart failure, and digitalis toxicity. AVNRT can cause angina or myocardial infarction in patients with coronary artery disease.

What Do I Do About It?

Because AVNRT may be short-lived or sustained, treatment depends on the duration of the tachycardia and severity of the patient's signs and symptoms. Assessment findings and

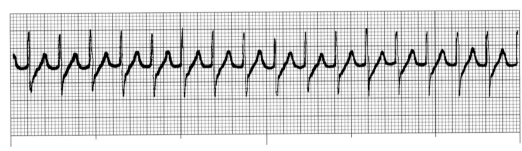

Figure 4-21   Atrioventricular nodal reentrant tachycardia (AVNRT).

Table 4-5	Characteristics of Atrioventricular Nodal Reentrant Tachycardia (AVNRT)
Rhythm	Ventricular rhythm is usually very regular
Rate	150 to 250 beats/min; typically 180 to 200 beats/min in adults
P waves	P waves are often hidden in the QRS complex; if the ventricles are stimulated first and then the atria, a negative (inverted) P wave will appear after the QRS in leads II, III, and aVF; when the atria are depolarized after the ventricles, the P wave typically distorts the end of the QRS complex.
PR interval	P waves are not seen before the QRS complex; therefore, the PR interval is not measurable
QRS duration	0.11 sec or less unless abnormally conducted

symptoms that may be associated with rapid ventricular rates may include the following:

- Chest pain or pressure
- Dizziness
- Dyspnea
- Heart failure
- Lightheadedness
- Nausea
- Nervousness, anxiety
- Palpitations (common)
- Signs of shock
- Syncope
- Weakness

If the patient is stable but symptomatic and the symptoms are the result of the rapid heart rate, apply a pulse oximeter and administer supplemental oxygen, if indicated. Obtain the patient's vital signs, establish IV access, and obtain a 12-lead ECG. While continuously monitoring the patient's ECG, attempt a vagal maneuver if there are no contraindications. AVNRT is usually responsive to vagal maneuvers. If vagal maneuvers do not slow the rate or cause conversion of the tachycardia to a sinus rhythm, the first antiarrhythmic given is adenosine.

An unstable patient is one who has signs and symptoms of hemodynamic compromise. Examples of these signs and symptoms include acute changes in mental status, chest pain or discomfort, hypotension, shortness of breath, pulmonary congestion, heart failure, acute myocardial infarction (MI), and signs of shock. If the patient is unstable, treatment should include application of a pulse oximeter and administration of supplemental oxygen (if indicated), IV access, and sedation (if the patient is awake and time permits), followed by synchronized cardioversion. To review animations on these topics, go to the Evolve site.

Recurrent AVNRT may require treatment with a long-acting calcium channel blocker or beta-blocker. Antiarrhythmics such as amiodarone may also be used. Recurrent episodes vary in frequency, duration, and severity from several times a day to every 2 to 3 years. Patients who are resistant to drug therapy or who do not wish to remain on lifelong medications for the dysrhythmia are candidates for radiofrequency catheter ablation. Catheter ablation has become the treatment of choice in the management of patients with symptomatic recurrent episodes of AVNRT. It is successful in permanently interrupting the circuit and curing the dysrhythmia in most cases.

Atrioventricular Reentrant Tachycardia

[Objective 13]

The next most common type of SVT is AVRT. Remember that the AV node is normally the only electrical connection between the atria and the ventricles. AVRT involves a pathway of impulse conduction outside the AV node and the bundle of His. The term **preexcitation** is used to describe rhythms that originate from above the ventricles but in which the impulse travels via a pathway other than the AV node and the AV bundle. As a result, the supraventricular impulse excites the ventricles earlier than would be expected if the impulse traveled by way of the normal conduction system.

During fetal development, strands of myocardial tissue form connections between the atria and the ventricles, outside of the normal conduction system. These strands normally become nonfunctional shortly after birth; however, in patients with preexcitation syndrome, these connections persist as congenital malformations of working myocardial tissue. Because these connections bypass part or all of the normal conduction system, they are called **accessory pathways** (Figure 4-22). Some people have more than one accessory pathway. The term **bypass tract** is used when one end of an accessory pathway is attached to normal conductive tissue.

Did You Know? _____

The electrophysiologic properties of accessory pathways vary among individuals and appear to be affected by age, autonomic stage, anatomic location, and the effects of medications.[3]

Unlike the AV node, an accessory pathway does not have the ability to slow or reduce the number of atrial impulses transmitted to the ventricles; therefore, patients with preexcitation syndromes are prone to tachydysrhythmias, including AVRT and AFib. The number of atrial impulses reaching the ventricles may approach 300 to 350 beats/min, which significantly increases the risk of development of ventricular fibrillation. The most common type of pre-excitation syndrome is called **Wolff-Parkinson-White (WPW) syndrome**. AFib has been noted to occur in 11.5% to 39% of patients with WPW.[3]

How Do I Recognize It?

The ECG characteristics of WPW described here are usually seen when the patient is *not* having a tachycardia. WPW syndrome usually goes undetected until it manifests in a patient as a tachycardia.

When WPW is associated with a sinus rhythm, the P wave looks normal. Remember that the AV node normally delays the impulse it receives from the SA node. The delay in conduction allows the atria to empty blood into the ventricles before the next ventricular contraction begins. In WPW, the PR interval is short (less than 0.12 sec) because the impulse travels very quickly across the accessory pathway, bypassing the normal delay in the AV node (Figure 4-23).

As the impulse crosses the insertion point of the accessory pathway in the ventricular muscle, that part of the ventricle is stimulated earlier (preexcited) than if the impulse had followed the normal conduction pathway through the bundle of His and Purkinje fibers. On the ECG, preexcitation of the ventricles can be seen as a **delta wave** in some leads. A delta wave is an initial slurred deflection at the beginning of the QRS complex that may be positive or negative and reflects the abnormal depolarization of the ventricles through the accessory pathway. (Figure 4-24).

ECG Pearl ⏦

Recognizing Wolff-Parkinson-White Syndrome
- Delta wave
- Short PR interval
- Widening of the QRS complex

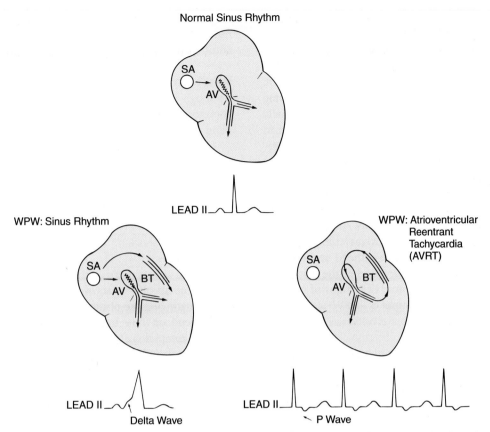

Figure 4-22   Conduction during sinus rhythm in the normal heart (top) spreads from the sinoatrial (SA) node to the atrioventricular (AV) node and then down the bundle branches. The jagged line indicates physiologic slowing of conduction in the AV node. With Wolff-Parkinson-White (WPW) syndrome (bottom left), an abnormal accessory conduction pathway called a *bypass tract* (BT) connects the atria and ventricles. With WPW, during sinus rhythm, the electrical impulse is conducted quickly down the BT, preexciting the ventricles before the impulse arrives via the AV node. Consequently, the PR interval is short and the QRS complex is wide, with slurring at its onset (delta wave). WPW predisposes patients to develop an atrioventricular reentrant tachycardia (AVRT) (bottom right) in which a premature atrial beat may spread down the normal pathway to the ventricles, travel back up the BT, and recirculate down the AV node again. This reentrant loop can repeat itself over and over, resulting in a tachycardia. Notice the normal QRS complex and often negative P wave in lead II during this type of BT tachycardia.

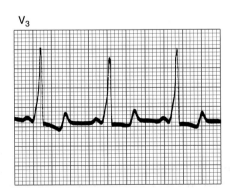

Figure 4-23   Lead V_3. Typical Wolff-Parkinson-White (WPW) syndrome pattern showing the short PR interval, delta wave, wide QRS complex, and secondary ST-segment and T-wave changes.

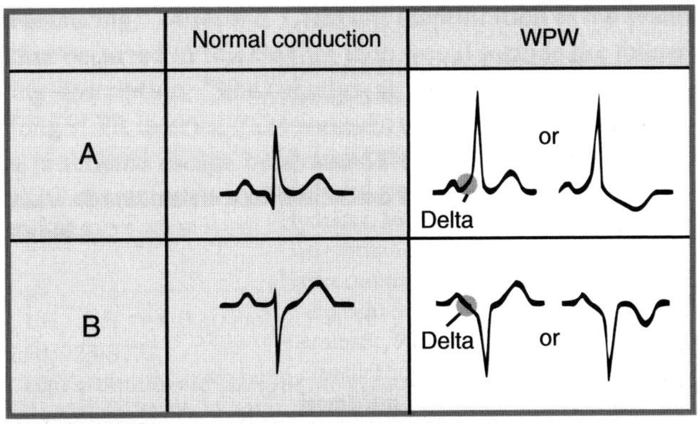

	Normal conduction	WPW
A		Delta ... or
B		Delta ... or

Figure 4-24   Characteristic findings in Wolff-Parkinson-White (WPW) syndrome (short PR interval, QRS widening, and delta wave) compared with normal conduction. **A,** The usual appearance of WPW in leads where the QRS complex is mainly upright. **B,** The usual appearance of WPW when the QRS is predominantly negative. Negative delta waves may simulate pathologic Q waves—mimicking myocardial infarction.

Normally, conduction through the Purkinje fibers is very fast. In WPW, the spread of the impulse is slow because it must spread from working cell to working cell in the ventricular muscle. This is because the accessory pathway bypasses the specialized cells of the heart's conduction system. Because the impulse spreads slowly through the working cells, the delay in conduction results in a QRS that is usually more than 0.12 sec in duration. The QRS complex seen in WPW is actually a combination of the impulse that preexcites the ventricles through the accessory pathway and the impulse that follows the normal conduction pathway through the AV node. As a result, the end (i.e., terminal) portion of the QRS usually looks normal. However, because the ventricles are activated abnormally, they repolarize abnormally. This is seen on the ECG as changes in the ST segment and T wave. The direction of the ST segment and T wave are usually opposite the direction of the delta wave and QRS complex, which can mimic ECG signs of myocardial ischemia or injury. An example of WPW is shown in Figure 4-25. The ECG characteristics of WPW are summarized in Table 4-6.

What Causes It?

WPW syndrome is more common among men than among women, and 60% to 70% of people with WPW syndrome have no associated heart disease. WPW syndrome is one of the most common causes of tachydysrhythmias in infants and children. Although the accessory pathway in WPW syndrome is believed to be congenital in origin, symptoms associated with preexcitation often do not appear until the patient is a teenager or during young adulthood.

What Do I Do About It?

Although some people with AVRT never have symptoms, common signs and symptoms associated with AVRT and a rapid ventricular rate include the following:
- Anxiety
- Chest discomfort
- Dizziness
- Lightheadedness
- Palpitations (common)
- Shortness of breath during exercise
- Signs of shock
- Weakness

If a delta wave is noted on the ECG but the patient is asymptomatic, no specific treatment is required.[1] If the patient is symptomatic because of the rapid ventricular rate, treatment will depend on how unstable the patient is, the width of the QRS complex (i.e., wide or narrow), and the regularity of the ventricular rhythm.[4] Consultation with a cardiologist is recommended when caring for a patient with AVRT. Medications such as adenosine, digoxin, diltiazem, and verapamil should be avoided. These medications are contraindicated because they slow or block conduction across the AV node, but they may speed up conduction through the accessory pathway, thereby resulting in a further *increase* in the ventricular rate. Although the potential for beta-blockers to enhance

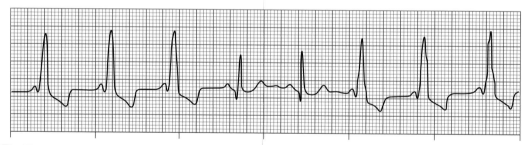

Figure 4-25 This rhythm strip shows an example of intermittent preexcitation. The first three beats show preexcitation. This is followed by abrupt normalization of the QRS complex in the next two beats. The preexcitation pattern returns for the final three beats.

Table 4-6	Characteristics of Wolff-Parkinson-White Syndrome
Rhythm	Regular, unless associated with atrial fibrillation
Rate	Usually 60 to 100 beats/min, if the underlying rhythm is sinus in origin
P waves	Normal and positive in lead II unless Wolff-Parkinson White (WPW) syndrome is associated with atrial fibrillation
PR interval	If P waves are observed, 0.12 sec or less, because the impulse travels very quickly across the accessory pathway, bypassing the normal delay in the AV node
QRS duration	Usually more than 0.12 sec; slurred upstroke of the QRS complex (delta wave) may be seen in one or more leads.

AV, atrioventricular.

conduction across an accessory pathway is controversial, caution should be exercised in the use of these drugs in patients with AFib associated with preexcitation.[5] If the patient is unstable, preparations should be made for synchronized cardioversion.

ATRIAL FLUTTER

[Objective 14]

Atrial flutter is an ectopic atrial rhythm in which an irritable site within the atria fires regularly at a very rapid rate (Figure 4-26).

How Do I Recognize It?

Atrial flutter has been classified into two types.

- Type I atrial flutter, which is also called *typical atrial flutter*, is caused by reentry. In this type of atrial flutter, an impulse circles around a large area of tissue, such as the entire right atrium. The atrial rate ranges from 250 to 350 beats/min.
- Type II atrial flutter is also called *atypical* or *very rapid atrial flutter*. The precise mechanism of type II atrial flutter has not been defined. Patients with this type of atrial flutter often develop AFib. In type II atrial flutter, the atrial rate ranges from 350 to 450 beats/min.

With atrial flutter, an irritable focus within the atrium typically depolarizes at a rate of 300 beats/min. If each impulse were transmitted to the ventricles, the ventricular rate would equal 300 beats/min. The healthy AV node protects the ventricles from these extremely fast atrial rates. Normally, the AV node cannot conduct faster than about 180 impulses/min. Thus, at an atrial rate of 300 beats/min, every other impulse arrives at the AV node while it is still refractory. The resulting ventricular response of 150 beats/min is called *2:1 conduction*. (The ratio of the atrial rate [300 beats/min] to the ventricular rate [150 beats/min] is 2 to 1.)

Atrial flutter with an atrial rate of 300 beats/min and a ventricular rate of 100 beats/min results in 3:1 conduction; 75 beats/min results in 4:1 conduction; 50 beats/min results in 6:1 conduction; and so on (Figure 4-27). Although conduction ratios in atrial flutter are often even (i.e., 2:1, 4:1, 6:1), variable conduction can also occur, which produces an irregular ventricular rhythm. In individuals with an accessory pathway, atrial flutter may be associated with 1:1 conduction because the AV node is bypassed, producing extremely rapid ventricular rates.

During episodes of atrial flutter, atrial waveforms are produced that resemble the teeth of a saw, or a picket fence; these are called *flutter waves* or *F waves*. Flutter waves are best observed in leads II, III, aVF, and V₁. Because P waves are not observed in atrial flutter, the PR interval is not measurable. The QRS complex is usually 0.11 sec or less because atrial flutter is a supraventricular rhythm, and the impulse is conducted normally through the AV junction and Purkinje fibers. However, if flutter waves are buried in the QRS complex or if an intraventricular conduction delay exists, the QRS will appear wide

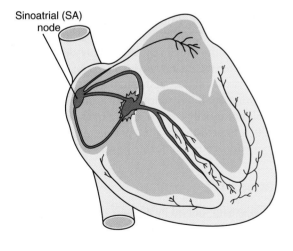

Sinus rhythm

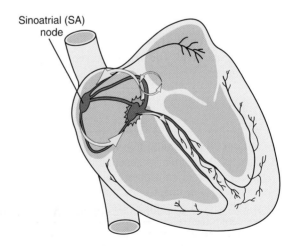

Atrial flutter

Figure 4-26   Atrial flutter. F, flutter wave.

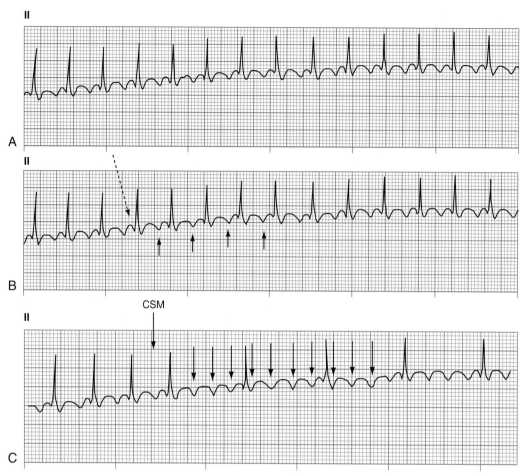

Figure 4-27 Atrial flutter. **A,** This rhythm strip shows a narrow-QRS tachycardia with a ventricular rate just under 150 beats/min. **B,** The same rhythm shown in **A** with arrows added indicating possible atrial activity. **C,** When carotid sinus massage (CSM) is performed, the rate of conduction through the atrioventricular (AV) node slows, revealing atrial flutter.

(i.e., greater than 0.11 sec). If the AV node blocks the impulses coming to it at a regular rate, the resulting ventricular rhythm will be regular. If the AV node blocks the impulses at an irregular rate, the resulting ventricular rhythm will be irregular.

ECG Pearl

Atrial flutter or atrial fibrillation (AFib) that has a ventricular rate of more than 100 beats/min is described as *uncontrolled*. The ventricular rate is considered rapid when it is 150 beats/min or more. New-onset atrial flutter or AFib is often associated with a rapid ventricular rate. Atrial flutter or AFib with a rapid ventricular response is commonly called *Aflutter with RVR* or *AFib with RVR*.

Atrial flutter or AFib that has a ventricular rate of less than 100 beats/min, is described as *controlled*. A controlled ventricular rate may be the result of a healthy atrioventricular (AV) node protecting the ventricles from very fast atrial impulses or of drugs used to control (i.e., block) conduction through the AV node, thereby decreasing the number of impulses that reach the ventricles.

When atrial flutter is present with 2:1 conduction, it may be difficult to tell the difference between atrial flutter and sinus tachycardia, AT, AVNRT, AVRT, or SVT. Vagal maneuvers may help to identify the rhythm by temporarily slowing AV conduction and revealing the underlying flutter waves. When vagal maneuvers are used in atrial flutter, the response is usually sudden slowing and then a return to the former rate. Vagal maneuvers will not usually convert atrial flutter because the reentry circuit is located in the atria, not the AV node. The ECG characteristics of atrial flutter are shown in Table 4-7.

What Causes It?

Atrial flutter is usually caused by a reentry circuit in which an impulse circles around a large area of tissue, such as the entire right atrium. It is usually a paroxysmal rhythm that is precipitated by a PAC. It may last for seconds to hours and occasionally persists for 24 hours or longer. Chronic atrial flutter is unusual. This is because the rhythm usually converts to sinus rhythm or AFib, either on its own or with treatment. Conditions associated with atrial flutter are shown in the Clinical Correlation box below.

Table 4-7	Characteristics of Atrial Flutter
Rhythm	Atrial regular; ventricular regular or irregular depending on AV conduction and blockade
Rate	With type I atrial flutter, the atrial rate ranges from 250 to 350 beats/min; with type II atrial flutter, the atrial rate ranges from 350 to 450 beats/min; the ventricular rate varies and is determined by AV blockade; the ventricular rate will usually not exceed 180 beats/min as a result of the intrinsic conduction rate of the AV junction
P waves	No identifiable P waves; saw-toothed "flutter" waves are present
PR interval	Not measurable
QRS duration	0.11 sec or less but may be widened if flutter waves are buried in the QRS complex or if abnormally conducted

AV, atrioventricular.

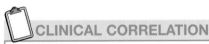

CLINICAL CORRELATION

Conditions Associated with Atrial Flutter
- Cardiac surgery
- Cardiomyopathy
- Chronic lung disease
- Complication of myocardial infarction
- Digitalis or quinidine toxicity
- Hyperthyroidism
- Ischemic heart disease
- Mitral or tricuspid valve stenosis or regurgitation
- Pericarditis or myocarditis
- Pulmonary embolism

What Do I Do About It?

Patients with atrial flutter commonly present with complaints of palpitations, difficulty breathing, fatigue, or chest discomfort. The severity of signs and symptoms associated with atrial flutter vary, depending on the ventricular rate, how long the rhythm has been present, and the patient's cardiovascular status. The faster the ventricular rate, the more likely the patient is to be symptomatic with this rhythm.

It is best to consult a cardiologist when considering treatment options. If atrial flutter is associated with a rapid ventricular rate and the patient is stable but symptomatic, treatment is usually aimed at controlling the ventricular rate with medications such as diltiazem or beta-blockers. Beta-blockers should generally be avoided in the presence of severe underlying pulmonary disease or heart failure.

Synchronized cardioversion should be considered for any patient with atrial flutter who has serious signs and symptoms because of the rapid ventricular rate (e.g., hypotension, signs of shock, or heart failure). If synchronized cardioversion is performed, atrial flutter can be successfully converted to a sinus rhythm with the use of low energy levels.

ATRIAL FIBRILLATION

[Objective 15]

AFib occurs because of altered automaticity in one or several rapidly firing sites in the atria or reentry involving one or more circuits in the atria (Figure 4-28). Irritable sites in the atria fire at a rate of 400 to 600 times per minute. These rapid impulses cause the muscles of the atria to quiver (i.e., fibrillate), thereby resulting in ineffectual atrial contraction, decreased stroke volume, a subsequent decrease in cardiac output, and a loss of atrial kick. AFib may occur alone or in association with other dysrhythmias, most commonly with atrial flutter or AT.[5] To review an animation on this topic, go to the Evolve site.

Did You Know?

Atrial fibrillation (AFib) is the most common sustained dysrhythmia in adults.[6] Although AFib occurs approximately 1.5 times more often in men then in women, the overall number of female patients with AFib exceeds the number of men with this condition because of greater longevity in women.[7]

How Do I Recognize It?

In AFib, the AV node attempts to protect the ventricles from the hundreds of impulses bombarding it per minute. It does this by blocking many of the impulses generated by the irritable sites in the atria. The ventricular rate and rhythm are determined by the degree of blocking by the AV node of these rapid impulses.

Look at the example of AFib in Figure 4-29. One of the first things you notice is that the ventricular rhythm is irregular. With AFib, atrial depolarization occurs very irregularly. This results in an irregular ventricular rhythm. The ventricular rhythm associated with AFib is described as irregularly irregular. Because the ventricular rhythm is irregular, we should give a ventricular rate range when describing the rhythm. In our example, the ventricular rate ranges from 63 to 100 beats/min.

Because of the quivering of the atrial muscle and because there is no uniform wave of atrial depolarization in AFib, there is no P wave. Instead, you see a baseline that looks erratic (i.e., wavy). This corresponds with the rapid atrial rate. These wavy deflections are called *fibrillatory waves* or *f waves*. Because there is no P wave, we cannot measure a PR interval. The QRS complex is narrow (i.e., measuring 0.08 to 0.10 second) because the impulse started above the bifurcation of the bundle of His and was conducted normally

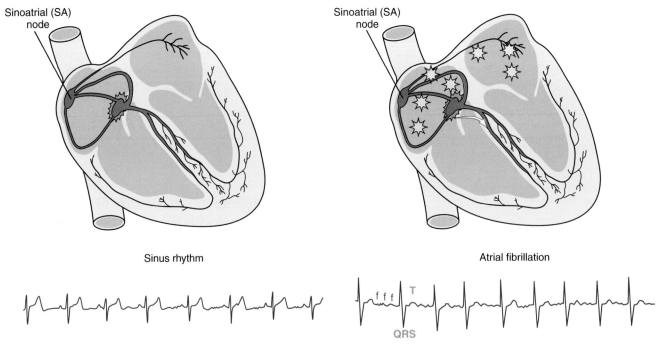

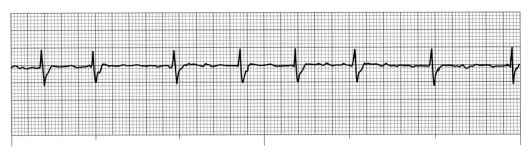

Figure 4-28   Atrial fibrillation. AV, atrioventricular; f, fibrillatory wave.

Figure 4-29   Atrial fibrillation (controlled) with a ventricular response of 63 to 100 beats/min.

through the AV node and bundle and Purkinje fibers. We cannot measure a QT interval because T waves are not clearly seen.

Suspect toxicity caused by digitalis, beta-blockers, or calcium channel blockers if AFib occurs with a slow, regular ventricular rate. This can occur when a patient who has AFib is prescribed medications to slow the ventricular rate. Excess medication can cause third-degree AV block (Figure 4-30). The ECG characteristics of AFib are shown in Table 4-8.

What Causes It?

Although most patients with AFib have some form of cardiovascular disease, AFib can occur in patients without detectable heart disease or related symptoms. Examples

of conditions that predispose patients to AFib appear in Table 4-9.

Patients who experience AFib are at increased risk of having a stroke. Because the atria do not contract effectively and expel all of the blood within them, blood may pool within them and form clots. A stroke can result if a clot moves from the atria and lodges in an artery in the brain. A clot may dislodge on its own or because of conversion of AFib to a sinus rhythm. To review an animation on this topic, go to the Evolve site.

What Do I Do About It?

AFib may occur as a self-limiting episode, it may come and go, or it may exist as a sustained rhythm. Patients who experience AFib may be symptomatic or asymptomatic. When symptoms are present, the severity of the signs and symptoms

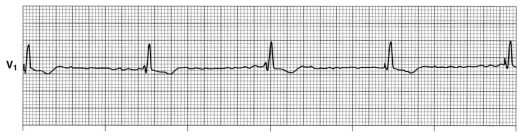

Figure 4-30   Atrial fibrillation with third-degree atrioventricular (AV) block. The ventricular rate is slow and regular because of the block.

Table 4-8	Characteristics of Atrial Fibrillation
Rhythm	Ventricular rhythm usually irregularly irregular
Rate	Atrial rate usually 400 to 600 beats/min; ventricular rate variable
P waves	No identifiable P waves, fibrillatory waves present; erratic, wavy baseline
PR interval	Not measurable
QRS duration	0.11 sec or less unless abnormally conducted

associated with AFib vary with the rate and irregularity of the ventricular response.[5] Examples of common symptoms include chest discomfort or pain, dizziness, fatigue, light-headedness, palpitations, shortness of breath, and syncope.

Obtaining a thorough medical history and patient assessment are important. When obtaining the patient's history, asking about the number of episodes of AFib, their frequency, the nature of the patient's symptoms, and possible triggers may help to determine the pattern of the dysrhythmia. The American College of Cardiology, the American Heart Association, and the European Society for Cardiology (ACC/AHA/ESC) Task Force recommends that the following terms be used to describe episodes of AFib that last more than 30 seconds and that are not caused by another reversible medical cause:[5]

- *First-detected*: The first diagnosed or known episode of AFib experienced by the patient. Determine if the patient is symptomatic or asymptomatic; attempt to determine the duration of the episode of AFib.
- *Recurrent*: Two or more detected episodes of AFib.
- *Paroxysmal*: Recurrent AFib that terminates spontaneously.
- *Persistent*: Recurrent AFib that is sustained beyond 7 days; termination with pharmacological therapy or electrical cardioversion does not change the designation. This category includes cases of long-standing AFib (e.g., greater than 1 year).
- *Permanent*: Paroxysmal or persistent AFib in which pharmacological cardioversion, electrical cardioversion, or both, is not attempted or is not successful.

Because the categories of paroxysmal and persistent AFib are not mutually exclusive, the ACC/AHA/ESC Task Force considers it practical to categorize a given patient by their most frequent presentation.

Treatment decisions are based on the ventricular rate, the duration of the rhythm, the patient's general health, and how he or she tolerates is tolerating the rhythm. It is best to consult a cardiologist when considering specific therapies. The

Table 4-9	Conditions That Predispose Patients to Atrial Fibrillation		
Cardiovascular Conditions	**Noncardiovascular Conditions**	**Iatrogenic Causes**
• Coronary artery disease	• Acute and chronic alcohol abuse	• Antihistamines
• Congenital heart disease (especially atrial septal defect in adults)	• Diabetes mellitus	• Bronchodilating beta agonists
• Dilated cardiomyopathy	• Electrocution	• Cardiac and noncardiac surgery
• Heart failure	• Hyperthyroidism	• Local anesthetics
• Hypertension	• Obesity	• Noncardiac diagnostic procedure
• Hypertrophic cardiomyopathy	• Pulmonary diseases (i.e., chronic obstructive pulmonary disease, pneumonia)	• Nonprescription cold remedies
• Pericardial disease	• Pulmonary embolism	
• Rheumatic heart disease		
• Valvular disease (especially mitral valve disease)		

two primary treatment strategies used to control symptoms associated with AFib are rate control and rhythm control. With rate control, the patient remains in AFib, but the ventricular rate is controlled to decrease acute symptoms, reduce signs of ischemia, and reduce or prevent signs of heart failure from developing. With rhythm control, sinus rhythm is reestablished.

CLINICAL CORRELATION

Some patients who have paroxysmal, persistent, or permanent atrial fibrillation (AFib) may demonstrate *tachycardia-bradycardia syndrome,* which is characterized by a rapid ventricular rate during episodes of AFib and bradycardia during periods of sinus rhythm. When these extremes in the ventricular rate occur in the same patient, the use of antiarrhythmic medications for rate control becomes difficult; catheter ablation or implantation of a permanent pacemaker may be necessary in these patients.[8]

AFib with a rapid ventricular response may produce signs and symptoms that include lightheadedness, palpitations, dyspnea, chest discomfort, and hypotension. If AFib is associated with a rapid ventricular rate and the patient is stable but symptomatic, treatment is usually aimed at controlling the ventricular rate with medications such as diltiazem, which is a calcium channel blocker, or beta-blockers. Beta-blockers should generally be avoided in the presence of severe underlying pulmonary disease or heart failure. Synchronized cardioversion should be considered if the patient with AFib has serious signs and symptoms because of the rapid ventricular rate. Anticoagulation is recommended before attempting to convert AFib to a sinus rhythm if AFib has been present for 48 hours or longer. Catheter ablation is recommended for selected patients with AFib, such as those who have AFib with WPW syndrome and a history of syncope caused by the rapid heart rate. A summary of atrial rhythm characteristics can be found in Tables 4-10 and 4-11. To review animations on these topics, go to the Evolve site.

Table **4-10**	Atrial Rhythms—Summary of Characteristics			
Characteristic	PACs	Wandering Atrial Pacemaker	Atrial Tachycardia	AVNRT
Rhythm	Regular with premature beats	May be irregular as pacemaker site shifts from SA node to ectopic atrial locations and AV junction	Regular	Ventricular rhythm is usually very regular
Rate (beats/min)	Usually within normal range, but depends on underlying rhythm	Usually 60 to 100; if rate greater than 100 beats/min, rhythm is called *multifocal atrial tachycardia*	150 to 250	150 to 250
P waves (lead II)	Premature, positive in lead II, one precedes each QRS, differ from sinus P waves, may be lost in preceding T wave	Size, shape, and direction may change from beat to beat	Atrial P waves differ from sinus P waves; isoelectric baseline usually present between P waves	P waves often hidden in QRS complex
PR interval	May be normal or prolonged	Varies	May be shorter or longer than normal	If P waves are seen, the PRI will usually measure 0.12 to 0.20 sec
QRS duration	0.11 sec or less unless abnormally conducted	0.11 sec or less unless abnormally conducted	0.11 sec or less unless abnormally conducted	0.11 sec or less unless abnormally conducted

AV, atrioventricular; *AVNRT,* atrioventricular nodal reentrant tachycardia; *PAC,* premature atrial complex; *PRI,* PR interval; *SA,* sinoatrial.

Table 4-11	Atrial Rhythms—Summary of Characteristics		
Characteristic	Atrial Flutter	Atrial Fibrillation (AFib)	Wolff-Parkinson-White (WPW) Syndrome
Rhythm	Atrial regular, ventricular regular or irregular	Ventricular rhythm usually irregularly irregular	Regular, unless associated with atrial fibrillation
Rate (beats/min)	Atrial rate 250 to 450, typically 300; ventricular rate variable—determined by AV blockade	Atrial rate 400 to 600; ventricular rate variable	60 to 100 if the underlying rhythm is sinus in origin
P waves (lead II)	No identifiable P waves; saw-toothed "flutter" waves present	No identifiable P waves; fibrillatory waves present; erratic, wavy baseline	Normal and positive unless WPW is associated with AFib
PR interval	Not measurable	Not measurable	If P waves are seen, less than 0.12 sec
QRS duration	0.11 sec or less unless abnormally conducted	0.11 sec or less unless abnormally conducted	Usually greater than 0.12 sec; delta wave may be seen in one or more leads

AV, atrioventricular.

REFERENCES

1. Hamdan MH: Cardiac arrhythmias. In Andreoli TE, Benjamin IJ, Griggs RC, et al: *Andreoli and Carpenter's Cecil essentials of medicine*, ed 8, Philadelphia, 2010, Saunders, pp 118–144.

2. Olgin JE: Approach to the patient with suspected arrhythmia. In Goldman L, Ausiello D, editors: *Cecil medicine*, ed 23, Philadelphia, 2008, Saunders, pp 394–400.

3. Fengler BT, Brady WJ, Plautz CU: Atrial fibrillation in the Wolff-Parkinson-White syndrome: ECG recognition and treatment in the ED, *Am J Emerg Med* 25(5):576–583, 2007.

4. Neumar RW, Otto CW, Link MS, et al: Part 8: adult advanced cardiovascular life support: 2010 American Heart Association guidelines for cardiopulmonary resuscitation and emergency cardiovascular care, *Circulation* 122(suppl 3):S729–S767, 2010.

5. Fuster V, Rydén LE, Cannom DS, et al: 2011 American College of Cardiology Foundation/American Heart Association/Heart Rhythm Society focused updates incorporated into the American College of Cardiology/American Heart Association/European Society of Cardiology 2006 guidelines for the management of patients with atrial fibrillation: a report of the American College of Cardiology Foundation/American Heart Association Task Force on Practice Guidelines, *J Am Coll Cardiol* 57:1330–1337, 2011.

6. Akhtar M: Cardiac arrhythmias with supraventricular origin. In Goldman L, Ausiello D, editors: *Cecil medicine*, ed 23, Philadelphia, 2008, Saunders, pp 405–414.

7. Indik JH, Alpert JS: The patient with atrial fibrillation, *Am J Emerg Med* 122(5):415–418, 2009.

8. Padanilam BJ, Prystowsky EN: Atrial fibrillation: goals of therapy and management strategies to achieve the goals, *Cardiol Clin* 27(1)(Feb):189–200, 2009.

STOP & REVIEW—CHAPTER 4

Multiple Choice

Identify the choice that best completes the statement or answers the question.

_____ 1. On the ECG, an impulse that begins in the atria and occurs earlier than the next expected sinus beat will appear as:
   a. A P wave that appears after the QRS complex.
   b. A QRS measuring more than 0.11 sec in duration.
   c. A P wave with a PR interval measuring more than 0.20 sec.
   d. A P wave that may appear in the T wave of the preceding beat.

_____ 2. In atrial fibrillation, the PR interval is usually:
   a. Not measurable.
   b. Within normal limits.
   c. Less than 0.20 sec in duration.
   d. More than 0.20 sec in duration.

_____ 3. Signs and symptoms experienced during a tachydysrhythmia are usually primarily related to:
   a. Atrial irritability.
   b. Vasoconstriction.
   c. Slowed conduction through the AV node.
   d. Decreased ventricular filling time and stroke volume.

_____ 4. A compensatory pause is a:
   a. Series of waveforms.
   b. Delay that occurs following a premature beat that resets the SA node.
   c. Period during the cardiac cycle during which cardiac cells can be stimulated to conduct an electrical impulse, if exposed to a stronger than normal stimulus.
   d. Period during the cardiac cycle during which cardiac cells cannot be stimulated to conduct an electrical impulse, no matter how strong the stimulus.

_____ 5. What is meant by the term "controlled" atrial fibrillation?
   a. The atrial rate is faster than 100 beats/min.
   b. The atrial rate is slower than 100 beats/min.
   c. The overall ventricular rate is faster than 100 beats/min.
   d. The overall ventricular rate is slower than 100 beats/min.

_____ 6. The most common type of supraventricular tachycardia (SVT) is:
   a. Atrial tachycardia.
   b. Atrial flutter.
   c. AV reentrant tachycardia (AVRT).
   d. AV nodal reentrant tachycardia (AVNRT).

_____ 7. Wolff-Parkinson-White syndrome is associated with a:
   a. Long PR interval, delta wave, and wide QRS complex.
   b. Short PR interval, delta wave, and wide QRS complex.
   c. Long PR interval, flutter waves, and narrow QRS complex.
   d. Short PR interval, flutter waves, and narrow QRS complex.

_____ 8. Which of the following dysrhythmias is most likely to be associated with a reduction in cardiac output and loss of atrial kick?
   a. Atrial fibrillation
   b. Sinus tachycardia
   c. Premature atrial complexes
   d. Wandering atrial pacemaker

_____ 9. All supraventricular dysrhythmias:
   a. Involve accessory pathways.
   b. Begin above the bifurcation of the bundle of His.
   c. Begin below the bifurcation of the bundle of His.
   d. Require the AV node's participation to sustain the dysrhythmia.

_____ 10. Which of the following ECG characteristics distinguishes atrial flutter from other atrial dysrhythmias?
   a. The presence of fibrillatory waves
   b. P waves of varying size and amplitude
   c. The presence of delta waves before the QRS
   d. The "saw-tooth" or "picket-fence" appearance of waveforms before the QRS

Questions 11—15 pertain to the following scenario.

A 35-year-old woman is complaining of palpitations.

_____ 11. The patient is alert and oriented to person, place, time, and event. Her blood pressure is 144/82 mm Hg and her ventilations are 18 breaths/min and unlabored. She appears anxious and states her "heart is racing." Which of the following statements is correct regarding assessment of this patient?
   a. Despite the patient's age, palpitations generally indicate the presence of cardiac disease.
   b. A complaint of palpitations is a cause for concern only if they are of sudden onset and their rhythm is irregular.
   c. A complaint of palpitations is always associated with evidence of a rhythm disturbance on the cardiac monitor.
   d. Information relayed by the patient can provide important clues about her cardiovascular status.

_____**12.** A pulse oximeter has been applied. The patient's oxygen saturation level on room air is 97%. The cardiac monitor reveals the rhythm shown in Figure 4-31. This rhythm, recorded in lead II, is:
  a. Sinus tachycardia
  b. AVNRT
  c. AVRT
  d. AFib

_____**13.** The PR interval in Figure 4-31:
  a. Is 0.06 sec.
  b. Is 0.12 sec.
  c. Is 0.20 sec.
  d. Cannot be measured.

_____**14.** The QT interval in Figure 4-31:
  a. Is 0.16 sec.
  b. Is 0.24 sec.
  c. Is 0.38 sec.
  d. Cannot be measured.

_____**15.** Intravenous access has been established. A repeat set of vital signs reveals the following: blood pressure, 140/82 mm Hg; pulse, 188 beats/min; ventilations, 20 breaths/min. The patient's anxiety has increased. She denies chest discomfort and shortness of breath. Her skin is pink and warm, but moist. Based on the information provided, you should anticipate orders for which of the following?
  a. Immediate sedation
  b. Attempt vagal maneuvers
  c. Synchronized cardioversion
  d. Administer intravenous atropine

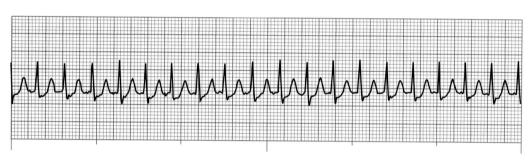

Figure 4-31

Matching

Match the key terms with their definitions by placing the letter of each correct answer in the space provided.
  a. Atrial kick
  b. Premature
  c. Beta-blockers
  d. Accessory pathway
  e. Trigeminy
  f. Bruit
  g. Adenosine
  h. Delta wave
  i. Uncontrolled
  j. Nonconducted PAC
  k. Atrial flutter
  l. Aberrantly conducted PAC
  m. Anticoagulant
  n. Erratic
  o. Atrial fibrillation
  p. Vagal maneuvers
  q. Palpitations
  r. Stroke
  s. Preexcitation
  u. Bigeminy
  t. Bypass tract

_____**16.** Term used when one end of an accessory pathway is attached to normal conductive tissue

_____**17.** Common complaint in a patient with a rapid heart rate

_____**18.** Term used to describe rhythms that originate from above the ventricles but in which the impulse travels by a pathway other than the AV node and bundle of His

_____**19.** Baseline appearance in atrial fibrillation

_____**20.** ECG finding associated with Wolff-Parkinson-White syndrome

_____**21.** Patients who experience AFib have increased risk of this.

_____**22.** Blood pushed into the ventricles because of atrial contraction

_____23. An extra bundle of working myocardial tissue that forms a connection between the atria and ventricles outside the normal conduction system

_____24. Methods used to stimulate the vagus nerve in an attempt to slow conduction through the AV node, resulting in slowing of the heart rate

_____25. This dysrhythmia has an irregularly irregular ventricular rhythm, no identifiable P waves.

_____26. Atrial flutter or fibrillation with a ventricular rate faster than 100 beats/min

_____27. Every other beat comes from somewhere other than the SA node.

_____28. An early P wave with no QRS following it

_____29. Earlier than expected

_____30. These should be avoided in the presence of severe underlying pulmonary disease.

_____31. Blowing or swishing sound within a vessel

_____32. The name given a PAC associated with a wide QRS complex

_____33. Drug of choice for AVNRT

_____34. This dysrhythmia has saw-tooth waveforms instead of P waves.

_____35. Every third beat comes from somewhere other than the SA node.

_____36. Before elective cardioversion, prophylactic treatment with a(n) _____ is recommended for the patient in atrial flutter or fibrillation.

Short Answer

37. Paroxysmal atrial tachycardia is visible on a patient's cardiac monitor. What does _paroxysmal_ mean?

_____

_____

_____

38. Explain why patients who experience atrial fibrillation are at increased risk of having a stroke.

_____

_____

_____

ATRIAL RHYTHMS—*PRACTICE RHYTHM STRIPS*

For each of the following rhythm strips, determine the atrial and ventricular rate and rhythm, measure the PR interval, QRS duration, and QT interval and then identify the rhythm. Note: These rhythm strips include sinus and atrial rhythms.

39. These rhythm strips are from an 89-year-old man complaining of weakness and nausea for 3 to 4 days. His blood pressure is 122/82 mm Hg. He has a history of diabetes.

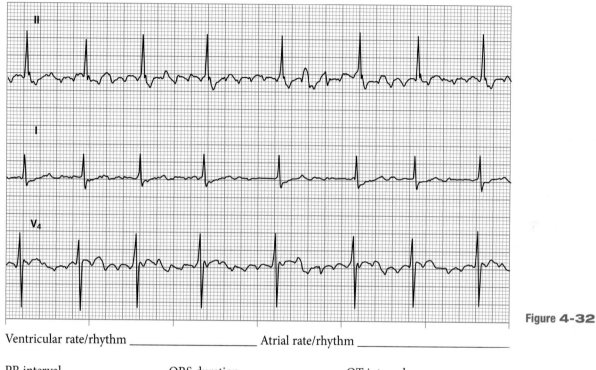

Figure 4-32

Ventricular rate/rhythm _____ Atrial rate/rhythm _____

PR interval _____ QRS duration _____ QT interval _____

Identification _____

40. This rhythm strip is from a 96-year-old man complaining of chest pain and palpitations. Medications include digoxin (Lanoxin) and warfarin (Coumadin).

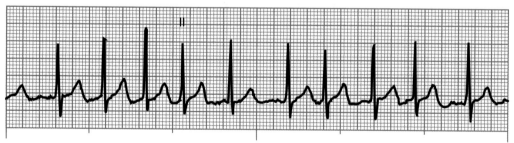

Figure 4-33

Ventricular rate/rhythm _____ Atrial rate/rhythm _____

PR interval _____ QRS duration _____ QT interval _____

Identification _____

41. This rhythm strip (lead II) is from a 57-year-old man with no cardiac history.

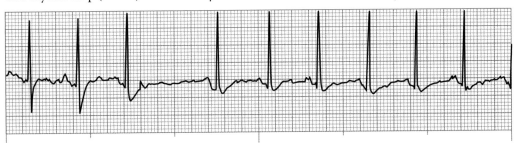

Figure **4-34**

Ventricular rate/rhythm _____ Atrial rate/rhythm _____

PR interval _____ QRS duration _____ QT interval _____

Identification _____

42. This rhythm strip (lead II) is from a 24-year-old woman complaining of weakness and fatigue.

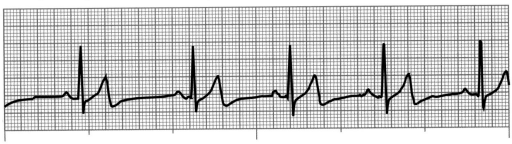

Figure **4-35**

Ventricular rate/rhythm _____ Atrial rate/rhythm _____

PR interval _____ QRS duration _____ QT interval _____

Identification _____

43. Identify the rhythm (lead II).

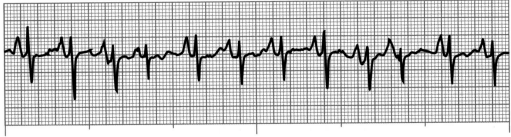

Figure **4-36**

Ventricular rate/rhythm _____ Atrial rate/rhythm _____

PR interval _____ QRS duration _____ QT interval _____

Identification _____

44. This rhythm strip (lead II) is from a 53-year-old woman with an altered level of responsiveness.

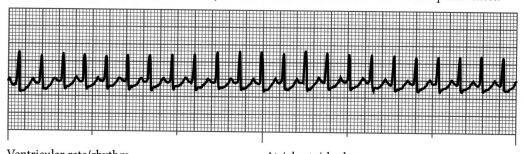

Figure 4-37

Ventricular rate/rhythm _____ Atrial rate/rhythm _____

PR interval _____ QRS duration _____ QT interval _____

Identification _____

45. This rhythm strip is from a 78-year-old woman complaining of left upper quadrant abdominal pain: blood pressure, 222/92 mm Hg; blood sugar, 323 mg/dL.

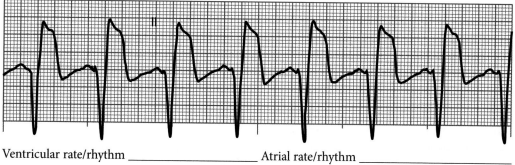

Figure 4-38

Ventricular rate/rhythm _____ Atrial rate/rhythm _____

PR interval _____ QRS duration _____ QT interval _____

Identification _____

46. Identify the rhythm (lead II).

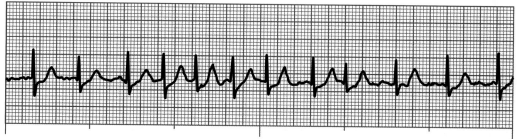

Figure 4-39

Ventricular rate/rhythm _____ Atrial rate/rhythm _____

PR interval _____ QRS duration _____ QT interval _____

Identification _____

47. This rhythm strip (lead II) is from an 82-year-old woman who had a ground level fall. Her blood pressure is 110/72 mm Hg and blood sugar is 156 mg/dL.

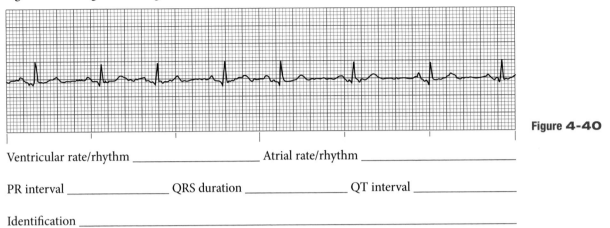

Figure 4-40

Ventricular rate/rhythm _____ Atrial rate/rhythm _____

PR interval _____ QRS duration _____ QT interval _____

Identification _____

48. These rhythm strips are from a 74-year-old woman with difficulty breathing.

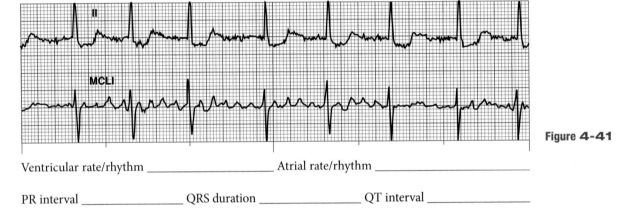

Figure 4-41

Ventricular rate/rhythm _____ Atrial rate/rhythm _____

PR interval _____ QRS duration _____ QT interval _____

Identification _____

49. Identify the rhythm (lead II).

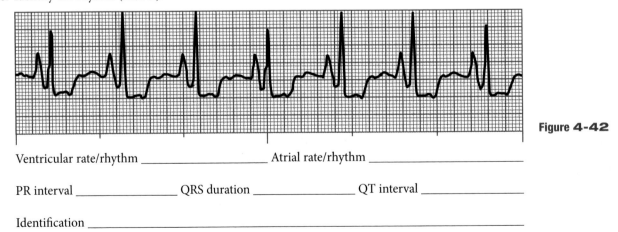

Figure 4-42

Ventricular rate/rhythm _____ Atrial rate/rhythm _____

PR interval _____ QRS duration _____ QT interval _____

Identification _____

50. Identify the rhythm (lead II).

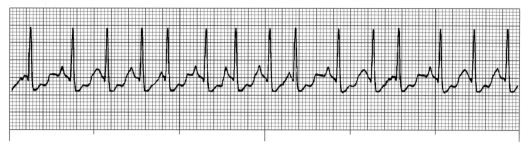

Figure 4-43

Ventricular rate/rhythm _____   Atrial rate/rhythm _____

PR interval _____ QRS duration _____ QT interval _____

Identification _____

51. Identify the rhythm (lead II).

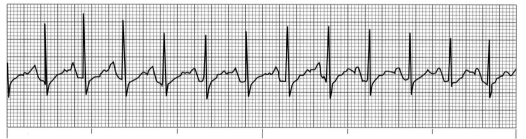

Figure 4-44

Ventricular rate/rhythm _____   Atrial rate/rhythm _____

PR interval _____ QRS duration _____ QT interval _____

Identification _____

52. This rhythm strip (lead II) is from a 17-year-old male who experienced a syncopal episode while playing baseball in 110° F heat for 4 hours. His blood pressure is 148/84 mm Hg; core temperature 101.8° F.

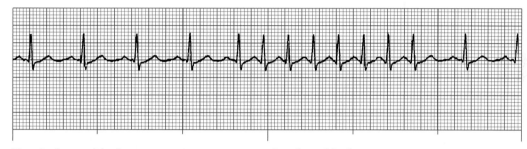

Figure 4-45

Ventricular rate/rhythm _____   Atrial rate/rhythm _____

PR interval _____ QRS duration _____ QT interval _____

Identification _____

53. This rhythm strip is from an 82-year-old man complaining of back pain. Top rhythm strip = lead II; bottom = lead MCL₁.

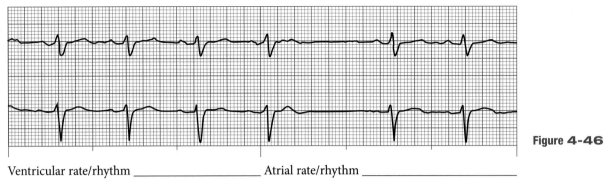

Figure **4-46**

Ventricular rate/rhythm _____ Atrial rate/rhythm _____

PR interval _____ QRS duration _____ QT interval _____

Identification _____

54. Identify the rhythm (lead II).

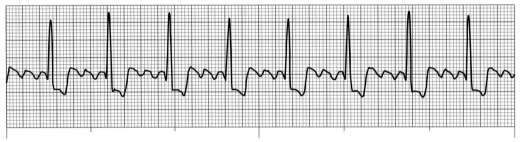

Figure **4-47**

Ventricular rate/rhythm _____ Atrial rate/rhythm _____

PR interval _____ QRS duration _____ QT interval _____

Identification _____

55. These rhythm strips are from a 35-year-old man complaining of a sudden onset of severe substernal chest pain. He has no significant past medical history and takes no medications. His initial blood pressure is 56/0 mm Hg.

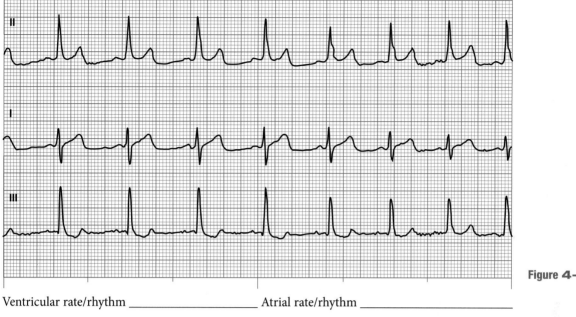

Figure 4-48

Ventricular rate/rhythm _____ Atrial rate/rhythm _____

PR interval _____ QRS duration _____ QT interval _____

Identification _____

56. This rhythm strip (lead II) is from a 67-year-old woman complaining of dizziness and a "funny feeling" in her chest. She denies chest pain and is not short of breath.

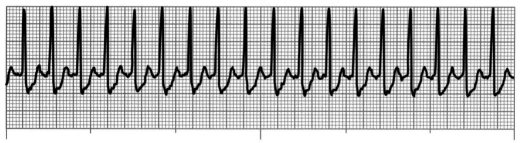

Figure 4-49

Ventricular rate/rhythm _____ Atrial rate/rhythm _____

PR interval _____ QRS duration _____ QT interval _____

Identification _____

57. These rhythm strips are from a 78-year-old man complaining of shortness of breath. He has a history of chronic obstructive pulmonary disease, coronary artery disease, and hypertension.

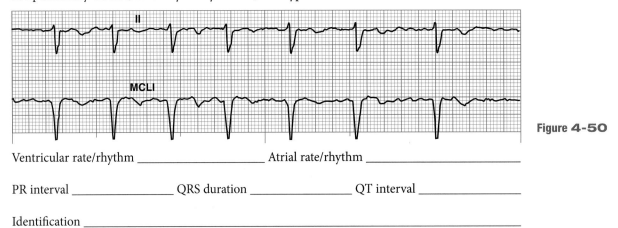

Figure 4-50

Ventricular rate/rhythm _____ Atrial rate/rhythm _____

PR interval _____ QRS duration _____ QT interval _____

Identification _____

58. Identify the rhythm (lead II).

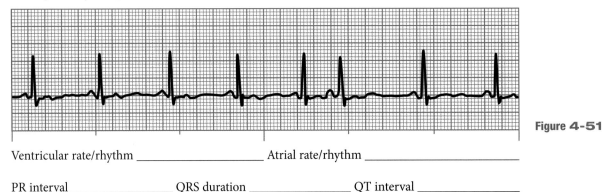

Figure 4-51

Ventricular rate/rhythm _____ Atrial rate/rhythm _____

PR interval _____ QRS duration _____ QT interval _____

Identification _____

59. Identify the rhythm (lead II).

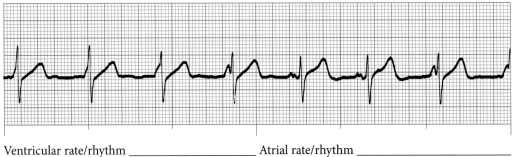

Figure 4-52

Ventricular rate/rhythm _____ Atrial rate/rhythm _____

PR interval _____ QRS duration _____ QT interval _____

Identification _____

60. This rhythm strip (lead II) is from a 71-year-old man complaining of shoulder pain that has been present for 3 weeks.

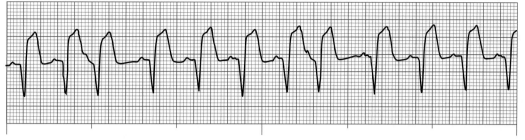

Figure 4-53

Ventricular rate/rhythm _____ Atrial rate/rhythm _____

PR interval _____ QRS duration _____ QT interval _____

Identification _____

61. These rhythm strips are from a 70-year-old woman with chest pain.

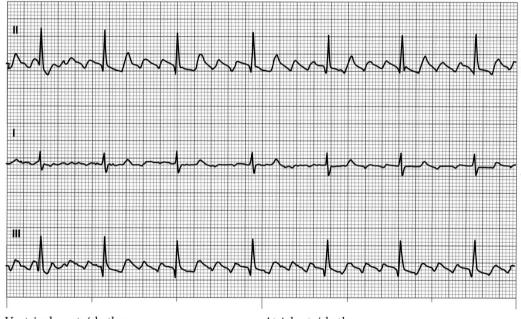

Figure 4-54

Ventricular rate/rhythm _____ Atrial rate/rhythm _____

PR interval _____ QRS duration _____ QT interval _____

Identification _____

62. Identify the rhythm (lead II).

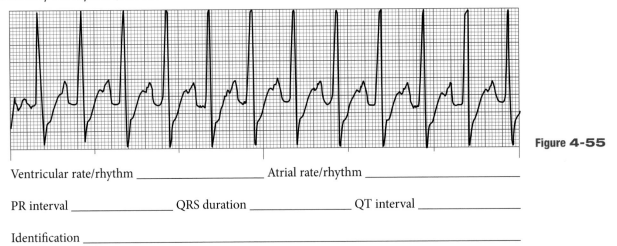

Figure 4-55

Ventricular rate/rhythm _____ Atrial rate/rhythm _____

PR interval _____ QRS duration _____ QT interval _____

Identification _____

63. This rhythm strip is from a 47-year-old woman with a sudden onset of left arm weakness/numbness while sitting at her desk.

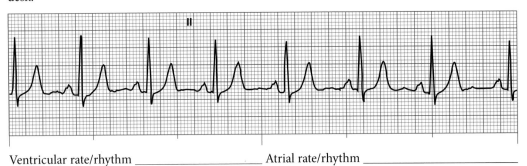

Figure 4-56

Ventricular rate/rhythm _____ Atrial rate/rhythm _____

PR interval _____ QRS duration _____ QT interval _____

Identification _____

64. Identify the rhythm (lead II).

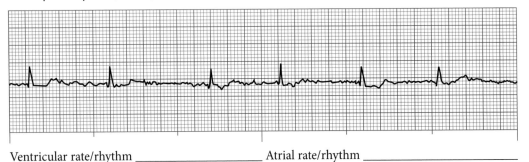

Figure 4-57

Ventricular rate/rhythm _____ Atrial rate/rhythm _____

PR interval _____ QRS duration _____ QT interval _____

Identification _____

65. This rhythm strip (lead II) is from a 72-year-old man complaining of nausea and lightheadedness. He suffered a stroke 2 months ago.

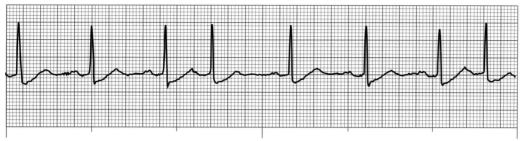

Figure 4-58

Ventricular rate/rhythm _____ Atrial rate/rhythm _____

PR interval _____ QRS duration _____ QT interval _____

Identification _____

66. This rhythm strip is from a 14-year-old complaining of chest pain.

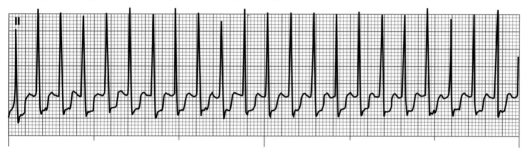

Figure 4-59

Ventricular rate/rhythm _____ Atrial rate/rhythm _____

PR interval _____ QRS duration _____ QT interval _____

Identification _____

67. The following rhythm strip is from the same 14-year-old as in Figure 4-59. This rhythm was observed after 6 mg of intravenous adenosine.

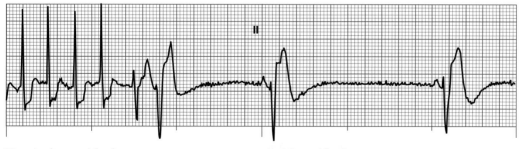

Figure 4-60

Ventricular rate/rhythm _____ Atrial rate/rhythm _____

PR interval _____ QRS duration _____ QT interval _____

Identification _____

STOP & REVIEW ANSWERS

Multiple Choice

1. ANS: D

When compared with the P-P intervals of the underlying rhythm, a premature atrial complex (PAC) is premature—occurring before the next expected sinus P wave. PACs are identified by early (premature) P waves, positive (upright) P waves (in lead II) that differ in shape from sinus P waves (atrial P waves may be flattened, notched, pointed, biphasic, or lost in the preceding T wave), and early P waves that may or may not be followed by a QRS complex.

OBJ: Describe the ECG characteristics, possible causes, signs and symptoms, and initial emergency care for PACs.

2. ANS: A

Because there are no P waves associated with atrial fibrillation, a PR interval cannot be measured.

OBJ: Describe the ECG characteristics, possible causes, signs and symptoms, and initial emergency care for atrial fibrillation.

3. ANS: D

Signs and symptoms experienced during a tachydysrhythmia are usually primarily related to a decrease in the length of time spent in diastole. Remember that as the heart rate increases, there is less time for the ventricles to fill and less blood for the ventricles to pump out with each contraction. Thus an excessively fast heart rate can lead to decreased cardiac output.

4. ANS: B

A compensatory pause is a delay that occurs following a premature beat that resets the sinoatrial (SA) node. A series of waveforms is called a *complex*. The period during the cardiac cycle during which cardiac cells can be stimulated to conduct an electrical impulse, if exposed to a stronger than normal stimulus describes the relative refractory period. The period during the cardiac cycle during which cardiac cells cannot be stimulated to conduct an electrical impulse, no matter how strong the stimulus describes the absolute refractory period.

OBJ: Explain the difference between a compensatory and noncompensatory pause.

5. ANS: D

Atrial flutter or atrial fibrillation that has a ventricular rate of less than 100 beats/min is described as "controlled." A controlled ventricular rate may be the result of a healthy atrioventricular (AV) node protecting the ventricles from very fast atrial impulses or medications used to control (block) conduction through the AV node, decreasing the number of impulses reaching the ventricles.

OBJ: Describe the ECG characteristics, possible causes, signs and symptoms, and initial emergency care for atrial fibrillation.

6. ANS: D

Atrioventricular nodal reentrant tachycardia (AVNRT), which is caused by reentry in the area of the AV node, is the most common type of supraventricular tachycardia (SVT).

OBJ: Describe the ECG characteristics, possible causes, signs and symptoms, and initial emergency care for atrioventricular nodal reentrant tachycardia (AVNRT).

7. ANS: B

The typical pattern associated with Wolff-Parkinson-White (WPW) syndrome is commonly referred to as a triad (meaning three) of ECG findings: (1) short PR interval, (2) delta wave, and (3) wide QRS complex. In addition, secondary ST-segment and T-wave changes are often present.

OBJ: Describe the ECG characteristics, possible causes, signs and symptoms, and initial emergency care for AVRT.

8. ANS: A

In atrial fibrillation, rapid impulses cause the muscles of the atria to quiver (fibrillate). This results in ineffectual atrial contraction, decreased stroke volume, a subsequent decrease in cardiac output, and loss of atrial kick.

OBJ: Describe the ECG characteristics, possible causes, signs and symptoms, and initial emergency care for atrial fibrillation.

9. ANS: B

A supraventricular rhythm is one that originates from a site above the bifurcation of the bundle of His, such as the SA node, atria, or AV junction.

10. ANS: D

In atrial flutter, atrial waveforms are produced that resemble the teeth of a saw, or a picket fence, called *flutter waves*. Flutter waves are best observed in leads II, III, aVF, and V_1.

OBJ: Describe the ECG characteristics, possible causes, signs and symptoms, and initial emergency care for atrial flutter.

11. ANS: D

Information relayed by the patient as part of the history can provide important clues to her cardiovascular (and pulmonary) status. Ask questions to find out the patient's description of her symptoms, when and how often they occur, how long they last, possible triggers, and what measures she has taken to relieve them. A complaint of palpitations warrants timely assessment and intervention, whether or not their rhythm is regular. It is important to determine if chest pain or discomfort, difficulty breathing, or shortness of breath accompany her palpitations. Some practitioners recommend having the patient "tap out" the rhythm of the palpitations to help determine rhythmicity. Palpitations that occur regularly with a sudden onset and end usually are caused by atrioventricular nodal reentrant tachycardia (AVNRT) or atrioventricular reentrant tachycardia (AVRT). Irregular palpitations may be a result of premature complexes, atrial fibrillation, or multifocal atrial tachycardia. Patients may report palpitations even when there is no evidence of a rhythm disturbance on the cardiac monitor. This occurs most often in patients with anxiety disorders. Although symptoms such as chest pain or discomfort, dyspnea, palpitations, edema, and syncope are classic symptoms of cardiac disease, they may also occur because of other organ system diseases (such as musculoskeletal, pulmonary, renal, and gastrointestinal). OBJ: Describe the ECG characteristics, possible causes, signs and symptoms, and initial emergency care for atrioventricular nodal reentrant tachycardia (AVNRT).

12. ANS: B

The rhythm shown is atrioventricular nodal reentrant tachycardia (AVNRT) at 188 beats/min. OBJ: Describe the ECG characteristics, possible causes, signs and symptoms, and initial emergency care for atrioventricular nodal reentrant tachycardia (AVNRT).

13. ANS: D

Because there are no P waves visible in Figure 4-31, the PR interval cannot be measured. OBJ: Define and describe the significance of each of the following as they relate to cardiac electrical activity: P wave, QRS complex, T wave, U wave, PR segment, TP segment, ST segment, PR interval, QRS duration, and QT interval.

14. ANS: B

The QT interval in Figure 4-31 measures 0.24 sec. OBJ: Define and describe the significance of each of the following as they relate to cardiac electrical activity: P wave, QRS complex, T wave, U wave, PR segment, TP segment, ST segment, PR interval, QRS duration, and QT interval.

15. ANS: B

The patient is symptomatic, but *stable*. Vagal maneuvers, such as asking the patient to cough or bear down, may be attempted. If vagal maneuvers were unsuccessful, anticipate orders for intravenous (IV) administration of adenosine. Sedation and cardioversion would be appropriate if the patient was *unstable* (showing signs of hemodynamic compromise). Because atropine is administered to increase heart rate and this patient is already tachycardic, it is contraindicated in this patient situation. OBJ: Describe the ECG characteristics, possible causes, signs and symptoms, and initial emergency care for atrioventricular nodal reentrant tachycardia (AVNRT).

Matching

16. ANS: T
17. ANS: Q
18. ANS: S
19. ANS: N
20. ANS: H
21. ANS: R
22. ANS: A
23. ANS: D
24. ANS: P
25. ANS: O
26. ANS: I
27. ANS: U
28. ANS: J
29. ANS: B
30. ANS: C
31. ANS: F
32. ANS: L
33. ANS: G
34. ANS: K
35. ANS: E
36. ANS: M

Short Answer

37. ANS:

The term *paroxysmal* is used to describe a rhythm that starts or ends suddenly. Some physicians use this term to describe the sudden onset or end of a patient's symptoms.

OBJ: Explain the terms *paroxysmal atrial tachycardia* (PAT) and *paroxysmal supraventricular tachycardia* (PSVT).

38. ANS:

Because the atria do not contract effectively and expel all of the blood within them, blood may pool within them and form clots. A clot may dislodge on its own or because of conversion to a sinus rhythm. A stroke can result if a clot moves from the atria and lodges in an artery in the brain.

OBJ: Describe the ECG characteristics, possible causes, signs and symptoms, and initial emergency care for atrial fibrillation.

39. Figure 4-32 answer

Ventricular rate/rhythm	64 to 83 beats/min; irregular
Atrial rate/rhythm	Unable to determine
PR interval	Unable to determine
QRS duration	0.08 sec
QT interval	Unable to determine
Identification	Atrial flutter at 64 to 83 beats/min

40. Figure 4-33 answer

Ventricular rate/rhythm	88 to 130 beats/min; irregular
Atrial rate/rhythm	Unable to determine
PR interval	Unable to determine
QRS duration	0.08 sec
QT interval	0.32 to 0.36 sec
Identification	Atrial fibrillation at 88 to 130 beats/min

41. Figure 4-34 answer

Ventricular rate/rhythm	57 to 100 beats/min; irregular
Atrial rate/rhythm	75 to 167 beats/min; irregular
PR interval	0.18 sec
QRS duration	0.08 sec
QT interval	0.28 to 0.30 sec; unable to clearly determine as a result of artifact
Identification	Sinus rhythm at 57 to 100 beats/min with a nonconducted premature atrial complex (PAC)

42. Figure 4-35 answer

Ventricular rate/rhythm	45 to 54 beats/min; irregular
Atrial rate/rhythm	45 to 54 beats/min; irregular
PR interval	0.18 sec
QRS duration	0.08 sec
QT interval	0.40 sec
Identification	Sinus bradyarrhythmia at 45 to 54 beats/min

43. Figure 4-36 answer

Ventricular rate/rhythm	115 to 167 beats/min; irregular
Atrial rate/rhythm	115 to 167 beats/min; irregular
PR interval	0.16 sec
QRS duration	0.08 to 0.10 sec
QT interval	0.40 sec
Identification	Sinus tachycardia at 115 to 167 beats/min with premature atrial complexes (PACs) (beats 4 and 10)

44. Figure 4-37 answer

Ventricular rate/rhythm	233 beats/min; regular
Atrial rate/rhythm	Unable to determine
PR interval	Unable to determine
QRS duration	0.06 sec
QT interval	0.24 sec
Identification	Atrioventricular nodal reentrant tachycardia (AVNRT) at 233 beats/min with ST-segment depression

45. Figure 4-38 answer

Ventricular rate/rhythm	86 beats/min; regular
Atrial rate/rhythm	86 beats/min; regular
PR interval	0.18 to 0.20 sec
QRS duration	0.10 sec
QT interval	0.40 to 0.44 sec
Identification	Sinus rhythm at 86 beats/min with ST-segment elevation

46. Figure 4-39 answer

Ventricular rate/rhythm	100 to 167 beats/min; irregular
Atrial rate/rhythm	Unable to determine
PR interval	Unable to determine
QRS duration	0.08 sec
QT interval	0.28 to 0.32 sec
Identification	Atrial fibrillation (uncontrolled) at 100 to 167 beats/min

47. Figure 4-40 answer

Ventricular rate/rhythm	79 to 88 beats/min; irregular
Atrial rate/rhythm	79 to 88 beats/min; irregular
PR interval	0.16 sec
QRS duration	0.06 sec
QT interval	0.32 sec
Identification	Sinus rhythm at 79 to 88 beats/min with premature atrial complexes (PACs) (beats 3 and 5)

48. Figure 4-41 answer

Ventricular rate/rhythm	75 to 107 beats/min; irregular
Atrial rate/rhythm	Unable to determine
PR interval	Unable to determine
QRS duration	0.08 sec
QT interval	Unable to determine
Identification	Atrial flutter at 75 to 107 beats/min

49. Figure 4-42 answer

Ventricular rate/rhythm	67 beats/min; regular
Atrial rate/rhythm	67 beats/min; regular
PR interval	0.16 sec
QRS duration	0.08 sec
QT interval	0.32 sec
Identification	Sinus rhythm at 67 beats/min with ST-segment depression and inverted T waves

50. Figure 4-43 answer

Ventricular rate/rhythm	115 to 215 beats/min; irregular
Atrial rate/rhythm	Unable to determine; irregular
PR interval	Varies
QRS duration	0.04 to 0.06 sec
QT interval	0.24 sec
Identification	Multifocal atrial tachycardia at 115 to 215 beats/min with ST-segment depression

51. Figure 4-44 answer

Ventricular rate/rhythm	96 to 214 beats/min; irregular
Atrial rate/rhythm	96 to 214 beats/min; irregular
PR interval	0.16 sec (sinus beats)
QRS duration	0.08 sec
QT interval	0.24 to 0.32 sec
Identification	Sinus rhythm at 96 beats/min with a premature atrial complex (PAC) precipitating a run of paroxysmal supraventricular tachycardia (PSVT) at 214 beats/min, back to a sinus rhythm at 96 beats/min

52. Figure 4-45 answer

Ventricular rate/rhythm	125 beats/min; regular
Atrial rate/rhythm	125 beats/min; regular
PR interval	0.16 sec
QRS duration	0.06 sec
QT interval	0.28 sec
Identification	Sinus tachycardia at 125 beats/min with ST-segment depression

53. Figure 4-46 answer

Ventricular rate/rhythm	42 to 75 beats/min; irregular
Atrial rate/rhythm	60 to 75 beats/min; irregular
PR interval	0.20 sec
QRS duration	0.12 sec
QT interval	0.36 sec
Identification	Sinus rhythm at 42 to 75 beats/min with a wide-QRS and a nonconducted premature atrial complex (PAC)

54. Figure 4-47 answer

Ventricular rate/rhythm	88 beats/min; regular
Atrial rate/rhythm	Unable to determine
PR interval	Unable to determine
QRS duration	0.06 sec
QT interval	Unable to determine
Identification	Atrial flutter at 88 beats/min with ST-segment depression

55. Figure 4-48 answer

Ventricular rate/rhythm	71 beats/min; regular
Atrial rate/rhythm	71 beats/min; regular
PR interval	0.14 sec
QRS duration	0.08 sec
QT interval	0.36 sec
Identification	Sinus rhythm at 71 beats/min with ST-segment elevation

56. Figure 4-49 answer

Ventricular rate/rhythm	186 beats/min; regular
Atrial rate/rhythm	Unable to determine
PR interval	Unable to determine
QRS duration	0.06 sec
QT interval	0.24 sec
Identification	Atrioventricular nodal reentrant tachycardia (AVNRT) at 186 beats/min with ST-segment depression

57. Figure 4-50 answer

Ventricular rate/rhythm	55 to 94 beats/min; irregular
Atrial rate/rhythm	Unable to determine
PR interval	Unable to determine
QRS duration	0.10 sec
QT interval	Unable to determine
Identification	Atrial fibrillation (controlled) at 55 to 94 beats/min

58. Figure 4-51 answer

Ventricular rate/rhythm	71 to 136 beats/min; irregular
Atrial rate/rhythm	71 to 136 beats/min; irregular
PR interval	0.12 sec
QRS duration	0.06 sec
QT interval	0.24 sec
Identification	Sinus rhythm at 71 to 136 beats/min with a premature atrial complex (PAC) (beat 6)

59. Figure 4-52 answer

Ventricular rate/rhythm	70 beats/min; regular
Atrial rate/rhythm	70 beats/min (sinus beats); unable to determine
PR interval	Varies
QRS duration	Varies
QT interval	0.44 sec
Identification	Underlying rhythm is sinus but pacemaker site varies; ventricular rate about 70 beats/min; patient with known Wolff-Parkinson-White (WPW) syndrome; note the delta waves

60. Figure 4-53 answer

Ventricular rate/rhythm	115 to 166 beats/min; irregular
Atrial rate/rhythm	115 to 166 beats/min; irregular
PR interval	0.12 sec (sinus beats)
QRS duration	0.08 sec (sinus beats)
QT interval	0.24 sec (sinus beats)
Identification	Sinus tachycardia at 115 to 166 beats/min with premature atrial complexes (PACs) and ST-segment elevation

61. Figure 4-54 answer

Ventricular rate/rhythm	81 beats/min; regular
Atrial rate/rhythm	Unable to determine
PR interval	Unable to determine
QRS duration	0.06 sec
QT interval	Unable to determine
Identification	Atrial flutter at 81 beats/min

62. Figure 4-55 answer

Ventricular rate/rhythm	116 beats/min; regular
Atrial rate/rhythm	116 beats/min; regular
PR interval	0.20 sec
QRS duration	0.10 sec
QT interval	0.30 sec
Identification	Sinus tachycardia at 116 beats/min with ST-segment depression

63. Figure 4-56 answer

Ventricular rate/rhythm	70 beats/min; regular
Atrial rate/rhythm	70 beats/min; regular
PR interval	0.18 sec
QRS duration	0.08 to 0.10 sec
QT interval	0.36 sec
Identification	Sinus rhythm at 70 beats/min with tall T waves

64. Figure 4-57 answer

Ventricular rate/rhythm	50 to 71 beats/min; irregular
Atrial rate/rhythm	Unable to determine
PR interval	Unable to determine
QRS duration	0.08 to 0.10 sec
QT interval	Unable to determine
Identification	Atrial fibrillation (controlled) at 50 to 71 beats/min

65. Figure 4-58 answer

Ventricular rate/rhythm	68 to 111 beats/min; irregular
Atrial rate/rhythm	68 to 111 beats/min; irregular
PR interval	0.20 sec (sinus beats)
QRS duration	0.06 sec (sinus beats)
QT interval	0.40 sec (sinus beats)
Identification	Sinus rhythm at 68 to 111 beats/min with two premature atrial complexes (PACs) (beats 4 and 8) and ST-segment depression

66. Figure 4-59 answer

Ventricular rate/rhythm	214 beats/min; regular
Atrial rate/rhythm	Unable to determine
PR interval	Unable to determine
QRS duration	0.06 sec
QT interval	Unable to determine
Identification	Atrioventricular nodal reentrant tachycardia (AVNRT) at 214 beats/min with ST-segment depression

67. Figure 4-60 answer

Ventricular rate/rhythm	214 beats/min (atrioventricular nodal reentrant tachycardia [AVNRT]) to 29 beats/min (sinus beats); regular to irregular as rhythm conversion occurs
Atrial rate/rhythm	Unable to determine (AVNRT) to 29 beats/min; unable to determine to irregular (sinus beats) as rhythm conversion occurs
PR interval	Unable to determine to 0.12 to 0.16 sec (sinus beats)
QRS duration	0.06 sec (AVNRT, last sinus beat)
QT interval	0.28 sec (sinus beats)
Identification	AVNRT at 214 beats/min with ST-segment depression with rhythm conversion evidenced by a sinus beat, a possible premature atrial complex (PAC), and then sinus bradycardia at 29 beats/min

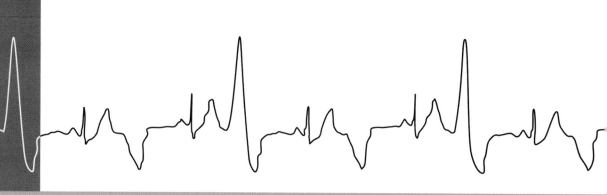

5 CHAPTER

Junctional Rhythms

LEARNING OBJECTIVES

After reading this chapter, you should be able to:

1. Describe the electrocardiogram (ECG) characteristics, possible causes, signs and symptoms, and initial emergency care for premature junctional complexes (PJCs).
2. Describe the ECG characteristics and possible causes for junctional escape beats.
3. Explain the difference between PJCs and junctional escape beats.
4. Describe the ECG characteristics, possible causes, signs and symptoms, and initial emergency care for a junctional escape rhythm.
5. Describe the ECG characteristics, possible causes, signs and symptoms, and initial emergency care for an accelerated junctional rhythm.
6. Describe the ECG characteristics, possible causes, signs and symptoms, and initial emergency care for junctional tachycardia.

KEY TERMS

Accelerated junctional rhythm: Dysrhythmia originating in the atrioventricular (AV) bundle with a rate between 61 and 100 beats/min

Atrioventricular bundle: The bundle of His

Atrioventricular node: A group of cells that conduct an electrical impulse through the heart; located in the floor of the right atrium immediately behind the tricuspid valve and near the opening of the coronary sinus

Bundle of His: Fibers located in the upper portion of the interventricular septum that conduct an electrical impulse through the heart

Junctional bradycardia: A rhythm that begins in the AV bundle with a rate of less than 40 beats/min

Junctional escape rhythm: A rhythm that begins in the AV bundle; characterized by a very regular ventricular rate of 40 to 60 beats/min

Junctional tachycardia: A rhythm that begins in the AV bundle with a ventricular rate of more than 100 beats/min

Retrograde: Moving backward; moving in the opposite direction to that which is considered normal

INTRODUCTION

The **atrioventricular node** (AV node) is a group of specialized cells located in the lower part of the right atrium, above the base of the tricuspid valve (Figure 5-1). The AV node's main job is to delay an electrical impulse. This allows the atria to contract and complete filling of the ventricles with blood before the next ventricular contraction.

After passing through the AV node, the electrical impulse enters the **bundle of His**. The bundle of His, also called the *common bundle* or the **atrioventricular bundle**, is located in the upper part of the interventricular septum. It connects the AV node with the right and left bundle branches. The bundle of His has pacemaker cells that are capable of discharging at a rhythmic rate of 40 to 60 beats/min. The AV node and the nonbranching portion of the bundle of His are called the *AV*

junction (Figure 5-2). The bundle of His conducts the electrical impulse to the bundle branches.

Remember that the sinoatrial (SA) node is normally the heart's pacemaker. The AV junction may assume responsibility for pacing the heart if:

- The SA node fails to discharge (such as sinus arrest).
- An impulse from the SA node is generated but blocked as it exits the SA node (such as SA block).
- The rate of discharge of the SA node is slower than that of the AV junction (such as a sinus bradycardia or the slower phase of a sinus arrhythmia).
- An impulse from the SA node is generated and is conducted through the atria but is not conducted to the ventricles (such as an AV block).

Rhythms that begin in the AV junction used to be called *nodal rhythms* until electrophysiologic studies proved the

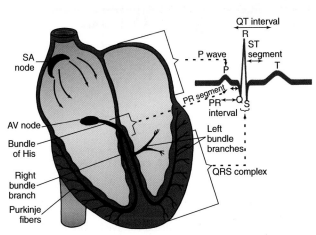

Figure 5-1 The atrioventricular (AV) node is located in the lower portion of the right atrium. The bundle of His is located in the upper part of the interventricular septum. SA, sinoatrial.

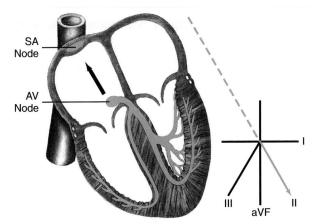

Figure 5-3 If the atrioventricular (AV) junction paces the heart, the electrical impulse must travel in a backward (retrograde) direction to activate the atria. SA, sinoatrial.

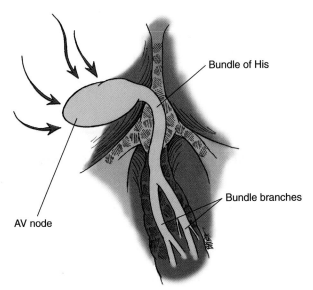

Figure 5-2 The atrioventricular (AV) junction.

AV node does not contain pacemaker cells. The cells nearest the bundle of His are actually responsible for secondary pacing function. Rhythms originating from the AV junction are now called *junctional dysrhythmias.*

If the AV junction paces the heart, the electrical impulse must travel in a backward (**retrograde**) direction to activate the atria. If a P wave is seen, it will be inverted in leads II, III, and aVF because the impulse is traveling away from the positive electrode (Figure 5-3). If the atria depolarize before the ventricles, an inverted P wave will be seen *before* the QRS complex (Figure 5-4) and the PR interval will usually measure 0.12 second or less. The PR interval is shorter than usual because an impulse that begins in the AV junction does not have to travel as far to stimulate the ventricles. If the atria and ventricles depolarize at the same time, a

P wave will not be visible because it will be hidden in the QRS complex. When the atria are depolarized after the ventricles, the P wave typically distorts the end of the QRS complex and an inverted P wave will appear *after* the QRS. The QRS duration associated with a rhythm that begins in the AV junction measures 0.11 second or less if conduction through the bundle branches, Purkinje fibers, and ventricles is normal.

ECG Pearl

P waves are usually positive (i.e., upright) in lead I. Inverted P waves may be seen in some, all, or none of the chest leads.

PREMATURE JUNCTIONAL COMPLEXES

How Do I Recognize Them?

[Objective 1]
A PJC occurs when an irritable site (i.e., focus) within the AV junction fires before the next SA node impulse is ready to fire. This interrupts the sinus rhythm. Because the impulse is conducted through the ventricles in the usual manner, the QRS complex will usually measure 0.11 second or less. PJCs are sometimes called *premature junctional extrasystoles.* A noncompensatory (incomplete) pause often follows a PJC. This pause represents the delay during which the SA node resets its rhythm for the next beat. PJCs may occur in patterns—couplets, bigeminy, trigeminy, and quadrigeminy.

You can usually tell the difference between a premature atrial complex (PAC) and a PJC by the P wave. A PAC typically has an upright P wave before the QRS complex in leads II, III, and aVF. A P wave may or may not be present with a PJC. If a P wave is present, it is inverted (retrograde) and

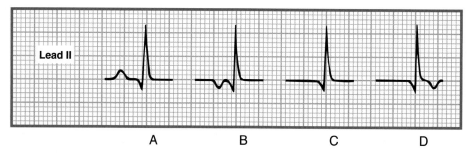

Figure 5-4   **A,** With a sinus rhythm, the P wave is positive (upright) in lead II because the wave of depolarization is moving toward the positive electrode. The P wave associated with a junctional beat (in lead II) may be: **B,** inverted (retrograde) and appear before the QRS; **C,** be hidden by the QRS, or **D,** appear after the QRS.

may precede or follow the QRS. PJCs can be misdiagnosed when the P wave of a PAC is buried in the preceding T wave.

Junctional complexes may come early (before the next expected sinus beat) or late (after the next expected sinus beat). If the complex is *early* it is called a *premature junctional complex.* If the complex is *late* it is called a *junctional escape beat.* To determine if a complex is early or late, we need to see at least two sinus beats in a row to establish the regularity of the underlying rhythm.

Let's look at Figure 5-5. Looking at the overall rhythm, it appears to be irregular. All QRS complexes appear to be narrow, so we assume that all impulses started from above the ventricles. Using a pen or pencil, mark an "S" for SA node above each normal looking P wave. Mark a "J" for junctional above those P waves that are inverted or absent. When you are finished, you should have a "J" marked over the P waves in beats 2, 5, 8, and 11. The rest of the P waves should be marked with an "S." Now take your calipers or a piece of paper and mark the third and fourth complexes in Figure 5-5. We already determined that these complexes came from the SA node. These beats reflect the underlying rhythm. Calculate the atrial and ventricular rate between these beats. It is 136 beats/min (1500 ÷ 11 small boxes). We now know that the underlying rhythm is a sinus tachycardia at 136 beats/min. Now move your calipers or paper to the right. If beat 5 occurred on time (i.e., when the next sinus beat was expected), it will line up with your calipers or paper. The fifth complex is early; it occurred *before* the next expected sinus beat, therefore this complex is a PJC. The

other beats that have an inverted P wave before the QRS are also PJCs.

A PJC is not an entire rhythm, it is a single beat. When identifying a rhythm, be sure to specify the underlying rhythm and the origin of the ectopic beat(s). In this rhythm strip we found that the underlying rhythm was a sinus tachycardia at 136 beats/min. All of the ectopic beats were early and came from the AV junction; therefore, we would identify this rhythm strip as, "Sinus tachycardia at 136 beats/min with frequent PJCs." The ECG characteristics of PJCs are shown in Table 5-1.

What Causes Them?

Premature junctional complexes are less common than either PACs or PVCs. Causes of PJCs include the following:

- Acute coronary syndromes
- Digitalis toxicity
- Electrolyte imbalance
- Heart failure
- Mental and physical fatigue
- Rheumatic heart disease
- Stimulants (e.g., caffeine, tobacco, cocaine)
- Valvular heart disease

What Do I Do About Them?

PJCs do not normally require treatment because most individuals who have PJCs are asymptomatic. However, PJCs

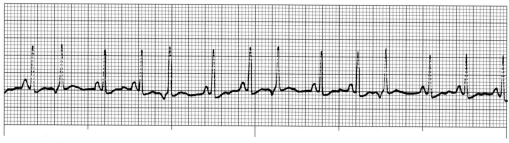

Figure 5-5   Sinus tachycardia at 136 beats/min with frequent premature junctional complexes (PJCs).

Table **5-1**	Characteristics of Premature Junctional Complexes
Rhythm	Regular with *premature* beats
Rate	Usually within normal range, but depends on underlying rhythm
P waves	May occur before, during, or after the QRS; if visible, the P wave is inverted in leads II, III, and aVF
PR interval	If a P wave occurs before the QRS, the PR interval will usually be 0.12 sec or less; if no P wave occurs before the QRS, there will be no PR interval
QRS duration	0.11 sec or less unless abnormally conducted

may lead to symptoms of palpitations or the feeling of skipped beats. Lightheadedness, dizziness, and other signs of decreased cardiac output can occur if PJCs are frequent. If PJCs occur because of ingestion of stimulants or digitalis toxicity, these substances should be withheld.

ECG Pearl

Keep in mind that inverted P waves are normal in lead V$_1$. To determine if a beat or rhythm came from the atrioventricular (AV) junction using this lead, look for a short PR interval. Use lead II, III, or aVF to confirm your findings.

JUNCTIONAL ESCAPE BEATS/RHYTHM

How Do I Recognize It?

[Objectives 2, 3, 4]

A junctional escape beat begins in the AV junction and appears *late* (i.e., after the next expected sinus beat). Junctional escape beats frequently occur during episodes of sinus arrest or follow pauses of nonconducted PACs. Look at Figure 5-6. Looking at the rhythm strip, you can see two normal looking beats on the left and two more on the far right. In the center

of the strip is an odd-looking beat that appears in the middle of a very long pause between beats 2 and 4. Looking more closely at beats 1, 2, 4, and 5 you can see an upright P wave before each QRS complex. These beats came from the SA node. When you calculate the atrial and ventricular rates between these beats, you will find that it is 71 beats/min (1500 ÷ 21 small boxes). On the basis of this information, we know that the underlying rhythm is sinus in origin. Using your calipers or a piece of paper, mark the first and second complexes. When you move the calipers or paper to the right, you can see that beat 3 came *late*; that is, after the next expected sinus beat.

Now let's try to figure out where beat 3 came from and why. If you put your finger over beat 3, can you explain what happened? The long pause between beats 2 and 4 is an episode of sinus arrest. Remember that if the SA node fails to initiate an impulse, an escape pacemaker site (i.e., the AV junction or ventricles) should assume responsibility for pacing the heart. Look closely at beat 3. The QRS complex is narrow, the ST segment is depressed, and there is no P wave before the QRS complex. If you compare the ST segment of beat 3 with the others in the rhythm strip, you can see that the ST segment in beat 3 is shaped differently. It appears that there is an inverted P wave in the ST segment of this beat. The narrow-QRS complex and absence of a positive P wave before the QRS complex tells us the beat came from the AV junction. Because the beat is *late*, it is a junctional escape beat. If beat 3 had been *early*, we would call it a PJC. What happened here? The SA node fired in beats 1 and 2. When the sinus did not fire again when it should have, the AV junction kicked in and fired. Thus a junctional escape beat is *protective*—preventing cardiac standstill. There is a noncompensatory pause after the junctional escape beat during which the SA node resets. This is followed by two sinus beats.

The ST segments of the beats in this rhythm strip are depressed. The PR interval of the sinus beats is prolonged, measuring 0.24 second. Complete identification of the events that occurred in this rhythm strip would include the following description, "Sinus rhythm at 71 beats/min with a prolonged PR interval (0.24 second), an episode of sinus arrest, a junctional escape beat, and ST-segment depression." The ECG characteristics of junctional escape beats are shown in Table 5-2.

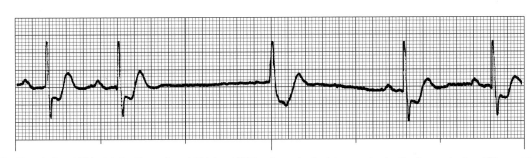

Figure 5-6   Sinus rhythm at 71 beats/min with a prolonged PR interval (0.24 sec), an episode of sinus arrest, a junctional escape beat, and ST-segment depression.

Table **5-2**	Characteristics of Junctional Escape Beats
Rhythm	Regular with *late* beats
Rate	Usually within normal range, but depends on underlying rhythm
P waves	May occur before, during, or after the QRS; if visible, the P wave is inverted in leads II, III, and aVF
PR interval	If a P wave occurs before the QRS, the PR interval will usually be 0.12 sec or less; if no P wave occurs before the QRS, there will be no PR interval
QRS duration	0.11 sec or less unless abnormally conducted

ECG Pearl

Junctional escape beats and rhythms occur when the sinoatrial (SA) node fails to pace the heart or atrioventricular (AV) conduction fails.

A junctional *rhythm* is several sequential junctional escape *beats*. The terms *junctional rhythm* and **junctional escape rhythm** are used interchangeably. Remember that the intrinsic rate of the AV junction is 40 to 60 beats/min. Because a junctional rhythm starts from above the ventricles, the QRS complex is usually narrow and its rhythm is very regular. If the AV junction paces the heart at a rate slower than 40 beats/min, the resulting rhythm is called a **junctional bradycardia**. This may seem confusing because the AV junction's normal pacing rate of 40 to 60 beats/min *is*

bradycardic. However, the term *junctional bradycardia* refers to a rate slower than normal for the AV junction. Figure 5-7 is a continuous rhythm strip. In A, you can see inverted (i.e., retrograde) P waves before the QRS complexes. In B, note the change in the location of the P waves. In the first beat, the retrograde P wave is seen before the QRS. In the second beat, no P wave is seen. In the remaining beats, the P wave is seen after the QRS complexes. The ECG characteristics of a junctional rhythm are shown in Table 5-3.

What Causes It?

Junctional escape beats frequently occur during episodes of sinus arrest or following pauses of nonconducted PACs. Junctional escape beats may also be observed in healthy individuals during sinus bradycardia. Causes of a junctional rhythm include the following:

- Acute coronary syndromes (particularly inferior wall myocardial infarction [MI])
- Effects of medications (e.g., beta-blockers, digitalis, diltiazem, quinidine, verapamil)
- Hypoxia
- Immediately after cardiac surgery
- Increased parasympathetic tone
- Rheumatic heart disease
- SA node disease
- Valvular disease

What Do I Do About It?

The patient may be asymptomatic with a junctional escape rhythm, or he or she may experience signs and symptoms that may be associated with the slow heart rate and decreased

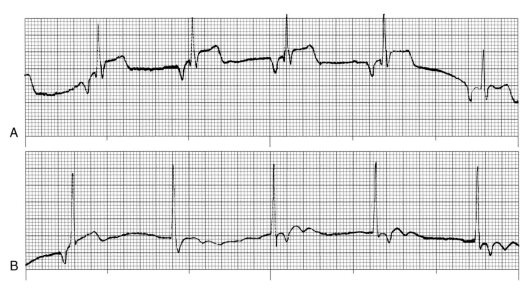

Figure 5-7   Junctional escape rhythm. Continuous strips. **A,** Note the inverted (retrograde) P waves before the QRS complexes. **B,** Note the change in the location of the P waves. In the first beat, the retrograde P wave is seen before the QRS. In the second beat, no P wave is seen. In the remaining beats, the P wave is seen after the QRS complexes.

Table **5-3**	Characteristics of Junctional Escape Rhythm
Rhythm	Very regular
Rate	40 to 60 beats/min
P waves	May occur before, during, or after the QRS; if visible, the P wave is inverted in leads II, III, and aVF
PR interval	If a P wave occurs before the QRS, the PR interval will usually be 0.12 sec or less; if no P wave occurs before the QRS, there will be no PR interval
QRS duration	0.11 sec or less unless abnormally conducted

Table **5-4**	Characteristics of Accelerated Junctional Rhythm
Rhythm	Very regular
Rate	61 to 100 beats/min
P waves	May occur before, during, or after the QRS; if visible, the P wave is inverted in leads II, III, and aVF
PR interval	If a P wave occurs before the QRS, the PR interval will usually be 0.12 sec or less; if no P wave occurs before the QRS, there will be no PR interval
QRS duration	0.11 sec or less unless abnormally conducted

cardiac output. Treatment depends on the cause of the dysrhythmia and the patient's presenting signs and symptoms. Signs and symptoms may include weakness, chest pain or pressure, syncope, an altered level of consciousness, and hypotension. If the dysrhythmia is caused by digitalis toxicity, this medication should be withheld. If the patient's signs and symptoms are related to the slow heart rate, treatment should include application of a pulse oximeter and administration of supplemental oxygen if indicated. Establish intravenous (IV) access, obtain a 12-lead ECG, and administer IV atropine. Reassess the patient's response and continue monitoring the patient.

ACCELERATED JUNCTIONAL RHYTHM

How Do I Recognize It?

[Objective 5]
If the AV junction speeds up and fires at a rate of 61 to 100 beats/min, the resulting rhythm is called an **accelerated junctional rhythm**. This rhythm is caused by enhanced automaticity of the bundle of His. The only ECG difference between a junctional rhythm and an accelerated junctional rhythm is the increase in the ventricular rate. An example of an accelerated junctional rhythm is shown in Figure 5-8. The ECG characteristics of this rhythm are shown in Table 5-4.

What Causes It?

Causes of this dysrhythmia include acute MI, cardiac surgery, chronic obstructive pulmonary disease, digitalis toxicity, hypokalemia, and rheumatic fever.

What Do I Do About It?

The patient is usually asymptomatic because the ventricular rate is 61 to 100 beats/min; however, the patient should be monitored closely. If the rhythm is caused by digitalis toxicity, this medication should be withheld.

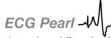 *ECG Pearl*

Junctional Dysrhythmias at a Glance
- Junctional rhythm: 40 to 60 beats/min
- Accelerated junctional rhythm: 61 to 100 beats/min
- Junctional tachycardia: 101 to 180 beats/min

JUNCTIONAL TACHYCARDIA

How Do I Recognize It?

[Objective 6]
Junctional tachycardia is an ectopic rhythm that begins in the pacemaker cells found in the bundle of His. When

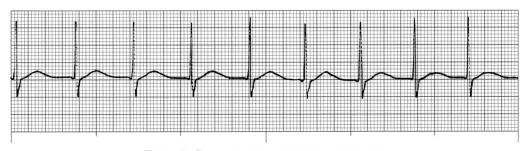

Figure 5-8 Accelerated junctional rhythm at 93 beats/min.

three or more sequential PJCs occur at a rate of more than 100 beats/min, a junctional tachycardia exists. *Nonparoxysmal* (i.e., gradual onset) *junctional tachycardia* usually starts as an accelerated junctional rhythm, but the heart rate gradually increases to more than 100 beats/min. The usual ventricular rate for nonparoxysmal junctional tachycardia is 101 to 140 beats/min. *Paroxysmal junctional tachycardia*, which is also known as *focal* or *automatic junctional tachycardia*, is an uncommon dysrhythmia that starts and ends suddenly and that is often precipitated by a PJC. The ventricular rate for paroxysmal junctional tachycardia is generally faster, at a rate of 140 beats/min or more. When the ventricular rate is greater than 150 beats/min, it is difficult to distinguish junctional tachycardia from AV nodal reentrant tachycardia and AV reentrant tachycardia. An example of junctional tachycardia is shown in Figure 5-9. The ECG characteristics of this rhythm are shown in Table 5-5.

What Causes It?

Junctional tachycardia is rare in adults. When it occurs, it is probably caused by enhanced automaticity. Junctional tachycardia may occur because of an acute coronary syndrome, digitalis toxicity, heart failure, or theophylline administration.

What Do I Do About It?

With sustained ventricular rates of 150 beats/min or more, the patient may complain of a "racing heart" and severe anxiety. Because of the fast ventricular rate, the ventricles may be unable to fill completely, which results in decreased cardiac output. The more rapid the rate, the greater the incidence of symptoms because of increased myocardial oxygen demand. Junctional tachycardia associated with an acute coronary syndrome may do the following:
- Cause heart failure, hypotension, or cardiogenic shock
- Extend the size of an MI

Table 5-5	Characteristics of Junctional Tachycardia
Rhythm	Very regular
Rate	101 to 180 beats/min
P waves	May occur before, during, or after the QRS; if visible, the P wave is inverted in leads II, III, and aVF
PR interval	If a P wave occurs before the QRS, the PR interval will usually be 0.12 sec or less; if no P wave occurs before the QRS, there will be no PR interval
QRS duration	0.11 sec or less unless abnormally conducted

- Increase myocardial ischemia
- Increase the frequency and severity of chest pain
- Predispose the patient to ventricular dysrhythmias

Treatment depends on the severity of the patient's signs and symptoms, and expert consultation is advised. If the patient tolerates the rhythm, observation is often all that is needed. If the patient is symptomatic because of the rapid rate, initial treatment should include application of a pulse oximeter and administration of supplemental oxygen, if indicated. Establish IV access and obtain a 12-lead ECG. Because it is often difficult to distinguish junctional tachycardia from other narrow-QRS tachycardias, vagal maneuvers and, if necessary, IV adenosine may be used to help determine the origin of the rhythm. If the rhythm is the result of digitalis toxicity, the drug should be withheld. In some cases, an antibody called *DigiFab* may be indicated in the treatment of digitalis toxicity, depending on the patient's clinical condition. If the rhythm is the result of theophylline administration, the infusion should be slowed or stopped. A beta-blocker or calcium channel blocker may be ordered (if no contraindications exist) to slow conduction through the AV node and thereby slow the ventricular rate. A summary of junctional rhythm characteristics can be found in Table 5-6.

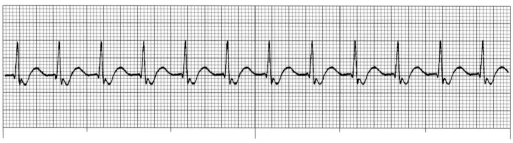

Figure 5-9   Junctional tachycardia at 120 beats/min.

Table 5-6	Junctional Rhythms—Summary of Characteristics				
Characteristic	PJCs	Junctional Escape Beat	Junctional Escape Rhythm	Accelerated Junctional Rhythm	Junctional Tachycardia
Rhythm	Regular with *premature* beats	Regular with *late* beats	Regular	Regular	Regular
Rate (beats/min)	Usually within normal range, but depends on underlying rhythm	Usually within normal range, but depends on underlying rhythm	40 to 60	61 to 100	101 to 180
P waves (leads II, III, aVF)	May occur before, during, or after the QRS; if visible, the P wave is inverted	May occur before, during, or after the QRS; if visible, the P wave is inverted	May occur before, during, or after the QRS; if visible, the P wave is inverted	May occur before, during, or after the QRS; if visible, the P wave is inverted	May occur before, during, or after the QRS; if visible, the P wave is inverted
PR interval	If a P wave occurs before the QRS, the PR interval will usually be 0.12 sec or less; if no P wave occurs before the QRS, there will be no PR interval	If a P wave occurs before the QRS, the PR interval will usually be 0.12 sec or less; if no P wave occurs before the QRS, there will be no PR interval	If a P wave occurs before the QRS, the PR interval will usually be 0.12 sec or less; if no P wave occurs before the QRS, there will be no PR interval	If a P wave occurs before the QRS, the PR interval will usually be 0.12 sec or less; if no P wave occurs before the QRS, there will be no PR interval	If a P wave occurs before the QRS, the PR interval will usually be 0.12 sec or less; if no P wave occurs before the QRS, there will be no PR interval
QRS duration	0.11 sec or less unless abnormally conducted	0.11 sec or less unless abnormally conducted	0.11 sec or less unless abnormally conducted	0.11 sec or less unless abnormally conducted	0.11 sec or less unless abnormally conducted

PJC, premature junctional complex.

STOP & REVIEW—CHAPTER 5

True/False

Indicate whether the statement is true or false.

____1. PJCs are more common than PACs or PVCs.

____2. A PJC produces a positive (upright) P wave in leads II, III, and aVF that comes before, during, or after the QRS complex.

____ 3. The intrinsic rate of the AV junction is 20 to 40 beats/min.

Multiple Choice

Identify the choice that best completes the statement or answers the question.

____4. The term *junctional bradycardia* is used to describe a rhythm that is junctional in origin with:
   a. An atrial rate slower than 60 beats/min.
   b. A ventricular rate of 40 to 60 beats/min.
   c. An atrial rate of 40 to 60 beats/min.
   d. A ventricular rate slower than 40 beats/min.

____5. A _____ pause often follows a PJC and represents the delay during which the SA node resets its rhythm for the next beat.
   a. Noncompensatory (incomplete)
   b. Compensatory (complete)

____6. In rhythms originating from the AV junction, the QRS duration is typically _____ or less unless an intraventricular conduction delay exists.
   a. 0.04 second
   b. 0.11 second
   c. 0.14 second
   d. 0.20 second

____7. An accelerated junctional rhythm is identified by a regular ventricular response occurring at a rate of:
   a. 20 to 40 beats/min.
   b. 40 to 60 beats/min.
   c. 61 to 100 beats/min.
   d. 101 to 180 beats/min.

____ 8. Select the *incorrect* statement regarding junctional dysrhythmias.
   a. A junctional rhythm may be seen in acute coronary syndromes.
   b. An accelerated junctional rhythm is a potentially life-threatening dysrhythmia.
   c. The ventricular rhythm associated with a junctional rhythm is typically very regular.
   d. The QRS complex of a PJC is typically markedly different from the QRS complex of a beat conducted by the SA node.

____ 9. The primary waveform used to differentiate PJCs from PACs is the:
   a. P wave.
   b. Q wave.
   c. R wave.
   d. T wave.

____10. In a junctional rhythm viewed in lead II, where is the location of the P wave on the ECG if ventricular depolarization precedes atrial depolarization?
   a. Before the QRS complex
   b. During the QRS complex
   c. After the QRS complex

Questions 11–14 pertain to the following scenario.

A 63-year-old man is complaining of dizziness that began about 45 minutes ago while cleaning his garage. Because the patient's oxygen saturation level on room air was 90%, supplemental oxygen is being administered. The cardiac monitor has been applied and reveals the rhythm below. A coworker is attempting to establish intravenous access.

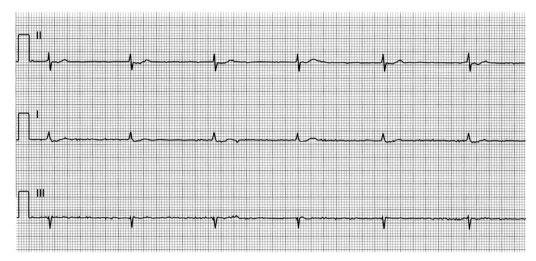

Figure 5-10

_____11. Which of the following statements is true regarding this patient's cardiac rhythm?
   a. The atrial rhythm is irregular.
   b. There are more P waves than QRS complexes.
   c. The ventricular rhythm is regular and the QRS is wide.
   d. The ventricular rhythm is regular and the QRS is narrow.

_____12. The patient's ventricular rate is:
   a. 30 beats/min.
   b. 45 beats/min.
   c. 60 beats/min.
   d. 75 beats/min.

_____13. The rhythm shown on the cardiac monitor is:
   a. Sinus bradycardia.
   b. Junctional bradycardia.
   c. Junctional escape rhythm.
   d. Accelerated junctional rhythm.

_____14. The patient's blood pressure is 82/50 mm Hg, ventilations 16 breaths/min. He states his normal blood pressure is about 130/80 mm Hg. The patient denies chest discomfort and states he takes no prescription medications. His skin is cool, pink, and moist and his breath sounds are clear. Intravenous access has been successfully established. Based on the information provided, which of the following statements is true regarding this patient situation?
   a. Because the patient is symptomatic with this rhythm, a vagal maneuver should be attempted.
   b. The patient is symptomatic with this rhythm. Obtain a 12-lead ECG and then administer atropine IV.
   c. Therapeutic interventions are not indicated because there is no evidence of ST-segment elevation on the cardiac monitor.
   d. Although the patient is complaining of dizziness, this symptom does not warrant any further intervention other than cardiac monitoring at this time.

Matching

Match the key terms with their definitions by placing the letter of each correct answer in the space provided.

a. Retrograde
b. Accelerated junctional rhythm
c. Nodal rhythms
d. Inverted P wave appears before the QRS complex in leads II, III, and aVF
e. Location of the AV node
f. Junctional tachycardia
g. Digitalis
h. Hidden within the QRS complex (not visible)
i. Location of the bundle of His
j. Premature junctional complex

_____15. Lower part of the right atrium, above the base of the tricuspid valve

_____16. Name given to a dysrhythmia that originates in the AV junction with a ventricular rate between 101 and 180 beats/min

_____17. Upper part of the interventricular septum

_____**18.** Location of the P wave on the ECG if atrial and ventricular depolarization occurs simultaneously

_____**19.** Term formerly used for dysrhythmias that originate in the AV junction

_____**20.** A beat originating within the AV junction that appears earlier than the next expected sinus beat

_____**21.** Name given to a dysrhythmia that originates in the AV junction with a ventricular rate between 61 and 100 beats/min

_____**22.** Occurring in a backward direction

_____**23.** Location of the P wave on the ECG if atrial depolarization precedes ventricular depolarization

_____**24.** Toxicity/excess of this medication is a common cause of junctional dysrhythmias

Short Answer

25. Fill in the blank areas in the table below to help you recall the primary differences among junctional rhythm, accelerated junctional rhythm, and junctional tachycardia.

ECG Finding	Junctional Rhythm	Accelerated Junctional Rhythm	Junctional Tachycardia
Rhythm	Regular	Regular	Regular
Rate (beats/min)			
P waves (lead II)			
PR interval			
QRS duration	0.11 sec or less unless abnormally conducted	0.11 sec or less unless abnormally conducted	0.11 sec or less unless abnormally conducted

JUNCTIONAL RHYTHMS—*PRACTICE RHYTHM STRIPS*

For each of the following rhythm strips, determine the atrial and ventricular rate and rhythm, measure the PR interval, QRS duration, and QT interval, and then identify the rhythm. Note: These rhythm strips include sinus, atrial, and junctional rhythms.

26. Identify the rhythm.

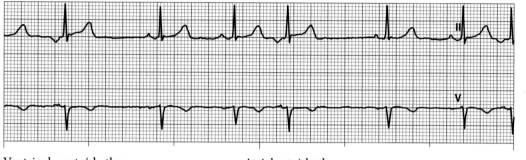

Figure 5-11

Ventricular rate/rhythm _____ Atrial rate/rhythm _____

PR interval _____ QRS duration _____ QT interval _____

Identification _____

27. Identify the rhythm.

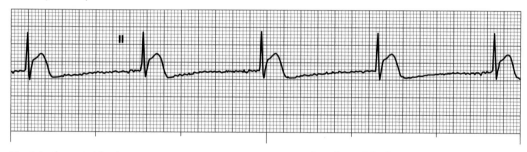

Figure 5-12

Ventricular rate/rhythm _____ Atrial rate/rhythm _____

PR interval _____ QRS duration _____ QT interval _____

Identification _____

28. This rhythm strip is from a 74-year-old woman complaining of difficulty breathing. Her blood pressure is 158/122 mm Hg. Identify the rhythm (lead II).

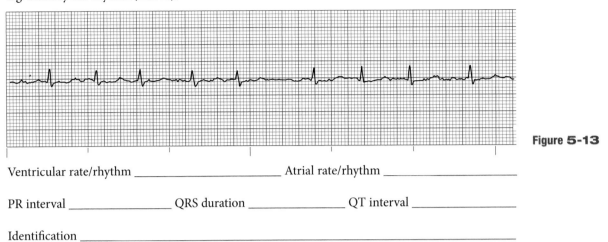

Figure 5-13

Ventricular rate/rhythm _____ Atrial rate/rhythm _____

PR interval _____ QRS duration _____ QT interval _____

Identification _____

29. This rhythm strip (lead II) is from a 63-year-old woman who is complaining of dizziness.

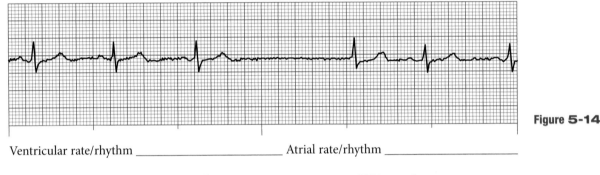

Figure 5-14

Ventricular rate/rhythm _____ Atrial rate/rhythm _____

PR interval _____ QRS duration _____ QT interval _____

Identification _____

30. Identify the rhythm (lead II).

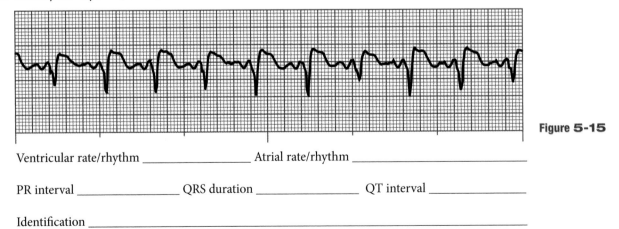

Figure 5-15

Ventricular rate/rhythm _____ Atrial rate/rhythm _____

PR interval _____ QRS duration _____ QT interval _____

Identification _____

31. Identify the rhythm (lead II).

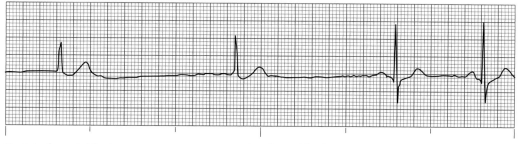

Figure 5-16

Ventricular rate/rhythm _____ Atrial rate/rhythm _____

PR interval _____ QRS duration _____ QT interval _____

Identification _____

32. Identify the rhythm.

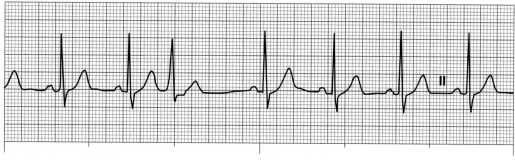

Figure 5-17

Ventricular rate/rhythm _____ Atrial rate/rhythm _____

PR interval _____ QRS duration _____ QT interval _____

Identification _____

33. Identify the rhythm.

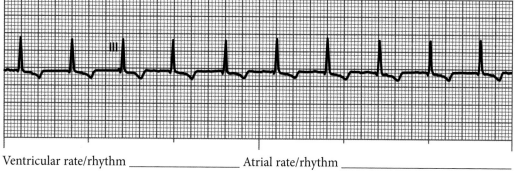

Figure 5-18

Ventricular rate/rhythm _____ Atrial rate/rhythm _____

PR interval _____ QRS duration _____ QT interval _____

Identification _____

34. Identify the rhythm.

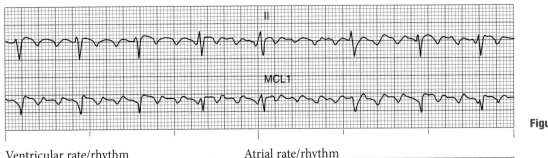

Figure 5-19

Ventricular rate/rhythm _____ Atrial rate/rhythm _____

PR interval _____ QRS duration _____ QT interval _____

Identification _____

35. Identify the rhythm (lead III).

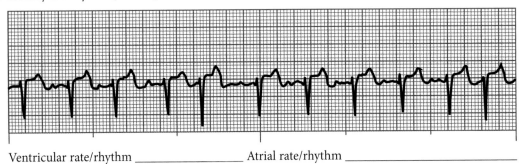

Figure 5-20

Ventricular rate/rhythm _____ Atrial rate/rhythm _____

PR interval _____ QRS duration _____ QT interval _____

Identification _____

36. Identify the rhythm (lead II).

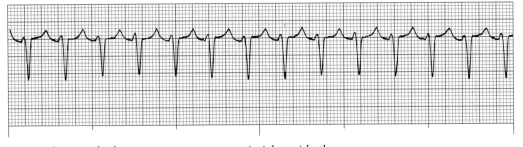

Figure 5-21

Ventricular rate/rhythm _____ Atrial rate/rhythm _____

PR interval _____ QRS duration _____ QT interval _____

Identification _____

37. This rhythm strip (lead II) is from an 88-year-old woman who experienced a syncopal episode. Her blood sugar level is 96 mg/dL. She takes verapamil. The patient's medical history includes a myocardial infarction 9 years ago, a stroke 5 years ago, hypertension, and diabetes.

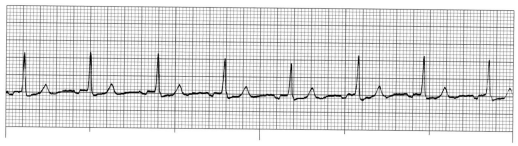

Figure 5-22

Ventricular rate/rhythm _____ Atrial rate/rhythm _____

PR interval _____ QRS duration _____ QT interval _____

Identification _____

38. Identify the rhythm.

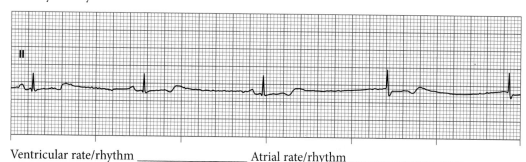

Figure 5-23

Ventricular rate/rhythm _____ Atrial rate/rhythm _____

PR interval _____ QRS duration _____ QT interval _____

Identification _____

39. Identify the rhythm (lead II).

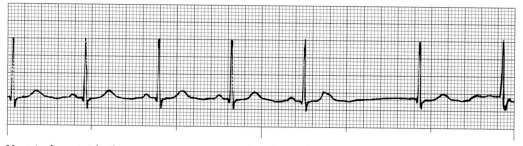

Figure 5-24

Ventricular rate/rhythm _____ Atrial rate/rhythm _____

PR interval _____ QRS duration _____ QT interval _____

Identification _____

40. Identify the rhythm (lead II).

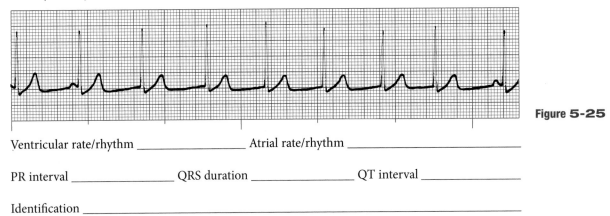

Figure 5-25

Ventricular rate/rhythm _____ Atrial rate/rhythm _____

PR interval _____ QRS duration _____ QT interval _____

Identification _____

41. This rhythm strip is from a 43-year-old woman who was complaining of palpitations. The patient has a history of supra-ventricular tachycardia and states that she cannot tolerate adenosine. This rhythm was observed on the cardiac monitor after diltiazem administration. Identify the rhythm.

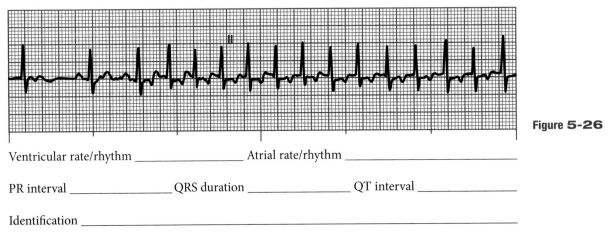

Figure 5-26

Ventricular rate/rhythm _____ Atrial rate/rhythm _____

PR interval _____ QRS duration _____ QT interval _____

Identification _____

42. This rhythm strip (lead I) is from an unresponsive 51-year-old man who has a history of esophageal varices and gastroin-testinal bleeding. His blood pressure is 182/100 mg Hg.

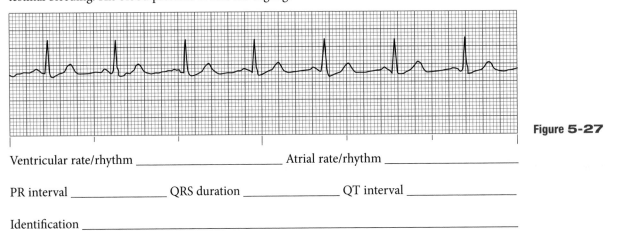

Figure 5-27

Ventricular rate/rhythm _____ Atrial rate/rhythm _____

PR interval _____ QRS duration _____ QT interval _____

Identification _____

43. Identify the rhythm (lead II).

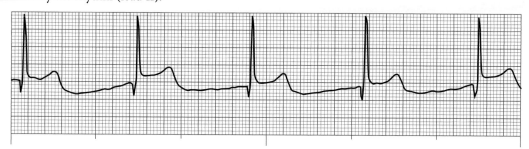

Figure 5-28

Ventricular rate/rhythm _____ Atrial rate/rhythm _____

PR interval _____ QRS duration _____ QT interval _____

Identification _____

44. This rhythm strip (lead II) is from a 53-year-old man complaining of chest pressure and shortness of breath. His blood pressure is 130/86 mm Hg, and his ventilatory rate is 20 breaths/min. He has a history of a spinal cord injury and coronary artery disease.

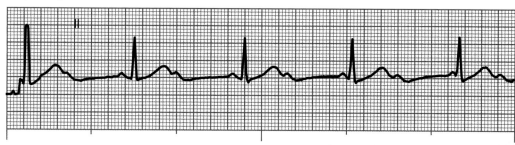

Figure 5-29

Ventricular rate/rhythm _____ Atrial rate/rhythm _____

PR interval _____ QRS duration _____ QT interval _____

Identification _____

45. These rhythm strips are from a 76-year-old woman who was complaining of weakness.

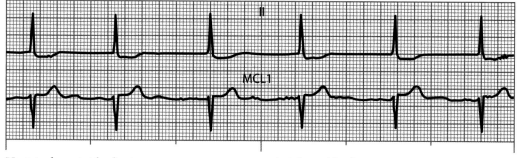

Figure 5-30

Ventricular rate/rhythm _____ Atrial rate/rhythm _____

PR interval _____ QRS duration _____ QT interval _____

Identification _____

STOP & REVIEW ANSWERS

True/False

1. ANS: F

2. ANS: F

3. ANS: F

The atrioventricular (AV) node and the nonbranching portion of the bundle of His are called the *AV junction.*

Multiple Choice

4. ANS: D

If the AV junction paces the heart at a rate slower than 40 beats/min, the resulting rhythm is called a *junctional bradycardia.* This may seem confusing because the AV junction's normal pacing rate (40 to 60 beats/min) *is* bradycardic. However, the term *junctional bradycardia* refers to a rate slower than normal for the AV junction.
OBJ: Describe the ECG characteristics, possible causes, signs and symptoms, and initial emergency care for a junctional escape rhythm.

5. ANS: A

A noncompensatory (incomplete) pause often follows a premature junctional complex (PJC). This pause represents the delay during which the sinoatrial (SA) node resets its rhythm for the next beat.
OBJ: Explain the difference between a compensatory and noncompensatory pause.

6. ANS: B

The QRS duration associated with a rhythm that begins in the AV junction measures 0.11 second or less if conduction through the bundle branches, Purkinje fibers, and ventricles is normal.
OBJ: Describe the ECG characteristics, possible causes, signs and symptoms, and initial emergency care for a junctional escape rhythm.

7. ANS: C

An accelerated junctional rhythm is a dysrhythmia originating in the AV bundle with a ventricular rate between 61 and 100 beats/min.
OBJ: Describe the ECG characteristics, possible causes, signs and symptoms, and initial emergency care for an accelerated junctional rhythm.

8. ANS: B

The patient who has an accelerated junctional rhythm is usually asymptomatic because the ventricular rate is 61 to 100 beats/min, which is the same rate as a sinus rhythm.
OBJ: Describe the ECG characteristics, possible causes, signs and symptoms, and initial emergency care for an accelerated junctional rhythm.

The bundle of His has pacemaker cells that are capable of discharging at a rhythmic rate of 40 to 60 beats/min.
OBJ: Describe the location, function, and (where appropriate), the intrinsic rate of the following structures: Sinoatrial (SA) node, AV bundle, and Purkinje fibers.

9. ANS: A

You can usually tell the difference between a premature atrial complex (PAC) and a PJC by the P wave. A PAC typically has an upright P wave before the QRS complex in leads II, III, and aVF. A P wave may or may not be present with a PJC. If a P wave is present, it is inverted (retrograde) and may precede or follow the QRS. PJCs can be misdiagnosed when the P wave of a PAC is buried in the preceding T wave.
OBJ: Describe the ECG characteristics, possible causes, signs and symptoms, and initial emergency care for PJCs.

10. ANS: C

If the AV junction paces the heart, the electrical impulse must travel in a backward (retrograde) direction to activate the atria. If a P wave is seen, it will be inverted in leads II, III, and aVF because the impulse is traveling away from the positive electrode. If the atria depolarize before the ventricles, an inverted P wave will be seen *before* the QRS complex and the PR interval will usually measure 0.12 second or less. The PR interval is shorter than usual because an impulse that begins in the AV junction does not have to travel as far to stimulate the ventricles. If the atria and ventricles depolarize at the same time, a P wave will not be visible because it will be hidden in the QRS complex. When the atria are depolarized after the ventricles, the P wave typically distorts the end of the QRS complex and an inverted P wave will appear *after* the QRS.
OBJ: Describe the ECG characteristics, possible causes, signs and symptoms, and initial emergency care for a junctional escape rhythm.

11. ANS: D

In these rhythm strips, the atrial rate and rhythm cannot be determined because P waves are not visible. The ventricular rhythm is regular and the QRS is narrow, measuring 0.06 second.
OBJ: Describe the ECG characteristics, possible causes, signs and symptoms, and initial emergency care for a junctional escape rhythm.

12. ANS: B

The patient's ventricular rate is 45 beats/min (1500 small boxes divided by 33).

OBJ: Identify how heart rates, durations, and amplitudes may be determined from electrocardiographic recordings.

13. ANS: C

The cardiac monitor shows a junctional escape rhythm at 45 beats/min.

OBJ: Describe the ECG characteristics, possible causes, signs and symptoms, and initial emergency care for a junctional escape rhythm.

14. ANS: B

Although there is no evidence of ST-segment elevation on the cardiac monitor, this patient is symptomatic with his slow heart rate as evidenced by his dizziness and hypotension. Treatment of a symptomatic bradycardia should include application of a pulse oximeter and administration of supplemental oxygen (if indicated) and establishing intravenous (IV) access, which have already been done. Next, obtain a 12-lead ECG and then administer atropine IV. Reassess the patient's response to your interventions and continue to monitor the patient. Because vagal maneuvers are used to attempt to slow the heart rate of some *tachycardias* and this patient is *bradycardic*, vagal maneuvers are contraindicated in this situation.

Matching

15. ANS: E
16. ANS: F
17. ANS: I
18. ANS: H
19. ANS: C

20. ANS: J
21. ANS: B
22. ANS: A
23. ANS: D
24. ANS: G

Short Answer

25. ANS:

ECG Finding	Junctional Rhythm	Accelerated Junctional Rhythm	Junctional Tachycardia
Rhythm	Regular	Regular	Regular
Rate (beats/min)	**40 to 60**	**61 to 100**	**101 to 180**
P waves (lead II)	**May occur before, during, or after the QRS; if visible, the P wave is inverted**	**May occur before, during, or after the QRS; if visible, the P wave is inverted**	**May occur before, during, or after the QRS; if visible, the P wave is inverted**
PR interval	**If a P wave occurs before the QRS, the PR interval will usually be 0.12 sec or less; if no P wave occurs before the QRS, there will be no PR interval**	**If a P wave occurs before the QRS, the PR interval will usually be 0.12 sec or less; if no P wave occurs before the QRS, there will be no PR interval**	**If a P wave occurs before the QRS, the PR interval will usually be 0.12 sec or less; if no P wave occurs before the QRS, there will be no PR interval**
QRS duration	0.11 sec or less unless abnormally conducted	0.11 sec or less unless abnormally conducted	0.11 sec or less unless abnormally conducted

OBJ: Describe the ECG characteristics, possible causes, signs and symptoms, and initial emergency care for a junctional escape rhythm. Describe the ECG characteristics, possible causes, signs and symptoms, and initial emergency care for an accelerated junctional rhythm. Describe the ECG characteristics, possible causes, signs and symptoms, and initial emergency care for junctional tachycardia.

26. Figure 5-11 answer

Ventricular rate/rhythm	53 to 97 beats/min (sinus beats); irregular (every third beat is a premature junctional complex [PJC])
Atrial rate/rhythm	53 to 97 beats/min (sinus beats); irregular (every third beat is a PJC)
PR interval	0.12 to 0.16 sec (sinus beats)
QRS duration	0.06 sec (sinus beats)
QT interval	0.36 sec (sinus beats)
Identification	Sinus rhythm at 53 to 97 beats/min with PJCs (junctional trigeminy)

27. Figure 5-12 answer

Ventricular rate/rhythm	44 beats/min; regular
Atrial rate/rhythm	44 beats/min; regular
PR interval	0.14 sec
QRS duration	0.08 sec
QT interval	0.32 sec
Identification	Junctional rhythm at 44 beats/min; ST-segment elevation

28. Figure 5-13 answer

Ventricular rate/rhythm	65 to 103 beats/min; irregular
Atrial rate/rhythm	Unable to determine
PR interval	Unable to determine
QRS duration	0.06 to 0.08 sec
QT interval	Unable to determine
Identification	Atrial fibrillation at 65 to 103 beats/min

29. Figure 5-14 answer

Ventricular rate/rhythm	64 beats/min (sinus beats); regular except for the event
Atrial rate/rhythm	64 beats/min (sinus beats); regular except for the event
PR interval	0.16 to 0.18 sec
QRS duration	0.08 sec
QT interval	0.44 sec
Identification	Sinus rhythm at 64 beats/min with an episode of sinus arrest and a junctional escape beat

30. Figure 5-15 answer

Ventricular rate/rhythm	98 beats/min; regular
Atrial rate/rhythm	98 beats/min; regular
PR interval	0.12 sec
QRS duration	0.08 sec
QT interval	0.32 sec
Identification	Accelerated junctional rhythm at 98 beats/min; ST-segment elevation

31. Figure 5-16 answer

Ventricular rate/rhythm	30 beats/min (junctional beats) to 56 beats/min (sinus beats); irregular
Atrial rate/rhythm	30 beats/min (junctional beats) to 56 beats/min (sinus beats); irregular
PR interval	None (junctional beats) to 0.18 sec (sinus beats)
QRS duration	0.04 sec (junctional beats) to 0.08 sec (sinus beats)
QT interval	0.36 sec
Identification	Junctional bradycardia at 30 beats/min to sinus bradycardia at 56 beats/min

32. Figure 5-17 answer

Ventricular rate/rhythm	56 to 120 beats/min; irregular
Atrial rate/rhythm	56 to 120 beats/min; irregular
PR interval	0.16 sec
QRS duration	0.08 sec
QT interval	0.36 sec
Identification	Sinus rhythm at 56 to 120 beats/min with a premature junctional complex (PJC) (beat 3 is a PJC)

33. Figure 5-18 answer

Ventricular rate/rhythm	100 beats/min; regular
Atrial rate/rhythm	None
PR interval	None
QRS duration	0.08 sec
QT interval	0.28 sec
Identification	Accelerated junctional rhythm at 100 beats/min

34. Figure 5-19 answer

Ventricular rate/rhythm	58 to 79 beats/min; irregular
Atrial rate/rhythm	Unable to determine
PR interval	Unable to determine
QRS duration	0.10 sec
QT interval	Unable to determine
Identification	Atrial flutter at 58 to 79 beats/min

35. Figure 5-20 answer

Ventricular rate/rhythm	86 to 150 beats/min; irregular
Atrial rate/rhythm	86 to 150 beats/min; irregular
PR interval	0.20 sec
QRS duration	0.08 to 0.10 sec
QT interval	0.24 to 0.28 sec
Identification	Sinus rhythm at 86 to 150 beats/min with two premature junctional complexes (PJCs); ST-segment elevation (beats 5 and 11 are PJCs)

36. Figure 5-21 answer

Ventricular rate/rhythm	138 beats/min; regular
Atrial rate/rhythm	Unable to determine
PR interval	Unable to determine
QRS duration	0.10 sec
QT interval	0.36 sec
Identification	Narrow-QRS tachycardia, probably junctional tachycardia, at 138 beats/min

37. Figure 5-22 answer

Ventricular rate/rhythm	75 beats/min; regular
Atrial rate/rhythm	75 beats/min; regular
PR interval	0.16 sec
QRS duration	0.08 sec
QT interval	0.32 sec
Identification	Accelerated junctional rhythm at 75 beats/min

38. Figure 5-23 answer

Ventricular rate/rhythm	33 beats/min (sinus beats); 32 beats/min (junctional beats)
Atrial rate/rhythm	33 beats/min (sinus beats); unable to determine (junctional beats)
PR interval	0.20 sec (sinus beats)
QRS duration	0.04 to 0.06 sec
QT interval	0.40 sec
Identification	Sinus bradycardia at 33 beats/min to junctional bradycardia at 32 beats/min

39. Figure 5-24 answer

Ventricular rate/rhythm	45 to 70 beats/min; irregular
Atrial rate/rhythm	45 to 70 beats/min; irregular
PR interval	0.16 sec
QRS duration	0.08 sec
QT interval	0.36 sec
Identification	Sinus rhythm at 45 to 70 beats/min with a nonconducted premature atrial complex (PAC) (note distortion of the T wave of the beat preceding the pause) and a junctional escape beat

40. Figure 5-25 answer

Ventricular rate/rhythm	79 beats/min; regular (junctional beats)
Atrial rate/rhythm	Not measurable in junctional beats
PR interval	Not measurable in junctional beats
QRS duration	0.06 sec
QT interval	0.32 sec
Identification	Sinus rhythm changing to an accelerated junctional rhythm at 79 beats/min, back to a sinus rhythm

41. Figure 5-26 answer

Ventricular rate/rhythm	188 beats/min; regular during the tachycardia
Atrial rate/rhythm	Unable to determine
PR interval	Unable to determine
QRS duration	0.08 sec
QT interval	Unable to determine
Identification	Junctional beat, two sinus beats, changing to a narrow-QRS tachycardia that is probably junctional tachycardia at 188 beats/min

42. Figure 5-27 answer

Ventricular rate/rhythm	75 beats/min; regular
Atrial rate/rhythm	75 beats/min; regular
PR interval	0.12 sec
QRS duration	0.08 sec
QT interval	0.40 sec
Identification	Sinus rhythm at 75 beats/min

43. Figure 5-28 answer

Ventricular rate/rhythm	45 beats/min; regular
Atrial rate/rhythm	None
PR interval	None
QRS duration	0.08 sec
QT interval	0.48 sec
Identification	Junctional rhythm at 45 beats/min; ST-segment elevation

44. Figure 5-29 answer

Ventricular rate/rhythm	58 beats/min; regular
Atrial rate/rhythm	58 beats/min; regular
PR interval	0.20 sec
QRS duration	0.06 sec
QT interval	0.36 sec
Identification	Sinus bradycardia at 58 beats/min

45. Figure 5-30 answer

Ventricular rate/rhythm	57 beats/min; regular
Atrial rate/rhythm	None
PR interval	None
QRS duration	0.06 to 08 sec
QT interval	0.34 sec
Identification	Junctional rhythm at 57 beats/min; ST-segment elevation

Ventricular Rhythms

6

CHAPTER

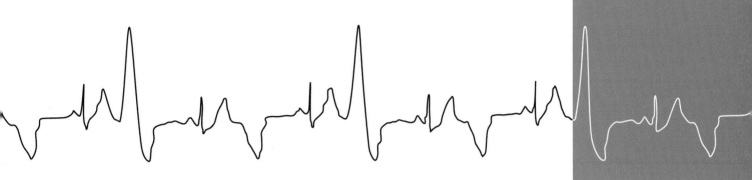

LEARNING OBJECTIVES

After reading this chapter, you should be able to:

1. Describe the electrocardiogram (ECG) characteristics, possible causes, signs and symptoms, and initial emergency care for premature ventricular complexes (PVCs).
2. Explain the terms *bigeminy*, *trigeminy*, *quadrigeminy*, and *run* when used to describe premature complexes.
3. Explain the difference between PVCs and ventricular escape beats.
4. Describe the ECG characteristics of ventricular escape beats.
5. Describe the ECG characteristics, possible causes, signs and symptoms, and initial emergency care for an idioventricular rhythm (IVR).
6. Explain the term *pulseless electrical activity* (PEA).
7. Describe the ECG characteristics, possible causes, signs and symptoms, and initial emergency care for an accelerated idioventricular rhythm (AIVR).

8. Explain the terms *sustained* and *nonsustained ventricular tachycardia* (VT), *monomorphic VT*, and *polymorphic VT* (PMVT).
9. Describe the ECG characteristics, possible causes, signs and symptoms, and initial emergency care for monomorphic VT.
10. Describe the ECG characteristics, possible causes, signs and symptoms, and initial emergency care for PMVT.
11. Describe the ECG characteristics, possible causes, signs and symptoms, and initial emergency care for ventricular fibrillation (VF).
12. State the purpose, indications, and procedure for defibrillation.
13. Describe the ECG characteristics, possible causes, signs and symptoms, and initial emergency care for asystole.

KEY TERMS

Accelerated idioventricular rhythm (AIVR): Dysrhythmia originating in the ventricles with a rate between 41 and 100 beats/min

Agonal rhythm: Dysrhythmia similar in appearance to an IVR but occurring at a rate of less than 20 beats/min; dying heart

Asystole: A total absence of ventricular electrical activity

Automated external defibrillator (AED): A machine with a sophisticated computer system that analyzes a patient's heart rhythm using an algorithm to distinguish shockable rhythms from nonshockable rhythms and providing visual and auditory instructions to the rescuer to deliver an electrical shock, if a shock is indicated.

Atrioventricular (AV) dissociation: Any dysrhythmia in which the atria and ventricles beat independently (e.g., VT, complete AV block)

Burst: Three or more sequential ectopic beats; also referred to as a salvo or run

Coarse ventricular fibrillation: VF with fibrillatory waves greater than 3 mm in height

Current: The flow of an electrical charge from one point to another

Defibrillation: Delivery of an electrical current across the heart muscle over a very brief period to terminate an abnormal heart rhythm; also called *unsynchronized countershock* or *asynchronous countershock* because the delivery of current has no relationship to the cardiac cycle.

Fine ventricular fibrillation: VF with fibrillatory waves less than 3 mm in height

Interpolated PVC: PVC that occurs between two normally conducted QRS complexes and that does not disturb the next ventricular depolarization or sinoatrial node activity

Fusion beat: Beat that occurs because of simultaneous activation of one cardiac chamber by two sites (foci); in pacing, the ECG waveform that results when an intrinsic depolarization and a pacing stimulus occur simultaneously and both contribute to depolarization of that cardiac chamber

Monomorphic: Having the same shape

Polymorphic: Varying in shape

Prophylaxis: Preventive treatment

Run: Three or more sequential ectopic beats; also referred to as a "salvo" or "burst"

Salvo: Three or more sequential ectopic beats; also referred to as a "run" or "burst"

Torsades de pointes (TdP): Type of polymorphic VT associated with a prolonged QT interval; the QRS changes in shape, amplitude, and width and appears to "twist" around the isoelectric line, resembling a spindle

Ventricular tachycardia (VT): Dysrhythmia originating in the ventricles with a ventricular response greater than 100 beats/min

INTRODUCTION

The ventricles are the heart's least efficient pacemaker (Figure 6-1). If the ventricles function as the heart's pacemaker, they normally generate impulses at a rate of 20 to 40 beats/min. The ventricles may assume responsibility for pacing the heart if the sinoatrial (SA) node fails to discharge, an impulse from the SA node is generated but blocked as it exits the SA node, the rate of discharge of the SA node is slower than that of the ventricles, or an irritable site in either ventricle produces an early beat or rapid rhythm.

The shape of the QRS complex is influenced by the site of origin of the electrical impulse. Normally an electrical impulse that begins in the SA node, atria, or AV junction results in depolarization of the right and left ventricles at about the same time. The resulting QRS complex is usually narrow, measuring 0.11 second or less in duration.

If an area of either ventricle becomes ischemic or injured, it can become irritable. This irritability affects the manner in which impulses are conducted. Ventricular beats and rhythms can start in any part of the ventricles and may occur because of reentry, enhanced automaticity, or triggered activity.[1,2] When an ectopic site within a ventricle assumes responsibility for pacing the heart, the electrical impulse bypasses the normal intraventricular conduction pathway. This results in stimulation of the ventricles at slightly different times. As a result, ventricular beats and rhythms usually have QRS complexes that are abnormally shaped and longer than normal (e.g., greater than 0.12 second). If the atria are depolarized after the ventricles, retrograde P waves may be seen.

Because ventricular depolarization is abnormal, ventricular repolarization is also abnormal, and results in changes in ST segments and T waves. The T waves are usually in a direction opposite that of the QRS complex; if the major QRS deflection is negative, the ST segment is usually elevated and

the T wave positive (i.e., upright). If the major QRS deflection is positive, the ST segment is usually depressed and the T wave is usually negative (i.e., inverted). P waves are usually not seen with ventricular dysrhythmias but if they are visible, they have no consistent relationship to the QRS complex (i.e., **AV dissociation**).

CLINICAL CORRELATION

When a ventricular rhythm is present, the appearance of ST segments and T waves in the opposite direction of the last portion of the QRS complex can complicate matters when looking for ECG signs of myocardial injury and infarction. For example, when the QRS complexes of a ventricular rhythm are negative, the ST segment is usually elevated. The resulting ST-segment elevation may be the result of abnormal repolarization, and not a result of any infarction-related causes. Assess the patient's clinical presentation and the results of other diagnostic studies, in addition to your ECG findings.

PREMATURE VENTRICULAR COMPLEXES

How Do I Recognize Them?

[Objective 1]

A PVC, which is also called a *premature ventricular extrasystole*, *ventricular premature beat*, or *premature ventricular depolarization*, arises from an irritable site (i.e., focus) within either ventricle. By definition, a PVC is *premature*, occurring earlier than the next expected sinus beat. The shape of the QRS of a PVC depends on the location of the irritable focus within the ventricles (Figure 6-2). The width of the QRS of a PVC is typically 0.12 second or greater because the PVC causes the ventricles to fire prematurely and in an abnormal manner (Figure 6-3). The T wave is usually in a direction that is opposite that of the QRS complex.

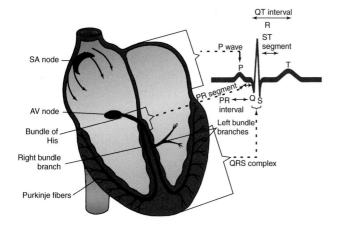

Figure 6-1   The ventricles are the heart's least efficient pacemaker. AV, atrioventricular; SA, sinoatrial.

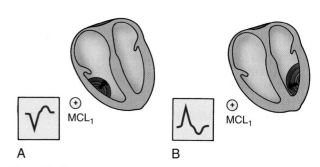

Figure 6-2   **A,** Right ventricular premature ventricular complex (PVC). The spread of depolarization is from right to left, away from the positive electrode in lead V₁ (MCL₁), resulting in a wide, negative QRS complex. **B,** Left ventricular PVC. The spread of depolarization is from left to right, toward the positive electrode in lead V₁ (MCL₁). The QRS complex is wide and upright.

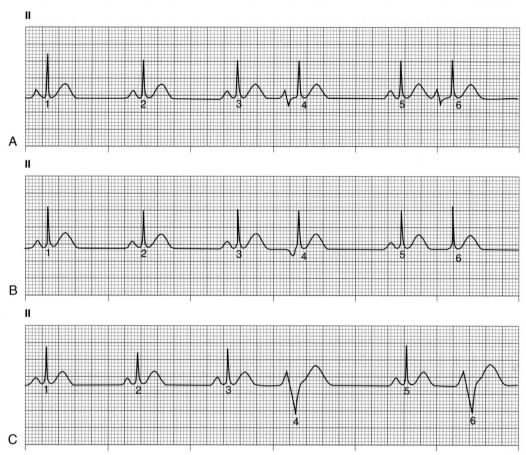

Figure 6-3   Premature beats. **A,** Sinus rhythm with premature atrial complexes (PACs). The fourth and sixth beats are preceded by premature P waves that look different from the normally conducted sinus beats. Note that the QRS complex that follows each of these PACs is narrow and identical in appearance to that of the sinus-conducted beats. **B,** Sinus rhythm with premature junctional complexes (PJCs). The fourth and sixth beats are PJCs. Beat 4 is preceded by an inverted P wave with a short PR interval. There is no identifiable atrial activity associated with beat 6. **C,** Sinus rhythm with premature ventricular complexes (PVCs). The fourth and sixth beats are very different in appearance from the normally conducted sinus beats. Beats 4 and 6 are PVCs. They are not preceded by P waves.

A **compensatory pause** often follows a PVC and occurs because the SA node is usually not affected by the PVC (Figure 6-4). The SA node discharges at its regular rate and rhythm, including the period during and after the PVC. It is important to note that the presence of a full compensatory pause does not reliably differentiate ventricular ectopy from atrial ectopy; this is because atrial ectopy may produce a similar compensatory pattern if it does not reset the SA node.[3] In addition, when backward (i.e., retrograde) conduction occurs and a PVC is conducted to the atria, as in slow sinus rates, the PVC can reset the SA node, thereby resulting in a noncompensatory pause.[2,3]

A **fusion beat** is a result of an electrical impulse from a supraventricular site (e.g., SA node) discharging at the same time as an ectopic site in the ventricles (Figure 6-5). Because fusion beats are a result of both supraventricular and ventricular depolarization, these beats do not resemble normally conducted beats, nor do they resemble true ventricular beats.

Patterns of Premature Ventricular Complexes

PVCs may occur alone or in groups (i.e., patterns). PVCs that occur infrequently with no identifiable pattern are

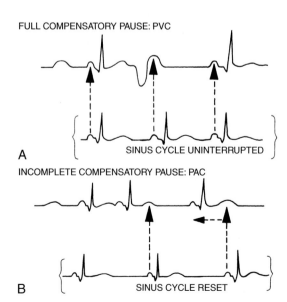

Figure 6-4   A premature ventricular complex (PVC) is often followed by a full compensatory pause. A premature atrial complex (PAC) is often followed by a noncompensatory (incomplete) pause.

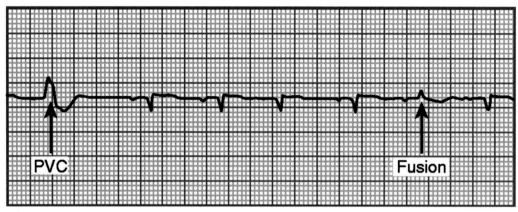

Figure 6-5   Ventricular fusion beat (second arrow). The QRS duration is only 0.08 second, and the shape represents the normal QRS and the previous premature ventricular complex (PVC).

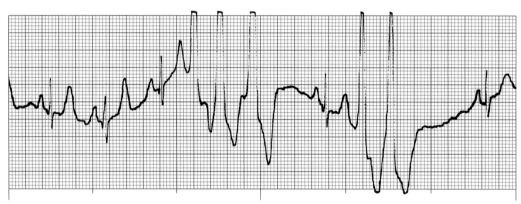

Figure 6-6   Sinus rhythm with a run of ventricular tachycardia (VT) and one episode of ventricular couplets.

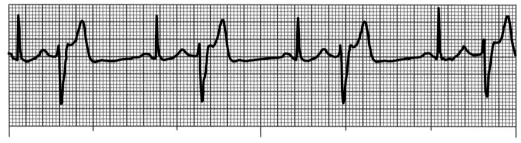

Figure 6-7   Sinus bradycardia with ventricular bigeminy.

called *isolated* PVCs. Two consecutive PVCs are called a *pair* or *couplet* (Figure 6-6). Couplets are also referred to as *two in a row* or *back-to-back* PVCs. The appearance of couplets indicates the ventricular ectopic site is very irritable. Three or more sequential PVCs are termed a **run** or **burst**, and three or more PVCs that occur in a row at a rate of more than 100 beats/min is considered a run of VT.

Ventricular bigeminy describes a rhythm in which every other beat is a PVC (Figure 6-7); with *ventricular trigeminy* every third beat is a PVC; and with *ventricular quadrigeminy*, every fourth beat is a PVC.

Types of Premature Ventricular Complexes
Uniform and Multiform Premature Ventricular Complexes
[Objective 2]

PVCs that look alike in the same lead and begin from the same anatomic site (i.e., focus) are called *uniform PVCs* (Figure 6-8). PVCs that look different from one another in the same lead are called *multiform PVCs* (Figure 6-9). The terms *unifocal* and *multifocal* are sometimes used to describe PVCs that are similar or different in appearance. Uniform PVCs are unifocal; that is, they arise from the same anatomic site within the ventricles. Multiform PVCs often, but do not

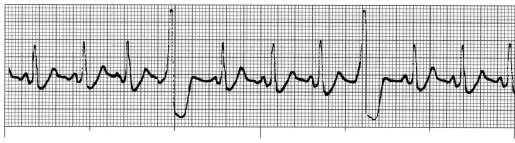

Figure 6-8   Sinus tachycardia with uniform premature ventricular complexes (PVCs).

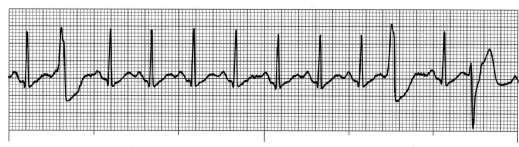

Figure 6-9   Sinus tachycardia with multiform premature ventricular complexes (PVCs).

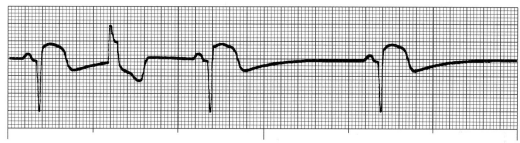

Figure 6-10   Sinus bradycardia with an interpolated premature ventricular complex (PVC) and ST-segment elevation.

always, arise from different anatomic sites; therefore, multiform PVCs are not necessarily multifocal.[4] In general, multiform PVCs are considered more serious than uniform PVCs because they suggest a greater area of irritable myocardial tissue.

Because a PVC can occur with any supraventricular dysrhythmia, it is important to first describe the patient's underlying rhythm and then to describe the ectopic beats that are present when identifying the rhythm (i.e., "Sinus tachycardia at 138 beats/min with frequent uniform PVCs" or "junctional rhythm at 50 beats/min with occasional multiform PVCs").

Interpolated Premature Ventricular Complexes

When a PVC occurs between two normally conducted QRS complexes without interfering with the normal cardiac cycle, it is called an **interpolated PVC** (Figure 6-10). An interpolated PVC does not have a full compensatory pause; rather it is "squeezed" between two normally conducted QRS complexes (i.e., the R-R intervals between sinus beats remain the same) and does not disturb the next ventricular depolarization or SA node activity. An interpolated PVC usually occurs when the PVC is very early or when the patient's underlying heart rate is relatively slow.

R-on-T Premature Ventricular Complexes

An R-on-T PVC occurs when the R wave of a PVC falls on the T wave of the preceding beat (Figure 6-11). Because ventricular repolarization is not yet complete during the last half of the T wave (i.e., the relative refractory period), it is possible that a PVC that occurs during this period of the cardiac cycle will precipitate VT or VF. The term *R-on-T phenomenon* refers to the start of a ventricular tachydysrhythmia as a result of an improperly timed electrical impulse on the T wave.[5] The general characteristics of PVCs are shown in Table 6-1.

What Causes Them?

PVCs are common, occurring in healthy individuals with apparently normal hearts, as well as in individuals with structural heart disease. PVCs can occur for no apparent cause and the frequency with which they occur increases with age. PVCs can occur at rest or they can be associated with exercise. Common causes of PVCs are shown in Box 6-1.

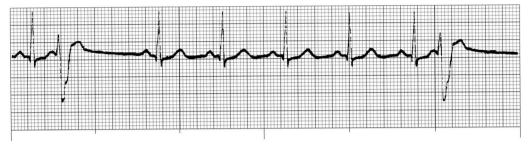

Figure 6-11 Sinus rhythm with two R-on-T premature ventricular complexes (PVCs).

Table 6-1	Characteristics of Premature Ventricular Complexes
Rhythm	Essentially regular with *premature* beats; if the premature ventricular complex (PVC) is an interpolated PVC, the rhythm will be regular
Rate	Usually within normal range, but depends on the underlying rhythm
P waves	Usually absent or, with retrograde conduction to the atria, may appear after the QRS (usually upright in the ST segment or T wave)
PR interval	None with the PVC because the ectopic beat originates in the ventricles
QRS duration	Usually 0.12 sec or greater; wide and bizarre; T wave is usually in the opposite direction of the QRS complex

Box 6-1	Common Causes of Premature Ventricular Complexes

Acid-base imbalance
Acute coronary syndromes
Cardiomyopathy
Digitalis toxicity
Electrolyte imbalance (e.g., potassium, magnesium)
Exercise
Heart failure
Hypoxia
Increase in catecholamines and sympathetic tone (e.g., emotional stress, anxiety)
Medications (e.g., sympathomimetic drugs)
Normal variant
Stimulants (e.g., caffeine, tobacco)
Valvular heart disease
Ventricular aneurysm

What Do I Do About Them?

The signs and symptoms associated with PVCs vary and generally depend on their frequency. Depending on their frequency, PVCs may or may not affect cardiac output. Some patients experiencing PVCs are asymptomatic; others may experience palpitations (i.e., sensations of a "racing heart,"

skipped beats, or "flip-flops"), weakness, lightheadedness, dizziness, fatigue, or a pounding sensation in the neck.

Treatment of PVCs depends on the cause, the patient's signs and symptoms, and on the clinical situation. Most patients experiencing PVCs do not require treatment with antiarrhythmic medications; rather, treatment of PVCs focuses on the search for, and treatment of, potentially reversible causes. For example, provide reassurance to the patient who is complaining of palpitations while searching for possible triggers for his or her PVCs (e.g., excessive caffeine ingestion, nicotine use, emotional stress). In the setting of an acute coronary syndrome, treatment is directed at ensuring adequate oxygenation, relieving pain, and rapidly identifying and correcting hypoxia, heart failure, and electrolyte or acid-base abnormalities.

CLINICAL CORRELATION

When premature ventricular complexes (PVCs) cause *serious* symptoms, antiarrhythmic medications (e.g., amiodarone, procainamide, lidocaine) are sometimes used to reduce the frequency with which they occur or to eliminate them. However, antiarrhythmics can cause a *proarrhythmic effect,* which means that they have the *potential* to cause serious adverse effects, more serious dysrhythmias, or both, than those that they were intended to treat. For example, the treatment of occasional PVCs, which are not life threatening, may initiate a life-threatening sustained ventricular tachydysrhythmia.

VENTRICULAR ESCAPE BEATS/ RHYTHM

How Do I Recognize It?

[Objectives 3, 4, 5]
Remember that premature beats are *early* and escape beats are *late.* We need to see at least two sinus beats in a row to establish the regularity of the underlying rhythm and to determine if a complex is early or late.

Although ventricular escape beats share some of the same physical characteristics as PVCs (e.g., wide QRS complexes, T waves deflected in a direction opposite the QRS), they

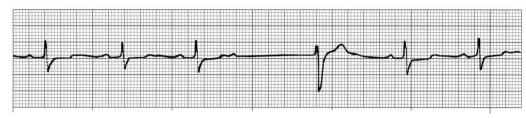

Figure 6-12 Sinus rhythm with a prolonged PR interval, nonconducted premature atrial complex, ventricular escape beat, and ST-segment depression.

differ in some very important areas. A PVC appears *early*, before the next expected sinus beat. PVCs often reflect irritability in some area of the ventricles. A ventricular escape beat occurs after a pause in which a supraventricular pacemaker failed to fire; thus, the escape beat is *late*, appearing after the next expected sinus beat. A ventricular escape beat is a *protective* mechanism, safeguarding the heart from more extreme slowing or even **asystole**. Because it is protective, you would not want to administer any medication that would "wipe out" the escape beat.

Take a look at Figure 6-12. When looking at this rhythm strip, one of the first things you notice is the beat with the wide QRS complex. Although this beat looks interesting, let us first examine the rhythm stripe systemically. The rhythm is essentially regular except for the single wide-QRS beat. There are upright P waves before beats 1, 2, 3, 5, and 6. When you calculate the atrial and ventricular rate, you find that the rate is 63 beats/min. Now we know that the underlying rhythm is a sinus rhythm at 63 beats/min. Next, let us examine the wide-QRS beat more closely and see what happened here. Look to the left of the wide-QRS beat and see if anything looks amiss. When you look closely at the T wave of beat 3, it has an extra "hump." If you take a moment to plot P waves across the strip, you will find that this extra hump is actually an early P wave that was not conducted. This is a nonconducted premature atrial complex (PAC). When plotting the P waves, you should have noticed that the wide-QRS beat occurred *late*—after the next expected sinus beat. This late beat is an escape beat. Because the QRS associated with it is *wide*, it is a *ventricular* escape beat. A *junctional* escape beat is also late, but it usually has a *narrow* QRS. Notice that the T wave of this beat is deflected in a direction opposite that of its QRS complex. When you look at the PR intervals and ST segment, you will find that the PR interval is longer than normal, measuring about 0.24 second. For now, we will simply say that it is prolonged. We will explore the reasons for this and give it a name in the next chapter. ST-segment depression is also present. Our identification of this rhythm would include a description like, "Sinus rhythm at 63 beats/min with a prolonged PR interval, nonconducted PAC, ventricular escape beat, and ST-segment depression." My goodness! That was one complicated rhythm strip! The ECG characteristics of ventricular escape beats are shown in Table 6-2.

An IVR, which is also called a *ventricular escape rhythm*, exists when three or more ventricular escape beats occur in a row at a rate of 20 to 40 beats/min (i.e., the intrinsic firing rate

Table 6-2	Characteristics of Ventricular Escape Beats
Rhythm	Essentially regular with *late* beats; the ventricular escape beat occurs *after* the next expected sinus beat
Rate	Usually within normal range, but depends on the underlying rhythm
P waves	Usually absent or, with retrograde conduction to the atria; may appear after the QRS (usually upright in the ST segment or T wave)
PR interval	None with the ventricular escape beat because the ectopic beat originates in the ventricles
QRS duration	0.12 sec or greater, wide and bizarre; the T wave is frequently in the opposite direction of the QRS complex

of the Purkinje fibers). The QRS complexes seen in IVR are wide and bizarre because the impulses begin in the ventricles, bypassing the normal conduction pathway. When the ventricular rate slows to a rate of less than 20 beats/min, some practitioners refer to the rhythm as an **agonal rhythm** or *dying heart*. An example of IVR is shown in Figure 6-13 and the characteristics of this rhythm are described in Table 6-3.

What Causes It?

A ventricular escape rhythm may occur when the SA node and the AV junction fail to initiate an electrical impulse, the rate of discharge of the SA node or AV junction becomes less than the intrinsic rate of the Purkinje fibers, or the impulses generated by a supraventricular pacemaker site are blocked. A ventricular escape rhythm may also occur as a result of an acute coronary syndrome, digitalis toxicity, or metabolic imbalances.

What Do I Do About It?

[Objective 6]
Because the ventricular rate associated with IVR is slow (i.e., 20 to 40 beats/min) with a loss of atrial kick, the patient may experience serious signs and symptoms as a result of decreased cardiac output. If the patient has a pulse and is

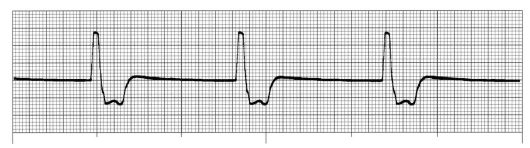

Figure 6-13   Idioventricular rhythm.

Table **6-3**	Characteristics of Idioventricular Rhythm
Rhythm	Ventricular rhythm is essentially regular
Rate	Ventricular rate 20 to 40 beats/min
P waves	Usually absent or, with retrograde conduction to the atria; may appear after the QRS (usually upright in the ST segment or T wave)
PR interval	None
QRS duration	0.12 sec or greater; the T wave is frequently in the opposite direction of the QRS complex

symptomatic because of the slow rate, treatment should include application of a pulse oximeter and administration of supplemental oxygen if indicated. Establish intravenous (IV) access, obtain a 12-lead ECG, and administer IV atropine. Reassess the patient's response and continue monitoring the patient. Transcutaneous pacing or a dopamine, epinephrine, or isoproterenol IV infusion may be tried if atropine is ineffective. Medications such as lidocaine should be avoided during the management of this rhythm because lidocaine may abolish ventricular activity, possibly causing asystole in a patient with a ventricular escape rhythm.

If the patient is not breathing and has no pulse despite the appearance of organized electrical activity on the cardiac monitor, PEA exists. The management of PEA should include cardiopulmonary resuscitation (CPR), giving oxygen, starting an IV, possible placement of an advanced airway, and an aggressive search for the underlying cause of the situation.

ACCELERATED IDIOVENTRICULAR RHYTHM

How Do I Recognize It?

[Objective 7]
An **accelerated idioventricular rhythm (AIVR)** exists when three or more ventricular beats occur in a row at a rate of

ECG Pearl

The memory aids PATCH-4-MD and the 5 Hs and 5 Ts may be used to recall the potentially reversible causes of cardiac emergencies, including cardiac arrest.

PATCH-4-MD
Pulmonary embolism—anticoagulants? Surgery?
Acidosis—ventilation, correct acid-base disturbances
Tension pneumothorax—needle decompression
Cardiac tamponade—pericardiocentesis
Hypovolemia—replace intravascular volume
Hypoxia—ensure adequate oxygenation and ventilation
Heat/cold (hyperthermia/hypothermia)—cooling/warming methods
Hypo-/hyperkalemia (and other electrolytes)—monitor serum glucose levels closely in concert with correcting electrolyte disturbances
Myocardial infarction—reperfusion therapy
Drug overdose/accidents—antidote/specific therapy

FIVE Hs AND FIVE Ts

Hypovolemia	**T**amponade, cardiac
Hypoxia	**T**ension pneumothorax
Hypothermia	**T**hrombosis: lungs (massive pulmonary embolism)
Hypo-/Hyperkalemia	**T**hrombosis: heart (acute coronary syndromes)
Hydrogen ion (acidosis)	**T**ablets/toxins: drug overdose

41 to 100 beats/min (Figure 6-14). Some cardiologists consider the ventricular rate range of AIVR to be 41 to 120 beats/min.

AIVR is usually considered a benign escape rhythm that appears when the sinus rate slows and disappears when the sinus rate speeds up. Episodes of AIVR usually last a few seconds to a minute. Because AIVR usually begins and ends gradually, it is also called *nonparoxysmal VT*. Fusion beats are often seen at the onset and end of the rhythm. The ECG characteristics of AIVR are shown in Table 6-4.

What Causes It?

AIVR is usually considered a benign escape rhythm. It is often seen during the first 12 hours of an acute myocardial

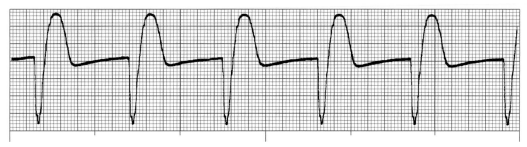

Figure 6-14   Accelerated idioventricular rhythm.

Table 6-4	Characteristics of Accelerated Idioventricular Rhythm
Rhythm	Ventricular rhythm is essentially regular
Rate	41 to 100 (41 to 120 per some cardiologists) beats/min
P waves	Usually absent or, with retrograde conduction to the atria, may appear after the QRS (usually upright in the ST segment or T wave)
PR interval	None
QRS duration	Greater than 0.12 sec; the T wave is frequently in the opposite direction of the QRS complex

infarction (MI), and it is particularly common after successful reperfusion therapy. AIVR has been observed in patients with the following:

- Acute myocarditis
- Cocaine toxicity
- Digitalis toxicity
- Dilated cardiomyopathy
- Hypertensive heart disease
- Subarachnoid hemorrhage

What Do I Do About It?

AIVR generally requires no treatment because the rhythm is protective and often transient, spontaneously resolving on its own; however, possible dizziness, lightheadedness, or other signs of hemodynamic compromise may occur because of the loss of atrial kick. If the patient is symptomatic

because of the loss of atrial kick, treatment should include application of a pulse oximeter and administration of supplemental oxygen if indicated. Establish IV access and obtain a 12-lead ECG. Atropine may be ordered in an attempt to block the vagus nerve and stimulate the SA node to overdrive the ventricular rhythm. *Atrial* (not ventricular) pacing may be attempted to suppress AIVR. Reassess the patient's response and continue monitoring the patient.

VENTRICULAR TACHYCARDIA

How Do I Recognize It?

[Objective 8]

Ventricular tachycardia (VT) exists when three or more sequential PVCs occur at a rate of more than 100 beats/min. VT may occur as a short run that lasts less than 30 seconds and spontaneously ends (i.e., *nonsustained VT*) (Figure 6-15). *Sustained VT* persists for more than 30 seconds and may require therapeutic intervention to terminate the rhythm (Figure 6-16). In patients with heart disease, nonsustained VT is often a predictor of high risk for sustained VT or VF.[6] VT may occur with or without pulses, and the patient may be stable or unstable with this rhythm.

Monomorphic Ventricular Tachycardia

[Objective 9]

VT, like PVCs, may originate from an ectopic focus in either ventricle. When the QRS complexes of VT are of the same shape and amplitude, the rhythm is called **monomorphic VT** (Figure 6-17). Monomorphic VT with a ventricular rate

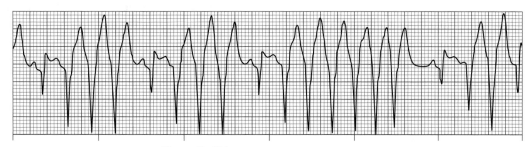

Figure 6-15   Nonsustained ventricular tachycardia.

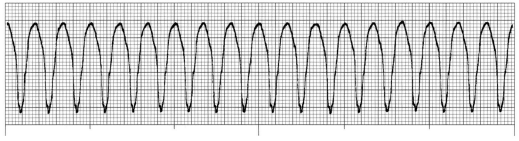

Figure 6-16   If this rhythm lasts longer than 30 seconds, it is called *sustained ventricular tachycardia*.

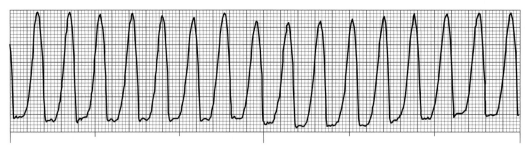

Figure 6-17   Monomorphic ventricular tachycardia.

greater than 200 beats/min is called *ventricular flutter* by some cardiologists. The ECG characteristics of monomorphic VT are shown in Table 6-5.

What Causes It?

Sustained monomorphic VT is often associated with underlying heart disease, particularly myocardial ischemia. It rarely occurs in patients without underlying heart disease. Common causes of VT include the following:

- Acid-base imbalance
- Acute coronary syndromes
- Cardiomyopathy
- Cocaine abuse
- Digitalis toxicity
- Electrolyte imbalance (e.g., hypokalemia, hyperkalemia, hypomagnesemia)
- Mitral valve prolapse

- Trauma (e.g., myocardial contusion, invasive cardiac procedures)
- Tricyclic antidepressant overdose
- Valvular heart disease

What Do I Do About It?

Signs and symptoms associated with VT vary. The patient who has sustained monomorphic VT may be stable for long periods. However, when the ventricular rate is very fast, or when myocardial ischemia is present, monomorphic VT can degenerate to polymorphic VT or VF. Syncope or near-syncope may occur because of an abrupt onset of VT. The patient's only warning symptom may be a brief period of lightheadedness.

During VT, the severity of the patient's symptoms are related to a number of factors including how rapid the ventricular rate is, how long the tachycardia has been present, the presence and extent of underlying heart disease, and the presence and severity of peripheral vascular disease.[6] Signs and symptoms of hemodynamic instability related to VT may include the following:

- Acute altered mental status
- Chest pain or discomfort
- Hypotension
- Pulmonary congestion
- Shock
- Shortness of breath

Table 6-5	Characteristics of Monomorphic Ventricular Tachycardia
Rhythm	Ventricular rhythm is essentially regular
Rate	101 to 250 (121 to 250 per some cardiologists) beats/min
P waves	Usually no seen; if present, they have no set relationship with the QRS complexes that appear between them at a rate different from that of the ventricular tachycardia (VT)
PR interval	None
QRS duration	0.12 sec or greater; often difficult to differentiate between the QRS and T wave

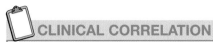

CLINICAL CORRELATION

Sustained ventricular tachycardia (VT) does not always produce signs of hemodynamic instability.

Treatment is based on the patient's signs and symptoms and the type of VT. If the rhythm is monomorphic VT (and the patient's symptoms are caused by the tachycardia):

- CPR and defibrillation are used to treat the pulseless patient with VT.
- Stable but symptomatic patients are treated with oxygen (if indicated), IV access, and ventricular antiarrhythmics (e.g., procainamide, amiodarone, sotalol) to suppress the rhythm. Procainamide should be avoided if the patient has a prolonged QT interval or signs of heart failure. Sotalol should also be avoided if the patient has a prolonged QT interval.
- Unstable patients (usually a sustained heart rate of 150 beats/min or more) are treated with oxygen, IV access, and sedation (if the patient is awake and time permits) followed by synchronized cardioversion.

In all cases, an aggressive search must be made for the cause of the VT.

ECG Pearl

A supraventricular tachycardia (SVT) with an intraventricular conduction delay may be difficult to distinguish from ventricular tachycardia (VT). Keep in mind that VT is considered a potentially life-threatening dysrhythmia. If you are unsure whether a regular, wide-QRS tachycardia is VT or SVT with an intraventricular conduction delay, treat the rhythm as VT until proven otherwise. Obtaining a 12-lead ECG may help differentiate VT from SVT, but do not delay treatment if the patient is symptomatic.

Polymorphic Ventricular Tachycardia

[Objective 10]

With **polymorphic VT** (PMVT), the QRS complexes vary in shape and amplitude from beat to beat and appear to twist from upright to negative or negative to upright and back, resembling a spindle (Figure 6-18). PMVT is a dysrhythmia of intermediate severity between monomorphic VT and VF (Figure 6-19). The ECG characteristics of polymorphic VT are shown in Table 6-6.

What Causes It?

Several types of PMVT and their possible causes have been identified as follows:

- Polymorphic VT that occurs in the presence of a long QT interval (typically 0.45 second or more and often 0.50 second or more) is called **torsades de Pointes**. A long QT interval may be congenital, acquired (typically precipitated by antiarrhythmic drug use or hypokalemia, which are typically associated with bradycardia), or idiopathic (neither familial nor with an identifiable acquired cause).
- Polymorphic VT can occur in the presence of an abnormally short QT interval (typically less than 0.32 second). This type of polymorphic VT is called *short-QT PMVT*.
- Polymorphic VT that occurs in the presence of a normal QT interval is simply referred to as *polymorphic VT* or *normal-QT PMVT*.
- Polymorphic VT that is triggered by stress or exercise and that occurs in the absence of QT prolongation or structural heart disease is called *catecholaminergic PMVT*.
- Polymorphic VT that is associated with an ECG pattern that consists of right bundle branch-like conduction and ST-segment elevation in the right chest leads without evidence of QT prolongation or structural heart disease is called *Brugada syndrome*.
- Polymorphic VT that is caused by acute myocardial ischemia or infarction and that occurs in the absence of QT prolongation is called *ischemic PMVT*.
- Polymorphic VT without QT prolongation that cannot be attributed to one of the above mechanisms is called *idiopathic normal QT PMVT*.

What Do I Do About It?

The signs and symptoms associated with PMVT are usually related to the decreased cardiac output that occurs because of the fast ventricular rate. Signs of shock are often present. The patient may experience a syncopal episode or seizures. The rhythm may occasionally terminate spontaneously and recur after several seconds or minutes, or it may deteriorate

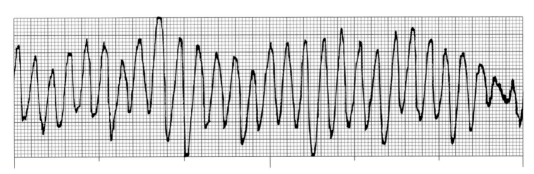

Figure 6-18 Polymorphic ventricular tachycardia. This rhythm strip is from a 77-year-old man 3 days post myocardial infarction (MI). His chief complaint at the onset of this episode was chest pain. He had a past medical history of a previous MI and an abdominal aortic aneurysm repair. The patient was given lidocaine and defibrillated several times without success. Laboratory results revealed a serum potassium (K+) level of 2.0. intravenous (IV) K+ was administered and the patient converted to a sinus rhythm with the next defibrillation.

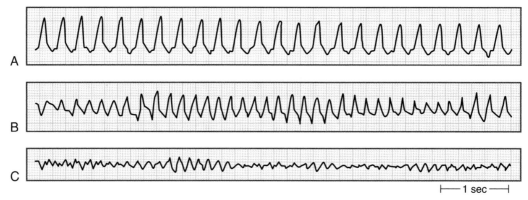

Figure 6-19   Ventricular tachydysrhythmias. **A,** Rhythm strip showing monomorphic ventricular tachycardia. **B,** Example of polymorphic ventricular tachycardia. **C,** Example of ventricular fibrillation. All tracings are from lead V₁.

Table 6-6	Characteristics of Polymorphic Ventricular Tachycardia
Rhythm	Ventricular rhythm may be regular or irregular
Rate	Ventricular rate 150 to 300 beats/min; typically 200 to 250 beats/min
P waves	None
PR interval	None
QRS duration	0.12 sec or more; there is a gradual alteration in the amplitude and direction of the QRS complexes; a typical cycle consists of 5 to 20 QRS complexes

to VF. The patient with sustained PMVT is rarely hemodynamically stable.

It is best to seek expert consultation when treating the patient with PMVT because of the diverse mechanisms of PMVT, for which there may or may not be clues as to its specific cause at the time of the patient's presentation. Treatment options vary and can be contradictory. For example, a medication that may be appropriate for the treatment of TdP may be contraindicated when treating another form of PMVT. In general, if the patient is symptomatic as a result of the tachycardia, treat ischemia (if it is present), correct electrolyte abnormalities, and discontinue

any medications that the patient may be taking that prolong the QT interval. If the patient is stable, the use of IV amiodarone (if the QT interval is normal), magnesium, or beta-blockers may be effective, depending on the cause of the PMVT. If the patient is unstable or has no pulse, proceed with defibrillation as for VF.

VENTRICULAR FIBRILLATION

How Do I Recognize It?

[Objective 11]

VF is a chaotic rhythm that begins in the ventricles. In VF, there is no organized depolarization of the ventricles. The ventricular muscle quivers, and as a result, there is no effective myocardial contraction and no pulse. The resulting rhythm looks chaotic with deflections that vary in shape and amplitude. No normal-looking waveforms are visible. VF with waves that are 3 or more mm high is called "coarse" VF (Figure 6-20). VF with low amplitude waves (i.e., less than 3 mm) is called "fine" VF (Figure 6-21). Table 6-7 lists the ECG characteristics of VF and Figure 6-22 illustrates a comparison of ventricular dysrhythmias.

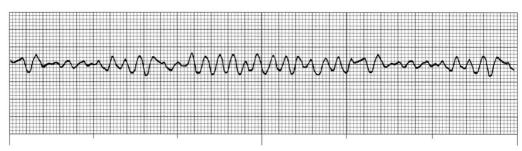

Figure 6-20   Ventricular fibrillation (VF) with waves that are 3 mm high or more is called "coarse" VF.

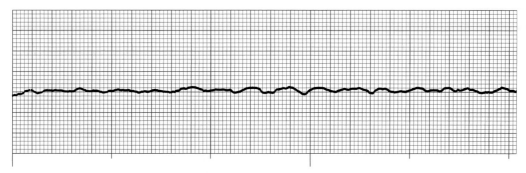

Figure 6-21   Ventricular fibrillation (VF) with low-amplitude waves (i.e., less than 3 mm) is called "fine" VF.

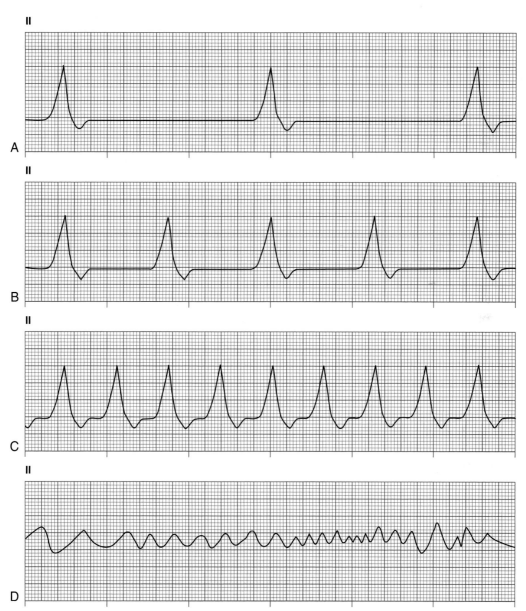

Figure 6-22   Comparison of ventricular dysrhythmias. **A,** Idioventricular rhythm at 38 beats/min. **B,** Accelerated idioventricular rhythm at 75 beats/min. **C,** Monomorphic ventricular tachycardia at 150 beats/min. **D,** Coarse ventricular fibrillation.

Table 6-7	Characteristics of Ventricular Fibrillation
Rhythm	Rapid and chaotic with no pattern or regularity
Rate	Cannot be determined because there are no discernible waves or complexes to measure
P waves	Not discernible
PR interval	Not discernible
QRS duration	Not discernible

What Causes It?

Factors that increase the susceptibility of the myocardium to fibrillate include the following:

- Acute coronary syndromes
- Dysrhythmias
- Electrolyte imbalance
- Environmental factors (e.g., electrocution)
- Hypertrophy
- Increased sympathetic nervous system activity
- Proarrhythmic effect of antiarrhythmics and other medications
- Severe heart failure
- Vagal stimulation

CLINICAL CORRELATION

Because artifact can mimic ventricular fibrillation (VF), *always* check the patient's pulse before beginning treatment.

What Do I Do About It?

The patient in VF is unresponsive, apneic, and pulseless. Because no drugs used for the treatment of cardiac arrest have been shown to improve survival to hospital discharge, the priorities of care in cardiac arrest as a result of pulseless VT or VF are high-quality CPR and defibrillation (Figure 6-23). Medications that may be used in the treatment of pulseless VT/VF include epinephrine, vasopressin, amiodarone, and lidocaine, if amiodarone is unavailable.[7]

ECG Pearl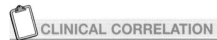

Cardiac Arrest Rhythms
- Asystole
- Pulseless electrical activity (PEA)
- Ventricular fibrillation (VF)
- Ventricular tachycardia (VT)

VF and VT are *shockable* rhythms, which means that delivering a shock to the heart by means of a defibrillator may result in termination of the rhythm. Asystole and PEA are *nonshockable* rhythms.

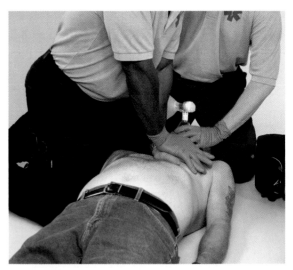

Figure 6-23 The priorities of care in cardiac arrest as a result of pulseless ventricular tachycardia or ventricular fibrillation are high-quality cardiopulmonary resuscitation (CPR) and defibrillation.

Defibrillation
[Objective 12]

Defibrillation is the delivery of an electrical **current** across the heart muscle over a very brief period to terminate an abnormal heart rhythm. Defibrillation is also called *unsynchronized countershock* or *asynchronous countershock*, because the delivery of current has no relationship to the cardiac cycle. The shock attempts to deliver a uniform electrical current of sufficient intensity to depolarize myocardial cells (including fibrillating cells) at the same time, thereby briefly "stunning" the heart. This provides an opportunity for the heart's natural pacemakers to resume normal activity. When the cells repolarize, the pacemaker with the highest degree of automaticity should assume responsibility for pacing the heart.

Manual defibrillation refers to the placement of paddles or pads on a patient's chest, the interpretation of the patient's cardiac rhythm by a trained healthcare professional, and the healthcare professional's decision to deliver a shock, if indicated. *Automated external defibrillation* refers to the placement of paddles or pads on a patient's chest and the interpretation of the patient's cardiac rhythm by an **automated external defibrillator** (AED). The AED has a sophisticated computer system that analyzes a patient's heart rhythm using an algorithm to distinguish shockable rhythms from nonshockable rhythms and providing visual and auditory instructions to the rescuer to deliver an electrical shock, if a shock is indicated. Defibrillation is indicated in the treatment of pulseless monomorphic VT, sustained polymorphic VT, and VF.

Defibrillation—Procedure

The procedure described below assumes that the patient is an adult and confirmed to be unresponsive, apneic, and pulseless. It also assumes that the patient's cardiac rhythm is pulseless VT or VF and that a four-person team is available to assist with procedures during the resuscitation effort.

While high-quality CPR continues, instruct a team member to expose the patient's chest and to remove any transdermal patches or ointment from the patient's chest, if present. Remove the defibrillation (i.e., combination) pads from their sealed package. Check the pads for the presence of adequate gel. Attach the pads to the hands-free defibrillation cable, and then attach the combination pads to the patient's chest in the position recommended by the manufacturer.

Turn the power to the monitor/defibrillator on and verify the presence of a shockable rhythm on the monitor. Select an appropriate energy level, using the energy levels recommended by the defibrillator manufacturer (Figure 6-24).

While the defibrillator is readied, instruct a team member to prepare the initial drugs that will be used during the resuscitation effort and to start an IV after the first shock is delivered. Charge the defibrillator by pressing the "CHARGE" button on the machine (Figure 6-25). All team members with the exception of the person performing chest compressions should *immediately* clear the patient as the machine charges. Listen as the machine charges. The sound usually changes when it reaches its full charge. To help minimize

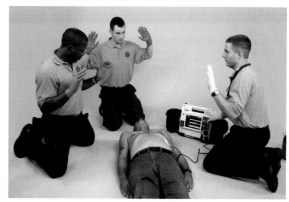

Figure 6-26   If a shockable rhythm is still present, call "Clear!" and ensure that everyone is clear of the patient before pressing the shock control to discharge energy to the patient.

interruptions in chest compressions, the person who is performing chest compressions should continue CPR while the machine is charging. When the defibrillator is charged, the chest compressor should *immediately* clear the patient.

If a shockable rhythm is still present, call "Clear!" Look around you (360 degrees) to be sure that everyone—including you—is clear of the patient, the bed, and any equipment that is connected to the patient (Figure 6-26). Press the "SHOCK" control to discharge energy to the patient. Release the shock control after the shock has been delivered. Instruct the team to resume chest compressions immediately without pausing for a rhythm or pulse check. Instruct team members to coordinate ventilations with chest compressions and to establish vascular access. Administer medications during CPR that are consistent with current resuscitation guidelines. Use the memory aids PATCH-4-MD or the 5 H's and 5 T's to help identify possible reversible causes of the arrest or factors that may be complicating the resuscitation effort. After 2 minutes of CPR, repeat the sequence, beginning with a rhythm check.

If defibrillation restores an organized rhythm, check for a pulse. If a pulse is present, check the patient's blood pressure and other vital signs and begin post–cardiac arrest care. If you are not sure if a pulse is present, resume CPR.[7] If a rhythm check reveals a nonshockable rhythm, resume CPR, consider possible causes of the arrest, and give medications and other emergency care as indicated.

ASYSTOLE (CARDIAC STANDSTILL)

How Do I Recognize It?

[Objective 13]

Asystole, which is also called *ventricular asystole*, is a total absence of ventricular electrical activity (Figure 6-27). There is no ventricular rate or rhythm, no pulse, and no cardiac output. Some atrial electrical activity may be evident. If atrial electrical activity is present, the rhythm is called *"P wave"*

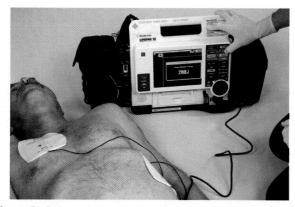

Figure 6-24   After verifying the presence of a shockable rhythm on the monitor, select an appropriate energy level, using the energy levels recommended by the defibrillator manufacturer.

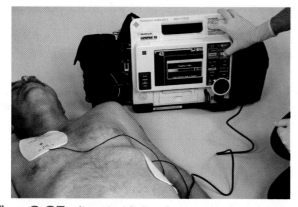

Figure 6-25   Charge the defibrillator. Because oxygen flow over the patient's chest during electrical therapy increases the risk of spark or fire, make sure that oxygen is not flowing over the patient's chest.

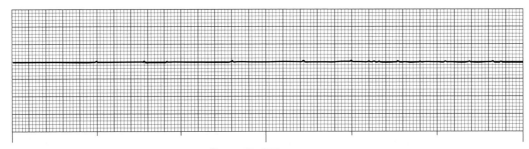

Figure 6-27   Asystole.

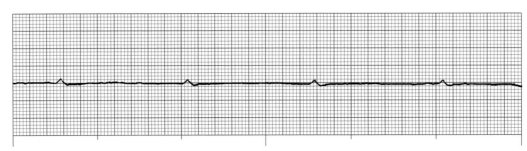

Figure 6-28   "P wave" asystole.

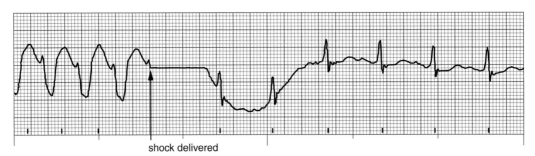

shock delivered

Figure 6-29   This rhythm strip is from a 62-year-old man complaining of palpitations. The patient's initial rhythm was monomorphic ventricular tachycardia. A synchronized shock was delivered, resulting in a sinus rhythm with a prolonged PR interval. Note the short period of asystole after the shock was delivered.

asystole or *ventricular standstill* (Figure 6-28). The ECG characteristics of asystole are shown in Table 6-8.

What Causes It?

Use the memory aids PATCH-4-MD and the 5 H's and 5 T's to recall possible reversible causes of asystole. In addition, ventricular asystole may occur temporarily following termination of a tachycardia with medications, defibrillation, or synchronized cardioversion (Figure 6-29).

What Do I Do About It?

When asystole is observed on a cardiac monitor, confirm that the patient is unresponsive and has no pulse, and then begin high-quality CPR. Additional care includes establishing

Table **6-8**	Characteristics of Asystole
Rhythm	Ventricular not discernible; atrial may be discernible
Rate	Ventricular not discernible but atrial activity may be observed (i.e., "P-wave" asystole)
P waves	Usually not discernible
PR interval	Not measurable
QRS duration	Absent

vascular access, considering the possible causes of the arrest, administering a vasopressor (e.g., epinephrine, vasopressin), and possibly inserting an advanced airway.[7]

A summary of all ventricular rhythm characteristics can be found in Table 6-9.

Table 6-9 Ventricular Rhythms—Summary of Characteristics

Characteristic	Premature Ventricular Complexes (PVCs)	Ventricular Escape Beat	Idioventricular Rhythm (IVR)	Accelerated Idioventricular Rhythm (AIVR)
Rhythm	Regular with *early* beats	Regular with *late* beats	Essentially regular	Essentially regular
Rate (beats/min)	Usually within normal range, but depends on underlying rhythm	Usually within normal range, but depends on underlying rhythm	20 to 40	41 to 100; some experts consider the rate 41 to 120
P waves (lead II)	Usually absent or, with retrograde conduction to the atria, may appear after the QRS (usually upright in ST segment or T wave)	Usually absent or, with retrograde conduction to the atria, may appear after the QRS (usually upright in ST segment or T wave)	Usually absent or, with retrograde conduction to the atria, may appear after the QRS (usually upright in ST segment or T wave)	Usually absent or, with retrograde conduction to the atria, may appear after the QRS (usually upright in ST segment or T wave)
PR interval	None	None	None	None
QRS duration	Usually 0.12 sec or greater	0.12 sec or greater	0.12 sec or greater	0.12 sec or greater

Characteristic	Monomorphic Ventricular Tachycardia	Polymorphic Ventricular Tachycardia	Ventricular Fibrillation	Asystole
Rhythm	Usually regular	Irregular	Chaotic	None
Rate (beats/min)	101 to 250; some experts consider the rate 121 to 250	150 to 300	Not discernible	None
P waves (lead II)	May be present or absent; if present, they have no set relationship to the QRS complexes, appearing between the QRSs at a rate different from that of the ventricular tachycardia (VT)	Independent or none	Absent	Atrial activity may be observed; P-wave asystole
PR interval	None	None	None	None
QRS duration	0.12 sec or greater	0.12 sec or greater	Not discernible	Absent

REFERENCES

1. Stevenson WG: Ventricular arrhythmias. In Goldman L, Schafer AI, editors: *Cecil medicine*, ed 24, Philadelphia, 2012, Saunders, pp 359–368.
2. Hamdan MH: Cardiac arrhythmias. In Andreoli TE, Benjamin IJ, Griggs RC, et al: *Andreoli and Carpenter's Cecil essentials of medicine*, ed 8, Philadelphia, 2010, Saunders, pp 118–114.
3. Crawford MV, Spence MI: Electrical complications in coronary artery disease: arrhythmias. In *Common sense approach to coronary care*, ed 6, St. Louis, 1995, Mosby, p 220.
4. Goldberger AL: Ventricular arrhythmias. In *Clinical electrocardiography: a simplified approach*, ed 7, St. Louis, 2006, Mosby, pp 189–202.
5. Spotts V: Temporary transcutaneous (external) pacing. In Lynn-McHale Wiegand DJ, editor: *AACN procedure manual for critical care*, ed 6, St. Louis, 2011, Saunders, pp 413–420.
6. Martin D, Wharton JM: Sustained monomorphic ventricular tachycardia. In Podrid PJ, Kowey PR, editors: *Cardiac arrhythmia: mechanisms, diagnosis, and management*, ed 2, Philadelphia, 2001, Lippincott Williams & Wilkins, pp 573–601.
7. Neumar RW, Otto CW, Link MS, et al: Part 8: adult advanced cardiovascular life support: 2010. American Heart Association guidelines for cardiopulmonary resuscitation and emergency cardiovascular care, *Circulation* 122:729–767, 2010.

STOP & REVIEW—CHAPTER 6

True/False

Indicate whether the statement is true or false.

____1. Torsades de pointes (TdP) is a type of monomorphic ventricular tachycardia.

____2. Uniform premature ventricular complexes (PVCs) are unifocal, but multiform PVCs are not necessarily multifocal.

____3. An accelerated junctional or an accelerated ventricular rhythm is faster than its intrinsic rate but slower than 100 beats/min.

Multiple Choice

Identify the choice that best completes the statement or answers the question.

____4. How would you differentiate between a junctional escape rhythm at 40 beats/min and an idioventricular rhythm at the same rate?
   a. It is impossible to differentiate a junctional escape rhythm from an idioventricular rhythm.
   b. The junctional escape rhythm will have a narrow QRS complex; the idioventricular rhythm will have a wide QRS complex.
   c. The rate (i.e., 40 beats/min) would indicate a junctional escape rhythm, not an idioventricular rhythm.
   d. The junctional escape rhythm will have a wide QRS complex; an idioventricular rhythm will have a narrow QRS complex.

____5. The term for three or more PVCs occurring in a row at a rate of more than 100/min is:
   a. Ventricular trigeminy.
   b. Ventricular fibrillation.
   c. A run of ventricular tachycardia.
   d. A run of ventricular escape beats.

Matching

Match the key terms with their definitions by placing the letter of each correct answer in the space provided.

a. Current
b. Fusion beat
c. Accelerated idioventricular rhythm
d. Compensatory pause
e. Ventricular tachycardia
f. Asystole
g. Monomorphic
h. Agonal rhythm
i. Defibrillation

j. Proarrhythmic
k. Atrioventricular dissociation
l. Multiform
m. Automated external defibrillator
n. Interpolated PVC
o. Polymorphic
p. R-on-T phenomenon
q. Idioventricular rhythm

____6. A dysrhythmia that is similar in appearance to an idioventricular rhythm but occurs at a rate of less than 20 beats/min

____7. Varying in shape

____8. A dysrhythmia that originates in the ventricles with a rate between 20 and 40 beats/min

____9. A machine with a sophisticated computer system that analyzes a patient's heart rhythm using an algorithm to distinguish shockable rhythms from nonshockable rhythms

____10. Antiarrhythmics can cause a _____ effect, which means that they have the *potential* to cause serious adverse effects, more serious dysrhythmias, or both, than those that they were intended to treat.

____11. Any dysrhythmia in which the atria and the ventricles beat independently

____12. A PVC that occurs between two normally conducted QRS complexes and that does not disturb the next ventricular depolarization or sinoatrial node activity

____13. A total absence of ventricular electrical activity

_____**14.** A beat that occurs because of the simultaneous activation of one cardiac chamber by two sites

_____**15.** The flow of an electrical charge from one point to another

_____**16.** A term used to describe PVCs that are different in appearance

_____**17.** A dysrhythmia that originates in the ventricles with a rate between 41 and 100 beats/min

_____**18.** The initiation of a ventricular tachydysrhythmia as a result of an improperly timed electrical impulse on the T wave

_____**19.** Delivery of an electrical current across the heart muscle over a very brief period to terminate an abnormal heart rhythm

_____**20.** A dysrhythmia that originates in the ventricles with a ventricular response greater than 100 beats/min

_____**21.** Having the same shape

_____**22.** This often follows a PVC and occurs because the sinoatrial node is usually not affected by the PVC.

Short Answer

23. Explain the difference between a PVC and a ventricular escape beat.

_____

_____

_____

24. How do coarse and fine ventricular fibrillation differ?

_____

_____

_____

VENTRICULAR RHYTHMS—*PRACTICE RHYTHM STRIPS*

For each of the following rhythm strips, determine the atrial and ventricular rate and rhythm, measure the PR interval, QRS duration, and QT interval, and then identify the rhythm. Note: These rhythm strips include sinus, atrial, junctional, and ventricular rhythms.

25. This rhythm strip is from a 63-year-old man who collapsed on the kitchen floor. He is unresponsive, apneic, and pulseless. His past medical history includes a coronary artery bypass graft 8 years ago and pacemaker implantation 5 years ago. Identify the rhythm (lead II).

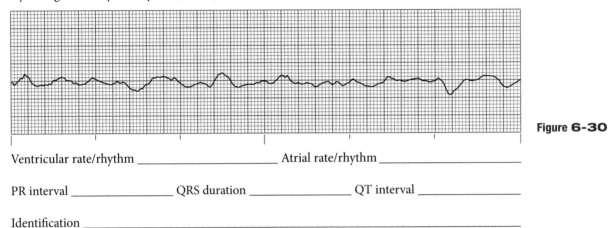

Figure 6-30

Ventricular rate/rhythm _____ Atrial rate/rhythm _____

PR interval _____ QRS duration _____ QT interval _____

Identification _____

26. Identify the rhythm (lead II).

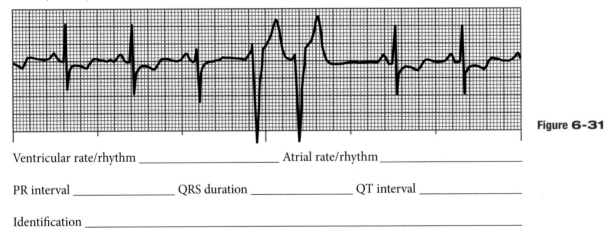

Figure 6-31

Ventricular rate/rhythm _____ Atrial rate/rhythm _____

PR interval _____ QRS duration _____ QT interval _____

Identification _____

27. This rhythm strip is from a 73-year-old woman who is complaining of chest pain. Identify the rhythm (lead II).

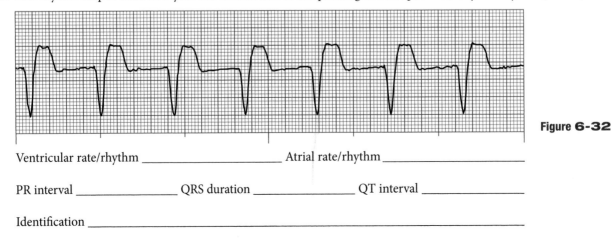

Figure 6-32

Ventricular rate/rhythm _____ Atrial rate/rhythm _____

PR interval _____ QRS duration _____ QT interval _____

Identification _____

28. Identify the rhythm (lead II).

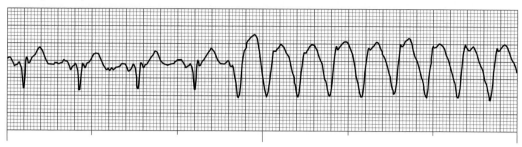

Figure 6-33

Ventricular rate/rhythm _____ Atrial rate/rhythm _____

PR interval _____ QRS duration _____ QT interval _____

Identification _____

29. This rhythm strip is from a 69-year-old man who is complaining of substernal chest pain. He rates his discomfort as 9/10. Identify the rhythm (lead II).

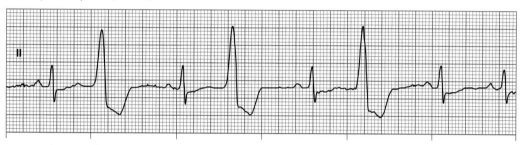

Figure 6-34

Ventricular rate/rhythm _____ Atrial rate/rhythm _____

PR interval _____ QRS duration _____ QT interval _____

Identification _____

30. This rhythm strip is from an 88-year-old woman complaining of dizziness. Her blood pressure is 176/68 mm Hg. Identify the rhythm (lead II).

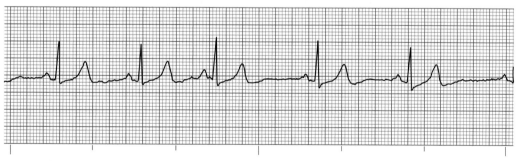

Figure 6-35

Ventricular rate/rhythm _____ Atrial rate/rhythm _____

PR interval _____ QRS duration _____ QT interval _____

Identification _____

31. Identify the rhythm (lead II).

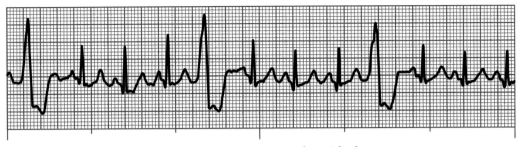

Figure 6-36

Ventricular rate/rhythm _____ Atrial rate/rhythm _____

PR interval _____ QRS duration _____ QT interval _____

Identification _____

32. Identify the rhythm (lead II).

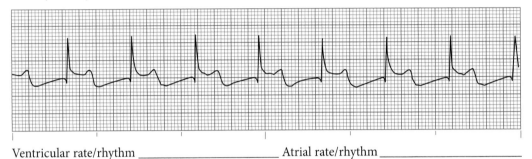

Figure 6-37

Ventricular rate/rhythm _____ Atrial rate/rhythm _____

PR interval _____ QRS duration _____ QT interval _____

Identification _____

33. This rhythm strip is from a 90-year-old unresponsive woman. She has a history of heart failure. Her medications include furosemide and albuterol. Identify the rhythm (lead II).

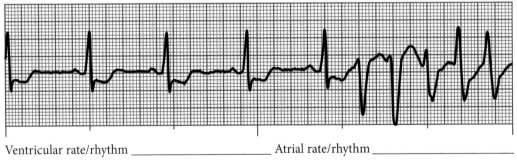

Figure 6-38

Ventricular rate/rhythm _____ Atrial rate/rhythm _____

PR interval _____ QRS duration _____ QT interval _____

Identification _____

34. This rhythm strip is from a 58-year-old man who was initially unresponsive, apneic, and pulseless. Identify the rhythm.

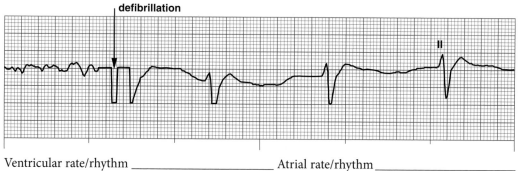

Figure 6-39

Ventricular rate/rhythm _____ Atrial rate/rhythm _____

PR interval _____ QRS duration _____ QT interval _____

Identification _____

35. Identify the rhythm (lead II).

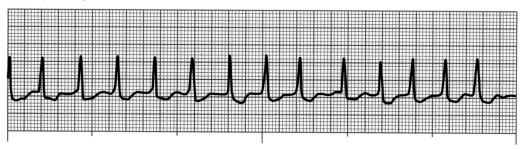

Figure 6-40

Ventricular rate/rhythm _____ Atrial rate/rhythm _____

PR interval _____ QRS duration _____ QT interval _____

Identification _____

36. Identify the rhythm (lead II).

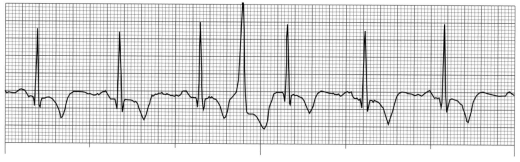

Figure 6-41

Ventricular rate/rhythm _____ Atrial rate/rhythm _____

PR interval _____ QRS duration _____ QT interval _____

Identification _____

37. Identify the rhythm (lead II).

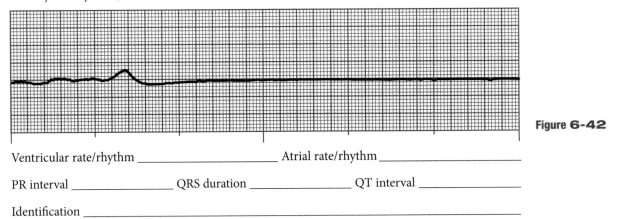

Figure **6-42**

Ventricular rate/rhythm _____ Atrial rate/rhythm _____

PR interval _____ QRS duration _____ QT interval _____

Identification _____

38. This rhythm strip is from a 70-year-old man who sustained second-degree burns over 20% of his body. He has a history of diabetes, coronary artery disease, and hypertension. His blood pressure is 150/79 mm Hg and his ventilatory rate is 13 breaths/min. Identify the rhythm (lead II).

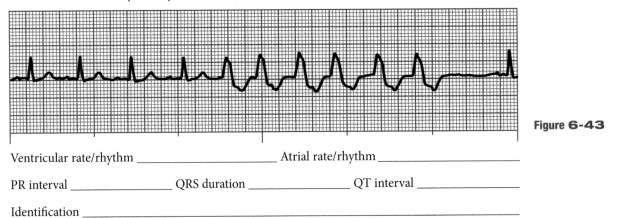

Figure **6-43**

Ventricular rate/rhythm _____ Atrial rate/rhythm _____

PR interval _____ QRS duration _____ QT interval _____

Identification _____

39. Identify the rhythm (lead II).

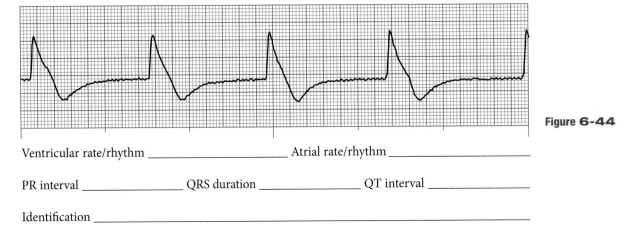

Figure **6-44**

Ventricular rate/rhythm _____ Atrial rate/rhythm _____

PR interval _____ QRS duration _____ QT interval _____

Identification _____

40. Identify the rhythm (lead II).

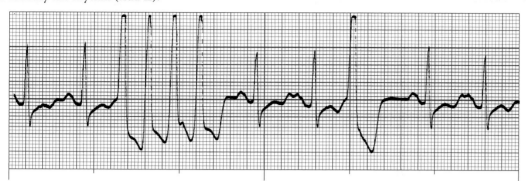

Figure 6-45

Ventricular rate/rhythm _____ Atrial rate/rhythm _____

PR interval _____ QRS duration _____ QT interval _____

Identification _____

41. This rhythm strip is from a 19-year-old male who walked into the emergency department after ingesting a number of unknown medications in a suicide attempt (per the patient). He became unresponsive 5 minutes after his arrival. Initial rhythms before the onset of this dysrhythmia were monomorphic VT and then third-degree AV block. After a brief episode of the rhythm shown here, the patient again converted to a third-degree AV block. His drug screen was negative. A transvenous pacemaker was inserted, and the patient was admitted to the critical care unit. Identify the rhythm (lead II).

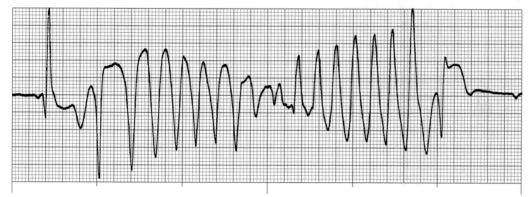

Figure 6-46

Ventricular rate/rhythm _____ Atrial rate/rhythm _____

PR interval _____ QRS duration _____ QT interval _____

Identification _____

42. This rhythm strip is from a 61-year-old woman who is complaining of shortness of breath. Her blood pressure is 176/110 mm Hg. Identify the rhythm (lead II).

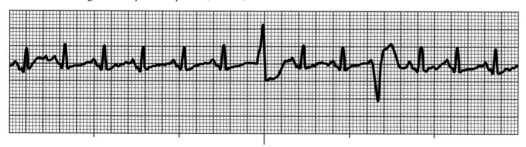

Figure 6-47

Ventricular rate/rhythm _____ Atrial rate/rhythm _____

PR interval _____ QRS duration _____ QT interval _____

Identification _____

43. Identify the rhythm (lead II).

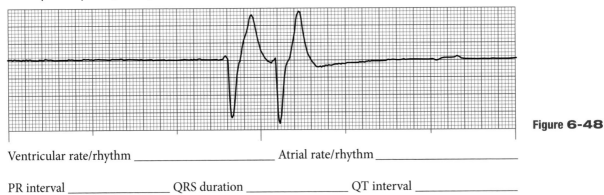

Figure **6-48**

Ventricular rate/rhythm _____ Atrial rate/rhythm _____

PR interval _____ QRS duration _____ QT interval _____

Identification _____

44. Identify the rhythm (lead II).

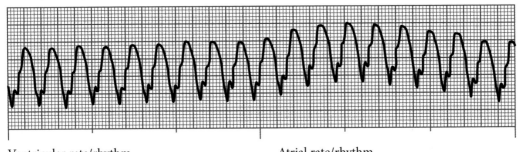

Figure **6-49**

Ventricular rate/rhythm _____ Atrial rate/rhythm _____

PR interval _____ QRS duration _____ QT interval _____

Identification _____

45. Identify the rhythm (lead II).

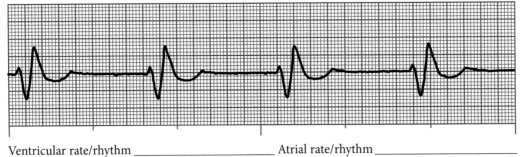

Figure **6-50**

Ventricular rate/rhythm _____ Atrial rate/rhythm _____

PR interval _____ QRS duration _____ QT interval _____

Identification _____

STOP & REVIEW ANSWERS

True/False

1. ANS: F

TdP is a type of polymorphic ventricular tachycardia that occurs in the presence of a long QT interval (typically 0.45 second or more and often 0.50 second or more).

OBJ: Describe the ECG characteristics, possible causes, signs and symptoms, and initial emergency care for polymorphic ventricular tachycardia.

2. ANS: T

Uniform premature ventricular complexes (PVCs) are unifocal; that is, they arise from the same anatomic site. Multiform PVCs often, but do not always, arise from different anatomic sites; therefore, multiform PVCs are not necessarily multifocal. In general, multiform PVCs are considered more serious than uniform PVCs because they suggest a greater area of irritable myocardial tissue.

OBJ: Describe the ECG characteristics, possible causes, signs and symptoms, and initial emergency care for premature ventricular complexes.

3. ANS: T

The intrinsic rate for an accelerated junctional rhythm is 61 to 100 beats/min. The intrinsic rate for an accelerated idioventricular rhythm (AIVR) is 41 to 100 beats/min. Some cardiologists consider the ventricular rate range of AIVR to be 41 to 120 beats/min.

OBJ: Describe the ECG characteristics, possible causes, signs and symptoms, and initial emergency care for an accelerated idioventricular rhythm.

Multiple Choice

4. ANS: B

The intrinsic rate of a junctional escape rhythm is 40 to 60 beats/min. A junctional escape rhythm has a narrow QRS complex. The intrinsic rate of an idioventricular rhythm is 20 to 40 beats/min. An idioventricular rhythm has a wide QRS complex.

OBJ: Describe the ECG characteristics, possible causes, signs and symptoms, and initial emergency care for an idioventricular rhythm.

5. ANS: C

Three or more sequential premature ventricular complexes (PVCs) are termed a run or burst, and three or more PVCs that occur in a row at a rate of more than 100 beats/min is considered a run of ventricular tachycardia.

OBJ: Explain the terms *bigeminy*, *trigeminy*, *quadrigeminy*, and *run* when used to describe premature complexes.

Matching

6. ANS: H
7. ANS: O
8. ANS: Q
9. ANS: M
10. ANS: J
11. ANS: K
12. ANS: N
13. ANS: F
14. ANS: B

15. ANS: A
16. ANS: L
17. ANS: C
18. ANS: P
19. ANS: I
20. ANS: E
21. ANS: G
22. ANS: D

Short Answer

23. ANS:

A premature ventricular complex (PVC) is premature and occurs before the next expected sinus beat. A ventricular escape beat is late, occurring after the next expected sinus beat.

OBJ: Explain the difference between PVCs and ventricular escape beats.

24. ANS:

Coarse ventricular fibrillation (VF) is 3 mm or more in amplitude. **Fine VF** is less than 3 mm in amplitude.

OBJ: Describe the ECG characteristics, possible causes, signs and symptoms, and initial emergency care for ventricular fibrillation.

25. **Figure 6-30 answer**

Ventricular rate/rhythm	77 to 120 beats/min; irregular
Atrial rate/rhythm	77 beats/min (sinus beats); irregular
PR interval	None
QRS duration	None
QT interval	None
Identification	Coarse ventricular fibrillation

26. **Figure 6-31 answer**

Ventricular rate/rhythm	77 to 120 beats/min; irregular
Atrial rate/rhythm	77 beats/min (sinus beats); irregular
PR interval	0.16 sec (sinus beats)
QRS duration	0.06 to 0.08 sec (sinus beats)
QT interval	0.32 to 0.36 sec (sinus beats)
Identification	Sinus rhythm at 77 to 120 beats/min with a pair of premature ventricular complexes (PVCs), ST-segment depression, inverted T waves

27. **Figure 6-32 answer**

Ventricular rate/rhythm	71 beats/min; regular
Atrial rate/rhythm	Unable to determine
PR interval	Unable to determine
QRS duration	0.12 sec
QT interval	0.38 sec
Identification	Accelerated idioventricular rhythm (AIVR) at 71 beats/min

28. **Figure 6-33 answer**

Ventricular rate/rhythm	94 beats/min (sinus beats) to 150 beats/min (ventricular tachycardia [VT]); regular (sinus beats); regular (ventricular beats)
Atrial rate/rhythm	94 beats/min (sinus beats); regular (sinus beats)
PR interval	0.16 sec (sinus beats)
QRS duration	0.10 sec (sinus beats); 0.14 sec (VT)
QT interval	0.32 to 0.36 sec (sinus beats)
Identification	Sinus rhythm at 94 beats/min, a fusion beat, and then monomorphic VT at 150 beats/min

29. **Figure 6-34 answer**

Ventricular rate/rhythm	86 beats/min, irregular
Atrial rate/rhythm	86 beats/min, irregular
PR interval	0.18 sec (sinus beats)
QRS duration	0.10 sec (sinus beats)
QT interval	0.40 sec (sinus beats)
Identification	Sinus rhythm at 86 beats/min with uniform premature ventricular complexes (PVCs)

30. **Figure 6-35 answer**

Ventricular rate/rhythm	48 to 67 beats/min; irregular
Atrial rate/rhythm	48 to 67 beats/min; irregular
PR interval	0.16 sec
QRS duration	0.08 sec
QT interval	0.42 sec
Identification	Sinus rhythm at 48 to 67 beats/min with a premature atrial complex (PAC)

31. **Figure 6-36 answer**

Ventricular rate/rhythm	115 beats/min; irregular (sinus beats)
Atrial rate/rhythm	115 beats/min; irregular (sinus beats)
PR interval	0.12 sec (sinus beats)
QRS duration	0.06 sec (sinus beats)
QT interval	0.34 sec (sinus beats)
Identification	Sinus tachycardia at 115 beats/min with ventricular quadrigeminy

32. **Figure 6-37 answer**

Ventricular rate/rhythm	79 beats/min; regular
Atrial rate/rhythm	None
PR interval	None
QRS duration	0.08 sec
QT interval	0.32 sec
Identification	Accelerated junctional rhythm at 79 beats/min with ST-segment elevation

33. **Figure 6-38 answer**

Ventricular rate/rhythm	65 beats/min (sinus beats) to approximately 167 beats/min (ventricular beats); regular to irregular
Atrial rate/rhythm	65 beats/min (sinus beats); regular (sinus beats)
PR interval	0.16 sec (sinus beats)
QRS duration	0.10 to 0.12 sec (sinus beats)
QT interval	0.32 sec (sinus beats)
Identification	Sinus rhythm at 65 beats/min with ST-segment depression to polymorphic ventricular tachycardia (VT) at 167 beats/min

34. Figure 6-39 answer

Ventricular rate/rhythm	None to 40 beats/min; irregular to regular
Atrial rate/rhythm	None
PR interval	None
QRS duration	None to 0.16 sec
QT interval	None to 0.36 sec
Identification	Ventricular fibrillation, a shock (defibrillation), idioventricular rhythm at 40 beats/min

35. Figure 6-40 answer

Ventricular rate/rhythm	115 to 167 beats/min; irregular
Atrial rate/rhythm	Unable to determine
PR interval	Unable to determine
QRS duration	0.08 sec
QT interval	Unable to determine
Identification	Uncontrolled atrial fibrillation at 115 to 167 beats/min

36. Figure 6-41 answer

Ventricular rate/rhythm	62 beats/min; essentially regular
Atrial rate/rhythm	62 beats/min; essentially regular
PR interval	0.20 sec
QRS duration	0.10 sec
QT interval	0.44 sec
Identification	Sinus rhythm at 62 beats/min with an interpolated premature ventricular complex (PVC) and inverted T waves

37. Figure 6-42 answer

Ventricular rate/rhythm	None
Atrial rate/rhythm	None
PR interval	None
QRS duration	None
QT interval	None
Identification	Asystole

38. Figure 6-43 answer

Ventricular rate/rhythm	96 beats/min (sinus beats); irregular
Atrial rate/rhythm	96 beats/min (sinus beats); irregular
PR interval	0.20 sec (sinus beats)
QRS duration	0.08 sec (sinus beats)
QT interval	0.34 sec (sinus beats)
Identification	Sinus rhythm at 96 beats/min with a run of monomorphic ventricular tachycardia (VT)

39. Figure 6-44 answer

Ventricular rate/rhythm	48 beats/min; regular
Atrial rate/rhythm	None
PR interval	None
QRS duration	0.24 sec
QT interval	0.48 to 0.52 sec
Identification	Accelerated idioventricular rhythm (AIVR) at 48 beats/min

40. Figure 6-45 answer

Ventricular rate/rhythm	30 to 94 beats/min (sinus beats); irregular
Atrial rate/rhythm	30 to 94 beats/min (sinus beats); irregular
PR interval	0.20 sec (sinus beats)
QRS duration	0.08 sec (sinus beats)
QT interval	0.40 sec (sinus beats)
Identification	Sinus rhythm at 30 to 94 beats/min with a premature ventricular complex (PVC) and a run of ventricular tachycardia (VT), ST-segment depression, and inverted T waves

41. Figure 6-46 answer

Ventricular rate/rhythm	230 to 330 beats/min; irregular
Atrial rate/rhythm	Unable to determine
PR interval	Unable to determine
QRS duration	Varies
QT interval	Unable to determine
Identification	Supraventricular beat and then polymorphic ventricular tachycardia (VT) at 230 to 330 beats/min

42. Figure 6-47 answer

Ventricular rate/rhythm	65 to 125 beats/min (sinus beats); irregular
Atrial rate/rhythm	65 to 125 beats/min (sinus beats); irregular
PR interval	0.12 sec (sinus beats)
QRS duration	0.06 sec (sinus beats)
QT interval	Unable to determine
Identification	Sinus tachycardia at 65 to 125 beats/min with multiform premature ventricular complexes (PVCs)

43. Figure 6-48 answer

Ventricular rate/rhythm	Two ventricular complexes to none
Atrial rate/rhythm	None
PR interval	None
QRS duration	0.14 sec to none
QT interval	0.48 sec to none
Identification	Agonal rhythm/asystole

44. Figure 6-49 answer

Ventricular rate/rhythm	188 beats/min; regular
Atrial rate/rhythm	None
PR interval	None
QRS duration	0.18 sec
QT interval	Unable to determine
Identification	Monomorphic ventricular tachycardia (VT) at 188 beats/min

45. Figure 6-50 answer

Ventricular rate/rhythm	38 beats/min; regular
Atrial rate/rhythm	None
PR interval	None
QRS duration	0.18 sec
QT interval	Unable to determine
Identification	Idioventricular rhythm (IVR) at 38 beats/min

Heart Blocks

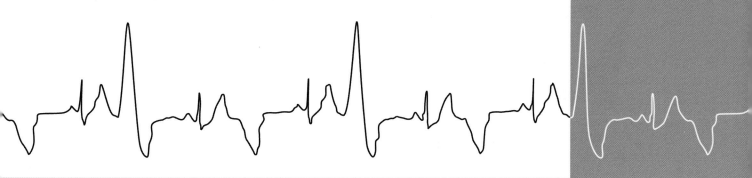

LEARNING OBJECTIVES

After reading this chapter, you should be able to:

1. Describe the electrocardiogram (ECG) characteristics, possible causes, signs and symptoms, and emergency management for first-degree atrioventricular (AV) block.
2. Describe the ECG characteristics, possible causes, signs and symptoms, and emergency management for second-degree AV block type I.
3. Describe the ECG characteristics, possible causes, signs and symptoms, and emergency management for second-degree AV block type II.

4. Describe 2:1 AV block and advanced second-degree AV block.
5. Describe the ECG characteristics, possible causes, signs and symptoms, and emergency management for third-degree AV block.
6. Describe the appearance of right and left bundle branch block as seen in lead V_1.

KEY TERMS

Atrioventricular (AV) block: A delay or interruption in impulse conduction from the atria to the ventricles that occurs because of a transient or permanent anatomic or functional impairment

Bundle branch block (BBB): A disruption in impulse conduction from the bundle of His through the right or left bundle branch to the Purkinje fibers; a BBB may be intermittent or permanent

INTRODUCTION

You have learned that the AV node and AV bundle have many important functions (Figure 7-1). First, a supraventricular impulse that enters the AV node is normally delayed, thereby allowing the atrial chambers to contract and empty blood into the ventricles before the next ventricular contraction begins. Second, the healthy AV node is able to filter some of the supraventricular impulses coming to it, thereby protecting the ventricles from excessively rapid rates. Third, the AV bundle has pacemaker cells that have an intrinsic rate of 40 to 60 beats/min and can function as an escape pacemaker if the sinoatrial (SA) node fails.

Depolarization and repolarization are slow in the AV node, which makes this area vulnerable to blocks in conduction. When a delay or interruption in impulse conduction from the atria to the ventricles occurs because of a

transient or permanent anatomic or functional impairment, the resulting dysrhythmia is called an **atrioventricular block**.

When analyzing a rhythm strip, disturbances in AV conduction can be detected by assessing PR intervals. Remember that the PR interval is made up of the P wave and the PR segment. The P wave reflects depolarization of the right and left atria. The PR segment reflects the spread of the electrical impulse through the AV node and the His-Purkinje network. The normal PR interval measures 0.12 to 0.20 second.

AV block is classified into (1) first-degree AV block, (2) second-degree AV block (types I and II), and (3) third-degree AV block (Figure 7-2). With first-degree AV block, impulses from the SA node to the ventricles are *delayed*; they are not blocked. With second-degree AV blocks, there is an *intermittent* disturbance in the conduction of impulses between the atria and the ventricles. With third-degree AV

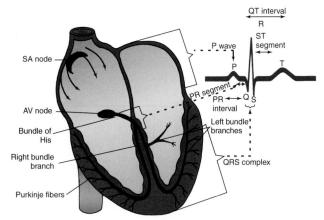

Figure 7-1 Interruptions in impulse transmission between the atria and ventricles can be detected by assessing PR intervals. AV, atrioventricular; SA, sinoatrial.

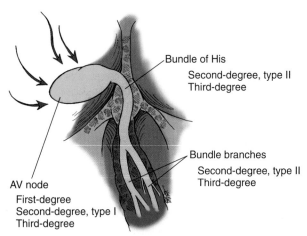

Figure 7-2 Common locations of atrioventricular (AV) blocks.

block, there is a *complete* block in the conduction of impulses between the atria and the ventricles.

First-degree AV block usually occurs because of a conduction delay within the AV node. Second- and third-degree AV blocks can occur at the level of the AV node, the bundle of His, or the bundle branches. AV blocks located at the bundle of His or bundle branches are called *infranodal* or *subnodal* AV blocks. Second and third-degree AV blocks may become serious enough to require the use of an escape pacemaker. Should such a pacemaker become a necessity, AV blocks that occur at the level of the AV node have a tremendous advantage. If required, there is usually a reliable junctional pacemaker available that can fire at 40 to 60 beats/min. However, when the location of an AV block is below the AV junction, the only available pacemaker may be a slow ventricular one, firing at 20 to 40 beats/min. Not only are ventricular pacemakers slow, they are prone to long pauses, making them less than reliable. Therefore, AV blocks at the level of the AV node usually have a more effective and

reliable escape pacemaker than do AV blocks at the bundle of His or below.

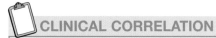

CLINICAL CORRELATION

The clinical significance of an atrioventricular (AV) block depends on the following:
- The degree of the block
- The rate of the escape pacemaker (junctional versus ventricular)
- The patient's response to that ventricular rate

FIRST-DEGREE ATRIOVENTRICULAR BLOCK

How Do I Recognize It?

[Objective 1]
With a first-degree AV block, all components of the cardiac cycle are usually within normal limits, with the exception of the PR interval. This is because electrical impulses travel normally from the SA node through the atria, but there is a delay in impulse conduction, usually at the level of the AV node (Figure 7-3). Despite its name, the SA node impulse is not blocked during a first-degree AV block; rather, each sinus impulse is *delayed* for the same period before it is conducted to the ventricles. This delay in AV conduction results in a PR interval that is longer than normal (i.e., more than 0.20 second in duration in adults) and constant before each QRS complex. Despite the prolonged PR interval, each P wave is followed by a QRS complex (i.e., there is a 1:1 relationship of P waves to QRS complexes).

When a PR interval is prolonged, it is usually between 0.21 and 0.48 second. A PR interval that is longer than 0.29 second is almost always associated with disease of the AV node.[1] Occasionally, a PR interval greater than 0.8 second may be seen. However, PR intervals as long as 1 second have been reported.[2,3]

When the QRS complex associated with a first-degree AV block is narrow, the conduction abnormality is most commonly in the AV node.[1,4] When the QRS complex associated with a first-degree AV block is wide, the conduction abnormality may be located in the AV node, the bundle of His, or the bundle branches.

Let's look at the rhythm shown in Figure 7-4. The ventricular rhythm is regular at a rate of 88 beats/min. Each QRS complex is preceded by an upright P wave. The atrial rhythm is also regular at a rate of 88 beats/min. On the basis of these findings, we now know that the underlying rhythm is a sinus rhythm at 88 beats/min. The QRS duration is within normal limits; however, the PR interval measures 0.28 second, which is longer than normal, and the interval is consistent before each QRS. The 1:1 relationship of P wave to QRS complex and a longer than normal PR interval fit the criteria for a first-degree AV block.

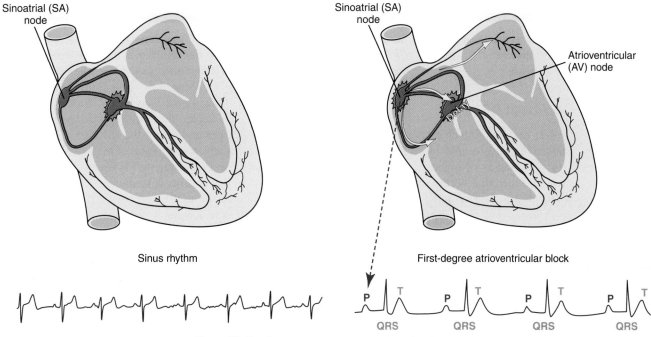

Figure 7-3 First-degree atrioventricular (AV) block. SA, sinoatrial.

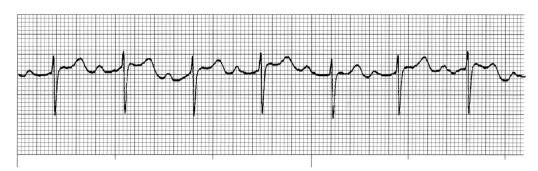

Figure 7-4 Sinus rhythm at 88 beats/min with a first-degree atrioventricular (AV) block and ST-segment elevation.

First-degree AV block is not a dysrhythmia itself; it is a condition that describes the prolonged (but constant) PR interval that is seen on the rhythm strip. Our identification of the rhythm strip in Figure 7-4 must include a description of the underlying rhythm, the ventricular rate, and then a description of anything that appears amiss. In this case, we will identify the rhythm as, "Sinus rhythm at 88 beats/min with a first-degree AV block and ST-segment elevation." The characteristics of first-degree AV block are shown in Table 7-1.

What Causes It?

First-degree AV block may be a normal finding in individuals with no history of cardiac disease, especially in athletes. In some people, mild prolongation of the PR interval may be a normal variant, especially with sinus bradycardia during rest or sleep. First-degree AV block may also occur because of the following:

- Acute myocardial infarction
- Acute myocarditis or endocarditis

Table 7-1	Characteristics of First-Degree Atrioventricular Block
Rhythm	Regular
Rate	Usually within normal range, but depends on underlying rhythm
P waves	Normal in size and shape; one positive (upright) P wave before each QRS
PR interval	Prolonged (i.e., more than 0.20 sec) but constant
QRS duration	Usually 0.11 sec or less unless abnormally conducted

- Cardiomyopathy
- Degenerative fibrosis and sclerosis of the conduction system
- Drug effect (e.g., amiodarone, beta-blockers, digoxin, diltiazem, procainamide, verapamil)
- Hyperkalemia

- Increased vagal tone (e.g., carotid massage, inferior infarction, vomiting)
- Ischemia or injury to the AV node or AV bundle
- Rheumatic heart disease
- Valvular heart disease

What Do I Do About It?

The patient with a first-degree AV block is often asymptomatic; however, marked first-degree AV block can lead to symptoms even in the absence of higher degrees of AV block.[5] First-degree AV block that occurs with acute myocardial infarction (MI) should be monitored closely.

SECOND-DEGREE ATRIOVENTRICULAR BLOCKS

Overview

The term *second-degree AV block* is used when one or more, but not all, sinus impulses are blocked from reaching the ventricles. Because the SA node is generating impulses in a normal manner, each P wave will occur at a regular interval across the rhythm strip (i.e., all P waves will plot through on time), although not every P wave will be followed by a QRS complex. This suggests that the atria are being depolarized normally, but not every impulse is being conducted to the ventricles (i.e., intermittent conduction). As a result, more P waves than QRS complexes are seen on the ECG.

Second-degree AV block is classified as type I or type II, depending on the behavior of the PR intervals associated with the dysrhythmia. The type I or type II designation is used to describe the *ECG pattern* of the PR intervals and should not be used to describe the anatomic site (i.e., location) of the AV block.[6] At least two consecutively conducted PR intervals must be observed to determine the pattern of the PR intervals.

Second-Degree Atrioventricular Block Type I

How Do I Recognize It?
[Objective 2]
Second-degree AV block type I is also known as *type I block*, *Mobitz I*, or *Wenckebach*. The term *Wenckebach phenomenon* is used to describe a progressive lengthening of conduction time in any cardiac conducting tissue that eventually results in the dropping of a beat or a reversion to the initial conduction time. With "classic" Wenckebach phenomenon, the PR interval after the dropped (i.e., blocked) beat is the shortest in the cycle and the largest increase in the PR interval occurs after the second conducted beat.[2,7] As each atrial impulse arrives earlier and earlier into the relative refractory period of the impaired AV node, more time is required to conduct the impulse to the ventricles. On the ECG, this is reflected as a progressive increase in the length of the PR intervals (Figure 7-5).

When an impulse finally arrives during the AV node's absolute refractory period, it fails to conduct to the ventricles and is seen on the ECG as a P wave that is not followed by a QRS complex.[4,8,9] Because the conduction delay in second-degree AV block type I is almost always a result of a lesion within the AV node, the QRS associated with this form of AV block is usually narrow. When a second-degree AV block type I occurs with a wide QRS complex, the block is within the AV node in 30% to 40% of cases and within the His-Purkinje system in 60% to 70% of cases, except in cases of MI.[6,10]

Second-degree AV block type I is characterized by a repeating pattern that consists of conducted P waves (i.e., each P wave is followed by a QRS) and then a P wave that is not conducted (i.e., the P wave is not followed by a QRS). In second-degree AV block type I, any P to QRS ratio may be seen. For example, an AV conduction ratio of 3:2 means that for every three P waves, two are followed by QRS complexes. Four conducted P waves to three QRS complexes results in 4:3 conduction; five conducted P waves to four QRS complexes results in 5:4 conduction; and so on. The P wave that is not conducted ends a *group* of beats. Because QRS complexes are periodically absent, the ventricular rhythm is irregular. The cycle then begins again. The repetition of this cyclic pattern is called *grouped beating*. It is important to note that the grouped beating pattern described occurs in less than 50% of patients who have second-degree AV block type I.[2]

Although *progressive lengthening* is a phrase that was used for many years to describe the behavior of the PR intervals associated with second-degree AV block type I, the use of this terminology is no longer recommended; rather, the term *inconstant* or *generally progressive* PR intervals is recommended.[6] Use of the term *inconstant* or *generally progressive* PR intervals is important because many type I AV blocks are atypical, missing one or more of the features of the classic Wenckebach phenomenon.[6,9] For example, the second conducted PR interval after a blocked impulse may fail to show the greatest increase in length; instead, the PR interval may actually shorten and then lengthen in the middle of a grouped beating pattern.[6] Alternately, the duration of the PR intervals may show no obvious change in the middle or for a few beats just before the end of a group.[6]

Let us look at the example of this type of AV block in Figure 7-6. For the purposes of our discussion, consider first labeling the QRS complexes on this rhythm strip 1 through 6. You can quickly see that the ventricular rhythm is irregular. Because it is irregular, calculate the rate between the shortest and longest R-R intervals. The rate range is about 43 to 60 beats/min. Now let us look at the atrial rhythm and calculate the atrial rate. Look to the left of each QRS and label each P wave in the rhythm strip. Place your calipers or a piece of paper on two P waves and begin moving from the left side of the strip to the right to see if the P waves occur on time. You will find that there is an "extra" P wave after beat 3. The extra P wave occurs on time, but there is no QRS after it. The remainder of the P waves occur on time. The atrial rate is about 68 beats/min.

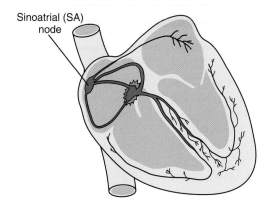

Sinoatrial (SA) node

Sinus rhythm

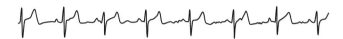

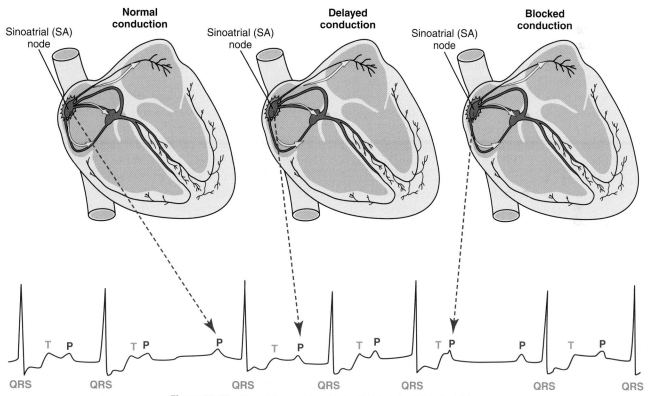

Normal conduction

Delayed conduction

Blocked conduction

Sinoatrial (SA) node

Sinoatrial (SA) node

Sinoatrial (SA) node

Figure 7-5 Second-degree atrioventricular (AV) block, type I. SA, sinoatrial.

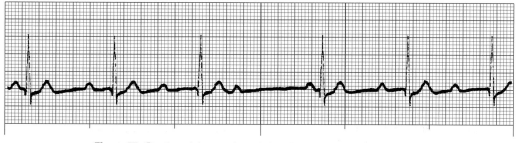

Figure 7-6 Second-degree atrioventricular (AV) block type I at 43 to 60 beats/min.

Although we are discussing AV blocks in this chapter, how do you know that the extra P wave with no QRS after it isn't a nonconducted premature atrial complex (PAC)? Well, the difference is in the timing of the P waves. If you have not been plotting P waves when analyzing a rhythm strip until now, it is *very* important that you do so when identifying AV blocks. In second and third-degree AV blocks there are more P waves than QRS complexes, and the P waves occur *on time*. This happens because the problem in second and third-degree AV blocks is not within the SA node. The problem occurs somewhere in the conduction system *below* the SA node. Therefore, the sinus fires regularly—as it is supposed to. The P wave that occurs after beat 3 is not a nonconducted PAC because all of the P waves are on time. By definition, the P wave of a nonconducted *premature atrial complex* is early.

The duration of the QRS complexes in Figure 7-6 are within normal limits. Now, look closely at the PR intervals and determine if a pattern exists. To do this, we need to see at least two PQRST cycles in a row that do not contain extra waveforms. Beats 1, 2, and 3 allow us to do this because there is one P wave before each QRS. When you compare the PR intervals of these beats, the PR interval of beat 1 is short. The PR interval of beat 2 is longer than that of beat 1, and the PR interval of beat 3 is longer than that of the first two beats. The PR intervals of beats 1 through 3 can be described as *inconstant* or *generally progressive*. The blocked sinus impulse appears on the ECG as a P wave with no QRS after it (i.e., a dropped beat). The cycle begins again after the dropped beat. The PR interval of the first conducted beat *after* the blocked sinus impulse (i.e., beat 4) is shorter than the PR interval of the conducted beat *before* the blocked beat (i.e., beat 3). This finding is an important one when identifying second-degree AV block type I. Our identification of this rhythm strip is, "Second-degree AV block type I at 43 to 60 beats/min." The ECG characteristics of second-degree AV block type I are shown in Table 7-2.

What Causes It?

Remember that the right coronary artery (RCA) supplies the AV node in 90% of the population. The RCA also supplies the inferior wall of the left ventricle and the right ventricle in most individuals. Blockage of the RCA, resulting in an inferior MI or right ventricular infarction, can also result in conduction delays such as first-degree AV block and second-degree AV block type I. Second-degree AV block type I can also occur in athletes, probably related to an increase in resting vagal tone,[2] and in healthy individuals during sleep. Other possible causes of this dysrhythmia include aortic valve disease, atrial-septal defect, medications (e.g., beta-blockers, digoxin, diltiazem, verapamil), mitral valve prolapse, and rheumatic heart disease.

What Do I Do About It?

The patient with this type of AV block is usually asymptomatic because the ventricular rate often remains nearly normal, and cardiac output is not significantly affected. If the patient is symptomatic and the dysrhythmia is a result of medications (e.g., digoxin, beta-blockers), these substances should be withheld. When it is associated with an acute inferior wall MI, this dysrhythmia is usually transient and resolves within 48 to 72 hours as the effects of parasympathetic stimulation disappear.

If the heart rate is slow and serious signs and symptoms occur because of the slow rate, treatment should include applying a pulse oximeter and administering oxygen (if indicated), obtaining the patient's vital signs, and establishing intravenous (IV) access. A 12-lead ECG should be obtained. Atropine, administered intravenously, is the drug of choice. Reassess the patient's response and continue monitoring the patient. When this rhythm occurs in conjunction with acute MI, the patient should be observed closely for increasing AV block.

Second-Degree Atrioventricular Block Type II

How Do I Recognize It?
[Objective 3]

Second-degree AV block type II is also called *type II block* or *Mobitz II* AV block. The conduction delay in second-degree AV block type II occurs below the AV node, within the His-Purkinje system. About 70% of the time, the block occurs below the bundle of His, which usually produces a wide QRS (i.e., more than 0.11 second in duration).[6] About 30% of the time, the block occurs in the bundle of His, which is associated with a narrow QRS.[6,7] Although second-degree AV block type II is less common than type I, type II is more serious and is a cause for concern because it has a greater potential to progress to a third-degree AV block.

As it is with second-degree AV block type I, there are more P waves than QRS complexes with second-degree AV block type II, and the P waves occur on time. The PR interval with type II block can be normal or prolonged; but

Table **7-2**	Characteristics of Second-Degree Atrioventricular Block Type I
Rhythm	Ventricular irregular; atrial regular (i.e., Ps plot through on time); grouped beating may be present
Rate	Atrial rate is greater than the ventricular rate
P waves	Normal in size and shape; some P waves are not followed by a QRS complex (i.e., more Ps than QRSs)
PR interval (PRI)	Inconstant; the PRI after a nonconducted P wave is shorter than the interval preceding the nonconducted beat
QRS duration	Usually 0.11 sec or less; complexes are periodically dropped

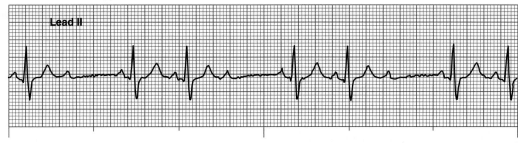

Figure 7-7 Second-degree atrioventricular (AV) block type II at 48 to 94 beats/min.

it is constant for the conducted beats. Most importantly, the PR intervals before and after a blocked sinus impulse (i.e., P wave) are *constant*.

Let's look at Figure 7-7. You can see right away that the ventricular rhythm is irregular. Because the ventricular rhythm is irregular, calculate the ventricular rate and provide a rate range. The ventricular rate ranges from about 48 to 94 beats/min. You can quickly see that there are more P waves than QRS complexes in this rhythm strip. Use your calipers or paper to plot the P waves and see whether they occur on time. Indeed, they occur regularly, although not every P wave is followed by a QRS complex. Now, calculate the atrial rate. It is about 94 beats/min. Each P wave occurs at a regular interval across the rhythm strip (i.e., all P waves plot through on time) because the SA node is generating impulses in a normal manner. Impulses generated by the SA node are conducted to the ventricles until a sinus impulse is suddenly blocked—appearing on the ECG as a P wave with no QRS after it (i.e., a dropped beat); this results in an irregular ventricular rhythm. Looking at the QRS complexes in Figure 7-7, you can see that they are slightly wider than normal, measuring about 0.12 second.

Now look closely at each of the PR intervals and compare them. Are they the same or different? In this rhythm strip, the PR intervals are the same and then a P wave suddenly appears with no QRS after it. When the PR intervals measure the same, we say that the PR intervals are *constant* or *fixed*. This is an important difference between second-degree AV block type I and second-degree AV block type II. In second-degree AV block type II, the PR interval may be within normal limits or prolonged, but it is constant for the conducted beats. Most importantly, the PR intervals before and after a blocked sinus impulse (i.e., P wave) are *constant*.

Our identification of the rhythm in Figure 7-7 is, "Second-degree AV block type II at a rate of 48 to 94 beats/min." The ECG characteristics of second-degree AV block type II are shown in Table 7-3.

ECG Pearl

Some experts believe that type II atrioventricular (AV) blocks are actually type I blocks that have changes in AV conduction that are so minute that they cannot be recorded or measured with standard equipment.[6]

Table 7-3	Characteristics of Second-Degree Atrioventricular Block Type II
Rhythm	Ventricular irregular; atrial regular (i.e., Ps plot through on time)
Rate	Atrial rate is greater than the ventricular rate; ventricular rate is often slow
P waves	Normal in size and shape; some P waves are not followed by a QRS complex (i.e., more Ps than QRSs)
PR interval	Within normal limits or prolonged but constant for the conducted beats; the PR intervals before and after a blocked P wave are *constant*
QRS duration	Within normal limits if the block occurs above or within the bundle of His; greater than 0.11 sec if the block occurs below the bundle of His; complexes are periodically absent after P waves

What Causes It?

You will recall that the conduction delay in second-degree AV block type II occurs below the AV node, within the His-Purkinje system, and that most of the time, the block occurs below the bundle of His. Because a branch of the left coronary artery supplies the bundle branches and the anterior wall of the left ventricle, disease of the left coronary artery or an anterior MI is often associated with conduction defects that occur within the bundle branches. Second-degree AV block type II may also occur because of acute myocarditis, aortic valve disease, cardiomyopathy, fibrosis of the conduction system, or rheumatic heart disease.

What Do I Do About It?

The patient's response to this rhythm is usually related to the ventricular rate. If the ventricular rate is within normal limits, the patient may be asymptomatic. More commonly, the ventricular rate is significantly slowed and serious signs and symptoms result because of the slow rate and decreased cardiac output. The greater the number is of nonconducted beats, the greater the impact is on the cardiac output.

If the heart rate is slow and serious signs and symptoms occur because of the slow rate, treatment should include applying a pulse oximeter and administering oxygen (if indicated), obtaining the patient's vital signs, and establishing IV access. A 12-lead ECG should be obtained. Although current resuscitation guidelines recommend IV administration of atropine to reduce vagal tone and improve conduction through the AV node, this is effective only if the site of the block is the AV node. If the block is below the AV node, atropine is unlikely to be effective. In this situation, atropine administration will usually not improve the block but rather will increase the rate of discharge of the SA node. This may trigger a situation in which even fewer impulses are conducted through to the ventricles and the ventricular rate is further slowed.

Because second-degree AV block type II may abruptly progress to third-degree AV block, the patient should be closely monitored for increasing AV block. When second-degree AV block type II occurs in the setting of an acute anterior MI, temporary or permanent pacing may be necessary.

ECG Pearl

Second-degree atrioventricular (AV) blocks can occur at two or more levels at the same time, making it difficult to distinguish between types I and II.[2]

2:1 Atrioventricular Block

How Do I Recognize It?

[Objective 4]

Before we discuss 2:1 AV block, let us review a few very important points regarding second-degree AV blocks. So far you have learned how important it is to plot P waves to make sure that they occur on time. If there are more P waves than QRS complexes and the P waves occur on time, you know that you have some type of AV block. The ventricular rhythm is irregular with both second-degree AV block type I and type II. The QRS complex with a second-degree AV block type I is usually narrow; it is usually wide with a second-degree AV block type II, although exceptions exist with both types of second-degree blocks.

You have also learned that there are differences in the PR interval patterns with second-degree AV block type I and

type II, and that these differences are important in differentiating between type I and type II AV block. To compare PR intervals, we must see at least two PQRST cycles in a row. More importantly, we must look at the PR interval of the conducted beat *after* a dropped QRS complex and compare it with the PR interval of the last conducted beat *before* the dropped QRS. With this information, you can then begin to differentiate what type of second-degree AV block it is. For example, if the PR interval after a dropped QRS complex is shorter than the PR interval before the dropped complex, a pattern consistent with second-degree AV block type I is present. If the PR interval after a dropped QRS complex is the same as the PR interval before the dropped complex, a pattern consistent with second-degree AV block type II exists.

With second-degree AV block in the form of 2:1 AV block, the level of the block can be located within the AV node or within the His-Purkinje system. With 2:1 AV block, there is one conducted P wave followed by a blocked P wave; thus, two P waves occur for every one QRS complex (i.e., 2:1 conduction). Because there are no two PQRST cycles in a row from which to compare PR intervals, 2:1 AV block cannot be conclusively classified as type I or type II. To determine the type of block with certainty, it is necessary to continue close ECG monitoring of the patient until the conduction ratio of P waves to QRS complexes changes to 3:2, 4:3, and so on, which would enable PR interval comparison.

If the QRS complex measures 0.11 second or less, the block is likely to be located in the AV node and a form of second-degree AV block type I (Figure 7-8). A 2:1 AV block associated with a wide QRS complex (i.e., more than 0.11 second) is usually associated with a delay in conduction below the bundle of His; thus, it is usually a type II block (Figure 7-9). The ECG characteristics of 2:1 AV block are shown in Table 7-4. The causes and emergency management for 2:1 AV block are those of type I or type II block previously described.

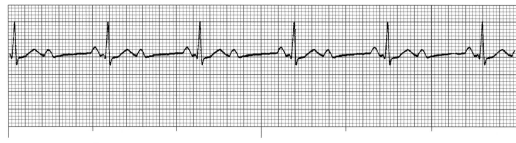

Figure 7-8   Second-degree 2:1 atrioventricular (AV) block with narrow QRS complexes.

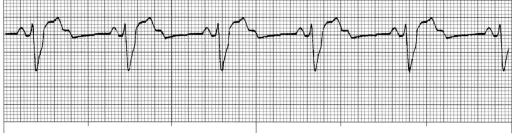

Figure 7-9   Second-degree 2:1 atrioventricular (AV) block with wide QRS complexes.

Table 7-4	Characteristics of Second-Degree 2:1 Atrioventricular Block
Rhythm	Ventricular regular; atrial regular (Ps plot through on time)
Rate	Atrial rate is twice the ventricular rate
P waves	Normal in size and shape; every other P wave is not followed by a QRS complex (i.e., more Ps than QRSs)
PR interval	Constant
QRS duration	May be narrow or wide; complexes are absent after every other P wave

Advanced Second-Degree Atrioventricular Block

[Objective 4]

The terms *advanced* or *high-grade* second-degree AV block may be used to describe three or more consecutive P waves that are not conducted. For example, with 3:1 AV block, every third P wave is conducted (i.e., followed by a QRS complex); with 4:1 AV block, every fourth P wave is conducted (Figure 7-10).

As is the case with 2:1 AV block, advanced second-degree AV block cannot be conclusively classified as type I or type II because there are no two PQRST cycles in a row from which to compare PR intervals. Monitoring of the patient's ECG for changes in P wave to QRS conduction ratios to enable PR interval comparison is essential. Because of the frequency with which impulses from the SA node to the Purkinje fibers are blocked, the presence of advanced AV block is a cause for concern and the development of third-degree AV block should be anticipated.

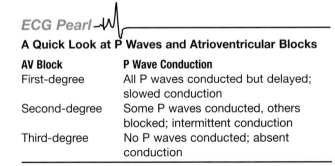

ECG Pearl

A Quick Look at P Waves and Atrioventricular Blocks

AV Block	P Wave Conduction
First-degree	All P waves conducted but delayed; slowed conduction
Second-degree	Some P waves conducted, others blocked; intermittent conduction
Third-degree	No P waves conducted; absent conduction

THIRD-DEGREE ATRIOVENTRICULAR BLOCK

How Do I Recognize It?

[Objective 5]

Second-degree AV blocks are types of *incomplete* blocks because at least some of the impulses from the SA node are conducted to the ventricles. With third-degree AV block, there is a *complete* block in conduction of impulses between the atria and the ventricles. The site of block in a third-degree AV block may be the AV node or, more commonly, the bundle of His or the bundle branches (Figure 7-11). A secondary pacemaker (either junctional or ventricular) stimulates the ventricles; therefore, the QRS may be narrow or wide, depending on the location of the escape pacemaker and the condition of the intraventricular conduction system.

Let's look at the rhythm strip in Figure 7-12, in which the P waves have been labeled. Determine the ventricular rhythm and then calculate the ventricular rate. You will find that the ventricular rhythm is regular and the ventricular rate is 30 beats/min. If the P waves were not labeled for you, it might have been difficult to locate all of the P waves in this rhythm strip. When locating P waves, it is often helpful to place your calipers, or to make marks on a piece of paper, on two clearly identifiable P waves and then move the calipers left and right across the strip, marking the remaining P waves as you go. For example, it would be a good idea to mark P waves 3 and 4 first in this rhythm strip because they are readily seen; then move to the left, identifying P waves 1 and 2, and then move to the right, identifying P waves 5 through 7. When all of the P waves have been identified, determine their regularity, and then determine their rate. You will find that the P waves occur regularly and that the atrial rate is 70 beats/min. Next, look closely at the PR intervals, which have been calculated for you in this rhythm strip. As you can see, there is no true PR interval because the atria and ventricle are beating independently of each other. Our identification of the dysrhythmia in Figure 7-12 is, "Third-degree AV block at 30 beats/min."

The ECG characteristics of third-degree AV block are shown in Table 7-5.

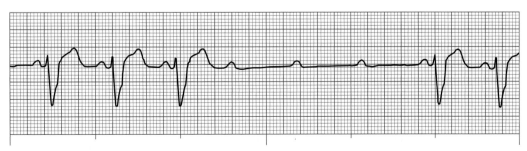

Figure 7-10 An example of advanced second-degree atrioventricular (AV) block.

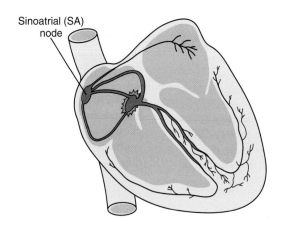

Sinus rhythm

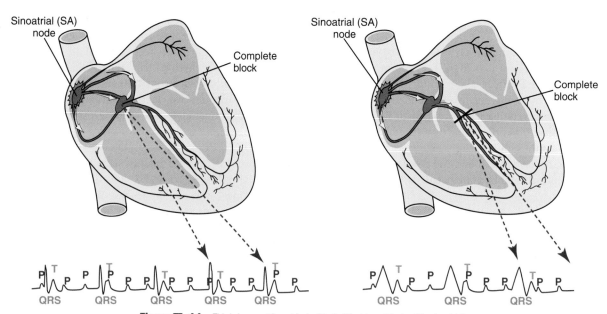

Figure 7-11   Third-degree atrioventricular block. AV, atrioventricular; SA, sinoatrial.

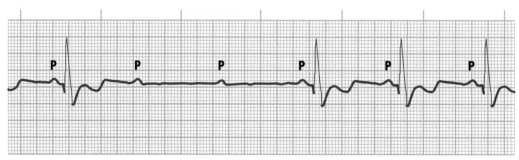

Figure 7-12   Third-degree atrioventricular block at 30 beats/min. PRI, PR interval.

Table 7-5	Characteristics of Third-Degree Atrioventricular Block
Rhythm	Ventricular regular; atrial regular (Ps plot through); no relationship between the atrial and ventricular rhythms (i.e., AV dissociation is present)
Rate	The ventricular rate is determined by the origin of the escape rhythm; the atrial rate is greater than (and independent of) the ventricular rate; ventricular rate is determined by the origin of the escape rhythm
P waves	Normal in size and shape; some P waves are not followed by a QRS complex (i.e., more Ps than QRSs)
PR interval	None: the atria and the ventricles beat independently of each other, thus there is no true PR interval
QRS duration	Narrow or wide, depending on the location of the escape pacemaker and the condition of the intraventricular conduction system

What Causes It?

Causes of third-degree AV block include the following:

- Acute MI
- Acute myocarditis
- Congenital heart disease
- Drug effect (e.g., amiodarone, beta-blockers, digoxin, diltiazem, procainamide, verapamil)
- Fibrosis of the conduction system
- Increased parasympathetic tone

Third-degree AV block that is associated with an inferior MI is thought to be the result of a block above the bundle of His. It often occurs after progression from first-degree AV block or second-degree AV block type I. The resulting rhythm is usually stable because the escape pacemaker is usually junctional (i.e., narrow QRS complexes) with a ventricular rate of more than 40 beats/min (Figure 7-13). Third-degree AV block that is associated with an anterior MI is usually preceded by second-degree AV block type II or an intraventricular conduction delay. The resulting rhythm is usually unstable because the escape pacemaker is usually ventricular (i.e., wide QRS complexes) with a ventricular rate of less than 40 beats/min (Figure 7-14).

What Do I Do About It?

The patient's signs and symptoms will depend on the origin of the escape pacemaker (i.e., junctional versus ventricular) and the patient's response to a slower ventricular rate. Possible rate-related signs and symptoms include dizziness, lightheadedness, generalized weakness, seizures, and *Adams-Stokes syndrome*, which is also known as *Stokes-Adams attacks*. Adams-Stokes syndrome is sudden, recurring episodes of loss of consciousness caused by the transient interruption of cardiac output by incomplete or complete heart block; the ventricular rate is inadequate to maintain cerebral perfusion and results in a syncopal episode.

If the patient is symptomatic as a result of the slow rate, treatment should include applying a pulse oximeter and administering oxygen (if indicated), obtaining the patient's vital signs, establishing IV access, and obtaining a 12-lead ECG. IV administration of atropine may be tried. If the disruption in AV nodal conduction is caused by increased parasympathetic tone, the administration of atropine may be effective in reversing excess vagal tone and improving AV node conduction. Other interventions that may be used in the treatment of third-degree AV block include epinephrine, dopamine, or isoproterenol IV infusions, or transcutaneous pacing. Frequent patient reassessment is essential. Most patients with third-degree AV block have an indication for permanent pacemaker placement.

Examples of most of the AV blocks discussed in this chapter appear in Figure 7-15. A summary of AV block characteristics can be found in Table 7-6.

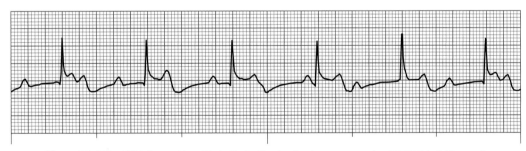

Figure 7-13   Third-degree atrioventricular block with a junctional escape pacemaker (QRS 0.04 to 0.06 second).

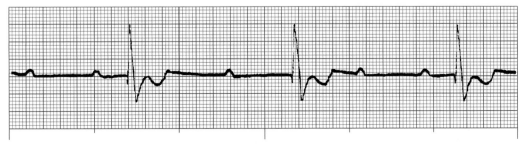

Figure 7-14   Third-degree atrioventricular block with a ventricular escape pacemaker (QRS 0.12–0.14 second).

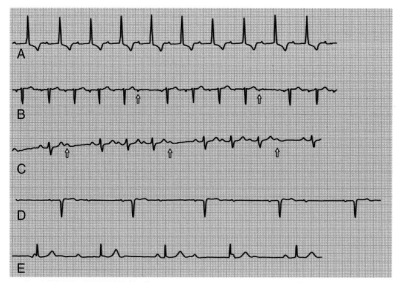

Figure 7-15   Atrioventricular (AV) blocks. **A,** First-degree AV block; the PR interval is constant and more than 0.20 second. **B,** Second-degree AV block type I. The PR intervals after the nonconducted P waves (arrows) are shorter than the interval preceding the nonconducted beat. **C,** Second-degree AV block type II. Nonconducted P waves are seen (arrows). The PR intervals before and after the nonconducted P waves are constant. **D,** 2:1 AV block during which every other P wave is conducted. **E,** Third-degree AV block with AV dissociation and a junctional escape rhythm.

Table **7-6**	Atrioventricular Blocks—Summary of Characteristics				
Characteristic	**First-Degree**	**Second-Degree Type I**	**Second-Degree Type II**	**Second-Degree 2:1 AV Block**	**Third-Degree**
Rhythm	Atrial regular, ventricular regular	Atrial regular, ventricular irregular	Atrial regular, ventricular irregular	Atrial regular, ventricular regular	Atrial regular, ventricular regular
Rate	Usually within normal range, but depends on underlying rhythm	Atrial rate greater than ventricular rate; both often within normal limits	Atrial rate greater than ventricular rate; ventricular rate often slow	Atrial rate greater than ventricular rate	Atrial rate greater than ventricular rate; ventricular rate determined by origin of escape rhythm
P waves (lead II)	Normal, one P wave precedes each QRS	Normal in size and shape; some P waves are not followed by a QRS complex (i.e., more Ps than QRSs)	Normal in size and shape; some P waves are not followed by a QRS complex (i.e., more P's than QRSs)	Normal in size and shape; every other P wave is not followed by a QRS complex (i.e., more Ps than QRSs)	Normal in size and shape; some P waves are not followed by a QRS complex (i.e., more P's than QRSs)
PR interval (PRI)	Greater than 0.20 sec and constant	Inconstant; the PRI after the nonconducted beat is shorter than the interval preceding the nonconducted beat	Within normal limits or prolonged but constant for the conducted beats; the PRIs before and after a blocked sinus impulse (i.e., P wave) are *constant*	Constant	None: the atria and ventricles beat independently of each other, thus there is no true PRI
QRS duration	Usually 0.11 sec or less unless an intraventricular conduction delay exists	Usually 0.11 sec or less and is periodically dropped	Within normal limits if the block occurs above or within the bundle of His; greater than 0.11 sec if the block occurs below the bundle of His; periodically absent after P waves	Narrow or wide depending on location of escape pacemaker and condition of intraventricular conduction system; absent after every other P wave	Narrow or wide depending on location of escape pacemaker and condition of intraventricular conduction system

AV, atrioventricular.

INTRAVENTRICULAR CONDUCTION DELAYS

Structures of the Intraventricular Conduction System

After passing through the AV node, the electrical impulse enters the bundle of His, which is normally the only electrical connection between the atria and the ventricles. The bundle of His conducts the electrical impulse to the right and left bundle branches (Figure 7-16). A **bundle branch block** (BBB) is a disruption in impulse conduction from the bundle of His through either the right or left bundle branch to the Purkinje fibers. A BBB may be intermittent or permanent, complete or incomplete.

The right bundle branch travels down the right side of the interventricular septum to conduct the electrical impulse to the right ventricle. Structurally, the right bundle branch is long, thin, and more fragile than the left. Because of its structure, a relatively small lesion in the right bundle branch can result in delays or interruptions in electrical impulse transmission.

The left bundle branch begins as a single structure that is short and thick and then divides into three divisions (fascicles) called the *anterior fascicle*, *posterior fascicle*, and the *septal fascicle*. The anterior fascicle spreads the electrical impulse to the anterior portions of the left ventricle. This fascicle is thin and vulnerable to disruptions in electrical impulse transmission. The posterior fascicle relays the impulse to the posterior portions of the left ventricle, and the septal fascicle relays the impulse to the mid-septum. The posterior fascicle is short, thick, and rarely disrupted because of its structure and dual blood supply from both the left anterior descending artery and the RCA.

Bundle Branch Activation[11]

The wave of normal ventricular depolarization moves from the endocardium to the epicardium. The left side of the interventricular septum, which is stimulated by the left posterior fascicle, is stimulated first. The electrical impulse (i.e., wave of depolarization) then traverses the septum to stimulate the right side. The left and right ventricles are then depolarized at the same time (Figure 7-17).

A delay or block can occur in any part of the intraventricular conduction system. If a delay or block occurs in one of the bundle branches, the ventricles will not be depolarized at the same time. The electrical impulse travels first down the unblocked branch and stimulates that ventricle. Because of the block, the impulse must then travel from cell to cell through the myocardium, rather than through the normal conduction pathway, to stimulate the other ventricle. The ventricle with the blocked bundle branch is the last to be depolarized.

How Do I Recognize It?[11]

Essentially two conditions must exist to suspect BBB. First, the QRS complex must have an abnormal duration (i.e., 0.12 second or more in width if a complete BBB), and second, the QRS complex must arise as the result of supraventricular activity (this excludes ventricular beats). If these two conditions are met, delayed ventricular conduction is assumed to be present, and BBB is the most common cause of this abnormal conduction.

When one of the bundles becomes blocked, the impulse that is normally conducted by that bundle branch is interrupted and does not depolarize the intended ventricle. Meanwhile, the other bundle branch is conducting its impulse and depolarizing its respective ventricle. How does the other ventricle depolarize? Very slowly. For the second ventricle to depolarize, the electrical impulses must trudge through myocardial cells, which are not specialized for electrical conduction. Thus the impulses from one ventricle must be transmitted, cell by cell, to the other ventricle. Because the impulses are wading through the muck and mire, and not travelling down the superhighway, ventricular depolarization takes longer to occur. This delay is evidenced in the form of a wide QRS complex. A QRS complex that is 0.12 second wide is a sign of abnormal ventricular conduction. However, BBB is not the only cause

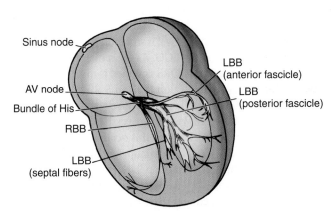

Figure 7-16   Cardiac conduction system. AV, atrioventricular; LBB, left bundle branch; RBB, right bundle branch.

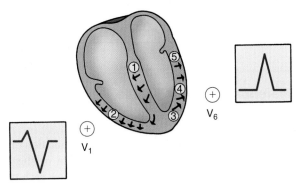

Figure 7-17   Sequence of normal ventricular depolarization and resulting QRS complex, as seen in leads V_1 and V_6.

of abnormal ventricular conduction; ventricular rhythms are another common cause of wide QRS complexes. Consequently an additional criterion must also be met to suspect BBB as the cause, as opposed to a ventricular rhythm. Because BBB implies that a supraventricular impulse was abnormally conducted, and ventricular rhythms are not the result of supraventricular activity, evidence of atrial activity producing the QRS complex rules out the possibility of a ventricular rhythm. Therefore the second criterion for BBB recognition is evidence of supraventricular activity producing the QRS complex.

Two important points must be remembered when examining any ECG. The first is not to trust your eyes. Complexes that are biphasic or triphasic can look narrower than they truly are. Some complexes appear narrow in some leads but, when measured, are just as wide as the other leads. *Measure the QRS complex duration. Do not trust only your eyes.* The second point is that the QRS complex may indeed be wider in one lead than it is in another. Variation in QRS duration from lead to lead is often seen and may produce confusion about whether the complex is or is not wide. As a rule, use the widest QRS complex to determine width. Be careful to accurately pinpoint the exact beginning and end of the QRS complex. This can be difficult to do and is sometimes impossible. Therefore, *when measuring for BBB, select the widest QRS complex with a discernible beginning and end.*

The criteria for BBB recognition may be found in any lead of the ECG. However, when differentiating right bundle branch block (RBBB) from left bundle branch block (LBBB), pay particular attention to the QRS morphology (i.e., shape) in specific leads. Lead V_1 is probably the single best lead to use when differentiating between RBBB and LBBB.

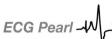

ECG Pearl

ECG Criteria for Bundle Branch Block Recognition

- QRS duration of 0.12 second or more in adults (if a *complete* right or left BBB); if a BBB pattern is discernible and the QRS duration is between 0.10 and 0.12 second in adults, it is called an *incomplete* right or left BBB. (If the QRS is wide but there is no BBB pattern, the term *wide QRS* or *intraventricular conduction delay* is used to describe the QRS).
- QRS complexes that are visible are produced by supraventricular activity (i.e., the QRS complex is not a paced beat, and it does not originate in the ventricles).

Differentiating Right Bundle Branch Block from Left Bundle Branch Block[11]

[Objective 6]

Once the presence of BBB is suspected, an examination of V_1 can reveal whether the block affects the right or the left bundle branch. Following are descriptions of how each type of block affects the direction of electrical current and produces its own, distinct QRS morphology.

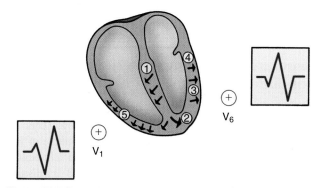

Figure 7-18 Sequence of ventricular depolarization for a right bundle branch block and resulting QRS complex, as seen in leads V_1 and V_6.

Right Bundle Branch Block[11]

With RBBB, the electrical impulse travels through the AV node and down the left bundle branch into the interventricular septum. The septum is activated by the left posterior fascicle and is depolarized in a left-to-right direction (Figure 7-18). Thus septal depolarization moves in a left-to-right direction, which is toward V_1, and produces an initial small R wave. As the left bundle continues to conduct impulses, the entire left ventricle is depolarized from right to left. This produces movement away from V_1 and results in a negative deflection (i.e., an S wave). Now the impulses that depolarized the left ventricle conduct through the myocardial cells and depolarize the right ventricle. This depolarization creates a movement of electrical activity in the direction of V_1, and so a second positive deflection is recorded (R'). The rSR' pattern is characteristic of RBBB. The rSR' pattern is sometimes referred to as an "M" or "rabbit ear" pattern.

Left Bundle Branch Block[11]

With LBBB, the septum is depolarized by the right bundle branch, as is the right ventricle. The septum is part of the left ventricle and is normally depolarized by the left bundle branch. Because the left bundle branch is blocked, depolarization of the septum by the right bundle branch occurs in an abnormal direction (i.e., from right to left); thus the wave of myocardial depolarization begins with the net movement of current going away from V_1 and is recorded as an initial negative deflection (Figure 7-19). The right ventricle is depolarized next. Because the wave of depolarization moves briefly toward the positive electrode in lead V_1, a small upright notch in the QRS complex is seen on the ECG. As the remainder of the left ventricle is depolarized, the QRS complex is inscribed in lead V_1 as a deep, negative deflection (i.e., an S wave), which is a reflection of the left ventricle's large muscle mass. Sometimes depolarization of the left ventricle overshadows that of the right ventricle on the ECG. When this occurs, a QS deflection is inscribed in lead V_1 and the small upright notch that is usually seen with right ventricular depolarization is absent.

Unfortunately not every BBB presents with a clear pattern as previously described, which makes the differentiation between right and left BBB less clear. Variant patterns of BBB as seen in lead V_1 appear in Figure 7-20.

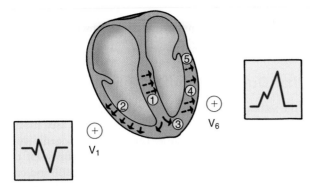

Figure 7-19   Sequence of ventricular depolarization for a left bundle branch block and resulting QRS complex, as seen in leads V_1 and V_6.

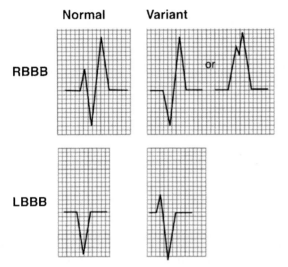

Figure 7-20   Variant patterns of bundle branch block as seen in lead V_1. LBBB, left bundle branch block; RBBB, right bundle branch block.

An Easier Way[11]

Remember that in the setting of BBB, the ventricles are not depolarized in their normal simultaneous manner. Instead, they are depolarized sequentially. The last ventricle to be depolarized is, of course, the ventricle with the blocked bundle branch. Therefore, if it is possible to determine the ventricle that was depolarized last, it becomes possible to determine the bundle branch that was blocked. For example, if the right ventricle was depolarized last, it is because the impulse travelled down the left bundle branch, depolarized the left ventricle first, then marched through and depolarized the right ventricle. It stands to reason that if one ventricle is depolarized late, its depolarization makes up the later portion of the QRS complex.

The final portion of the QRS complex is referred to as the *terminal force*. Examination of the terminal force of the QRS complex reveals the ventricle that was depolarized last, and, therefore, the bundle that was blocked. To identify the terminal force, first locate the J point. From the J point, move backward into the QRS and determine if the last electrical activity produced an upward or downward deflection. An example of the terminal force in both RBBB and LBBB is illustrated in

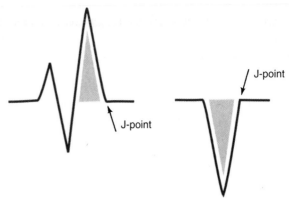

Figure 7-21   Determining the direction of the terminal force. In lead V_1, move from the J point into the QRS complex and determine whether the terminal portion (last 0.04 second) of the QRS complex is a positive (upright) or negative (downward) deflection.

Figure 7-21. If the right bundle branch is blocked, then the right ventricle will be depolarized last and the current will be moving from the left ventricle to the right. This will create a positive deflection of the terminal force of the QRS complex in V_1. If the left bundle branch is blocked, the left ventricle will be depolarized last, and the current will flow from right to left. This will produce a negative deflection of the terminal force of the QRS complex seen in V_1. Therefore, to differentiate RBBB from LBBB, look at V_1 and determine whether the terminal force of the QRS complex is a positive or negative deflection. If it is directed upward, an RBBB is present (i.e., the current is moving toward the right ventricle and toward V_1). A LBBB is present when the terminal force of the QRS complex is directed downward (i.e., the current is moving away from V_1 and toward the left ventricle). This rule is especially helpful when rSR′ and QS variants are present.

A simple way to remember this rule has been suggested by Mike Taigman and Syd Canan, and is demonstrated in Figure 7-22. They recognized the similarity between this rule

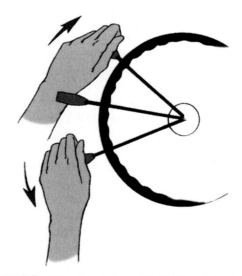

Figure 7-22   Differentiating between right and left bundle branch blocks. The "turn signal" theory is that right is up and left is down.

and the turn indicator on a car. When a right turn is made, the turn indicator is lifted up. Likewise, when a RBBB is present, the terminal force of the QRS complex points up. Conversely, left turns and LBBB are directed downward.

Exceptions[11]

Two notable exceptions must be mentioned to complete the discussion of BBB. The first involves the criteria used to recognize BBB, while the second relates to differentiating LBBB from RBBB.

The criteria used to recognize BBB are valid but lack some sensitivity and specificity. The sensitivity can be limited by junctional rhythms because there may be no discernible P waves when the AV junction is the pacemaker site. The AV junction is a supraventricular pacemaker, but this presents as an exception to the two-part rule of BBB recognition. Specificity is limited by Wolff-Parkinson-White (WPW) syndrome and other conditions that produce wide QRS complexes resulting from atrial activity. If the characteristic delta wave and shortened PR interval are recognized, WPW syndrome should be suspected.

As for differentiating LBBB from RBBB, a third category exists: nonspecific intraventricular conduction delay (NSIVCD). These blocks do not display the typical V_1 morphologies generally produced by BBB. Their origin may not be the result of a complete BBB but are often the result of several factors, of which incomplete BBB may be one. Atypical patterns of BBB can be attributed to NSIVCD.

What Causes It?[11]

Right BBB can occur in individuals with no underlying heart disease, but it occurs more commonly in the presence of organic heart disease, with coronary artery disease being the most common cause. Acute RBBB may occur secondary to a right ventricular infarction. Left BBB may be acute or chronic. Acute LBBB may occur secondary to an anteroseptal (more common) or inferior MI, acute heart failure, and acute pericarditis or myocarditis, among other causes.

Other causes of BBBs include aortic valve disease; congenital, hypertensive, and rheumatic heart disease; and trauma (e.g., cardiac surgery). Sometimes, the ECG will show occasional QRS complexes that have a right or left BBB morphology interspersed with normal QRS complexes. When the intermittent BBB is related to the patient's heart rate, it is referred to as a *rate-related BBB* (i.e., the R-R intervals of the QRS complexes that show BBB are shorter when compared with the R-R intervals of the normal QRS complexes).[12]

Nonischemic diseases, such as Lev disease and Lenègre disease, are also capable of producing a BBB. Lev disease produces BBB through a calcification of the heart's fibrous skeleton. The fibrous skeleton is the infrastructure to which the muscles and valves are attached. Portions of the conduction system are located near the fibrous skeleton or may pass through it. If the fibrous skeleton begins to calcify, part of the electrical conduction system may become "pinched," resulting in a block. Lenègre disease is a more diffuse sclerodegenerative disease that tends to affect the distal portions of the conduction system, but it may also affect the more proximal portions. This process occurs with age, is not related to ischemic heart disease, and is sometimes referred to as the "graying" of the electrical conduction system.

What Do I Do About It?[11]

In the setting of MI, a new onset of BBB is a significant finding. Infarct-induced BBB carries with it an increased mortality rate between 40% and 60%. The rate of cardiogenic shock increases as well, up to 70%. It is not the BBB itself that causes these outcomes; rather, the new onset BBB indicates extensive infarction, and it is the tissue lost to the infarct that produces the increase in mortality and cardiogenic shock.

Because the left anterior descending artery supplies much of the bundle branches, patients experiencing septal and anteroseptal infarctions are most likely to develop BBB. Of course, an infarcting patient presenting with BBB may have had it as a preexisting condition. Unless a previous ECG is available for comparison, or the BBB develops during the infarction, it can be difficult to determine which came first, the infarct or the BBB. BBB in the setting of infarction also identifies patients with a higher likelihood of developing third-degree AV block. Another significant aspect of BBB is its ability to mimic the infarct pattern on the ECG. For the patient who is experiencing chest discomfort, the presence of LBBB can complicate the diagnosis of an acute MI because LBBB can produce ST-segment elevation and wide Q waves that look remarkably similar to infarction. Close ECG monitoring and frequent patient reassessment is essential.

CLINICAL CORRELATION

When bundle branch block (BBB) is present, ST-segment elevation is often seen in leads with negatively deflected QRS complexes. Right bundle branch block (RBBB) rarely produces ST-segment elevation because most of the leads remain positively deflected. Occasionally, when the inferior leads (II, III, and aVF) happen to be negatively deflected, a RBBB may produce ST-segment elevation in those leads, and may occasionally mimic an inferior wall infarction. Although this combination is possible, left bundle branch block (LBBB) is by far the more common cause of ST-segment elevation.

The presence of a BBB in an asymptomatic patient requires no specific treatment. Right BBB generally requires no specific treatment; however, when RBBB occurs in the setting of an acute MI, close ECG monitoring for the development of symptomatic AV conduction system disturbances is essential.

Because of its association with organic heart disease, the patient with LBBB should be evaluated for cardiomyopathies, coronary disease, hypertension, valvular heart disease, and other conditions associated with LBBB. Insertion of a permanent pacemaker is generally required for patients with LBBB who develop second-degree AV block type II or third-degree AV block.

REFERENCES

1. Hamdan MH: Cardiac arrhythmias. In Andreoli TE, Benjamin IJ, Griggs RC, et al: *Andreoli and Carpenter's Cecil essentials of medicine*, ed 8, Philadelphia, 2010, Saunders, pp 118–114.
2. Olgin J, Zipes DP: Specific arrhythmias, diagnosis and treatment. In Bonow RO, Mann DL, Zipes DP, et al: *Braunwald's heart disease: a textbook of cardiovascular medicine*, ed 9, Philadelphia, 2012, Saunders, pp 771–823.
3. Rusterholz AP, Marriott H: How long can the P-R interval be? *Am J Noninvasive Cardiol* 8(11):11–13, 1994.
4. Paul S: Understanding advanced concepts in atrioventricular block, *Crit Care Nurse* 21(1):56–66, 2001.
5. Barold SS: Indications for permanent cardiac pacing in first-degree AV block: class I, II, or III? *PACE* 19(5):747–751, 1996.
6. Barold SS, Hayes DL: Second-degree atrioventricular block: a reappraisal, *Mayo Clin Proc* 76(1):44–57, 2001.
7. Zimelbaum P: Cardiac arrhythmias with supraventricular origin. In Goldman L, Schafer AI, editors: *Cecil medicine*, ed 24, Philadelphia, 2011, Saunders, pp 348–359.
8. Urden LD, Stacy KM, Lough ME: Cardiovascular diagnostic procedures. In *Critical care nursing: diagnosis and management*, ed 6, St. Louis, 2010, Mosby, pp 323–425.
9. Marriott H, Conover MB: AV block. In *Advanced concepts in arrhythmias*, ed 3, St. Louis, 1998, Mosby, pp 311–328.
10. MacKenzie R: Second-degree AV block, *J Insur Med* 36(4):327–332, 2004.
11. Phalen T, Aehlert B: Acute coronary syndromes imposters. In *The 12-lead ECG in acute coronary syndromes*, ed 3, St. Louis, 2012, Mosby, pp 145–152.
12. Litwin SE: Diagnostic tests and procedures in the patient with cardiovascular disease. In Andreoli TE, Benjamin IJ, Griggs RC, et al: *Andreoli and Carpenter's Cecil essentials of medicine*, ed 8, Philadelphia, 2010, Saunders, pp 46–57.

STOP & REVIEW—CHAPTER 7

True/False

Indicate whether the statement is true or false.

_____1. During a first-degree AV block, the PR intervals are completely variable because the atria and ventricles beat independently of each other.

_____2. A bundle branch block is a delay or interruption in impulse conduction from the atria to the ventricles that occurs because of a transient or permanent anatomic or functional impairment.

_____ 3. Second-degree AV blocks are examples of *incomplete* AV blocks.

_____ 4. The site of block in second-degree AV block type II is limited to the bundle branches.

_____ 5. With second-degree AV block type II, the PR intervals before and after a blocked sinus impulse (i.e., P wave) are constant.

Multiple Choice

Identify the choice that best completes the statement or answers the question.

_____6. Which of the following dysrhythmias may be a normal finding in individuals with no history of cardiac disease, especially in athletes?
   a. Atrial fibrillation
   b. First-degree AV block
   c. Third-degree AV block
   d. Ventricular tachycardia

_____7. An ECG rhythm strip shows a regular ventricular rhythm at a rate of 128 beats/min, one upright P wave before each QRS, a regular atrial rate, a constant PR interval of 0.24 second, and a QRS duration of 0.08 second. This rhythm is:
   a. Third-degree AV block.
   b. Second-degree AV block type I.
   c. Sinus tachycardia with first-degree AV block.
   d. Junctional tachycardia with a first-degree AV block.

_____8. Third-degree AV block is characterized by:
   a. Irregular P to P intervals.
   b. Irregular R to R intervals.
   c. Regular P to P intervals and regular R to R intervals.
   d. Regular P to P intervals and irregular R to R intervals.

_____9. An ECG rhythm strip reveals second-degree 2:1 AV block. Which of the following statements is correct regarding this rhythm?
   a. The ventricular rate is twice the atrial rate.
   b. The presence of constant PR intervals allows classification of the block as type I or type II.
   c. The PR intervals are generally progressive until a P wave appears without a QRS after it.
   d. This rhythm is characterized by P waves that are normal in size and shape, but every other P wave is not followed by a QRS.

_____10. The term *second-degree AV block type I* is synonymous with:
   a. Mobitz II.
   b. AV dissociation.
   c. Mobitz I or Wenckebach.
   d. Wolff-Parkinson-White phenomenon.

_____11. Which of the following dysrhythmias is more commonly seen with an inferior wall myocardial infarction?
   a. Sinus arrhythmia
   b. Second-degree AV block type I
   c. Second-degree AV block type II
   d. Third-degree AV block with a wide-QRS

_____12. An ECG rhythm strip reveals an irregular ventricular rhythm at a rate of 28 to 40 beats/min, more P waves than QRS complexes, regular P-P intervals, a constant PR interval of 0.16 second, and a QRS duration of 0.14 second. This rhythm is:
   a. 2:1 AV block.
   b. Third-degree AV block.
   c. Second-degree AV block type I.
   d. Second-degree AV block type II.

_____13. Which of the following is probably the single best lead to use when differentiating between right and left bundle branch block?
   a. Lead II
   b. Lead V_1
   c. Lead V_4
   d. Lead aVR

_____14. Of the following, which dysrhythmia has the greatest potential for sudden, third-degree AV block?
   a. Sinus bradycardia
   b. Junctional escape rhythm
   c. Second-degree AV block type I
   d. Second-degree AV block type II

_____15. The difference between second-degree type I and type II AV block is that with:
    a. Type I the P waves occur irregularly.
    b. Type I the ventricular rhythm is regular.
    c. Type II the QRS duration is consistently more than 0.12 second in duration.
    d. Type II the PR intervals before and after a blocked P wave are constant.

_____16. With a third-degree AV block, the PR interval:
    a. Shortens.
    b. Is absent.
    c. Is inconstant.
    d. Remains constant.

_____17. An ECG rhythm strip reveals an irregular ventricular rhythm at a rate of 46 to 54 beats/min, more P waves than QRS complexes with regular P-P intervals, PR intervals after nonconducted P waves are shorter than the interval preceding the nonconducted beats, and a QRS duration of 0.08 second. This rhythm is:
    a. 2:1 AV block.
    b. Third-degree AV block.
    c. Second-degree AV block type I.
    d. Second-degree AV block type II.

Matching

Match the terms with their definitions by placing the letter of each correct answer in the space provided.

a. Regular
b. Third-degree AV block
c. Between 0.10 and 0.12 second
d. Negative
e. PR interval pattern in second-degree AV block type II
f. Left bundle branch block
g. rSR'
h. First-degree AV block
i. 0.12 to 0.20 second
j. QS
k. Intraventricular conduction delay
l. Irregular
m. Terminal force
n. PR interval pattern in second-degree AV block type I
o. Positive

_____18. Normal duration of the PR interval

_____19. The PRI after the nonconducted P wave is shorter than the interval preceding the nonconducted beat.

_____20. A term used to describe a wide QRS that is not associated with a bundle branch block pattern

_____21. In adults, the QRS duration of an incomplete right or left bundle branch block

_____22. Ventricular rhythm pattern in 2:1 and third-degree AV block

_____23. The PR intervals before and after a blocked P wave are constant.

_____24. Deflection of the terminal force of the QRS complex in V_1 in right bundle branch block

_____25. AV block characterized by a PR interval greater than 0.20 second and one P wave for each QRS complex

_____26. The final portion of the QRS complex

_____27. QRS pattern that is characteristic of left bundle branch block

_____28. AV block characterized by regular P-P intervals, regular R-R intervals, and a PR interval with no consistent value or pattern

_____29. This can produce ST-segment elevation and wide Q waves that look remarkably similar to infarction.

_____30. Ventricular rhythm pattern in second-degree AV block types I and II

_____31. QRS pattern that is characteristic of right bundle branch block

_____32. Deflection of the terminal force of the QRS complex in V_1 in left bundle branch block

Short Answer

33. Indicate the ECG criteria for the following dysrhythmias.

	Second-Degree AV Block Type I	Third-Degree AV Block
Ventricular Rhythm	_____	_____
PR Interval	_____	_____
QRS Width	_____	_____

34. Indicate the ECG criteria for the following dysrhythmias.

	Second-Degree AV Block Type II	2:1 AV Block
Ventricular Rhythm	_____	_____
PR Interval	_____	_____
QRS Width	_____	_____

HEART BLOCKS—*PRACTICE RHYTHM STRIPS*

For each of the following rhythm strips, determine the atrial and ventricular rate and rhythm, measure the PR interval, QRS duration, and QT interval, and then identify the rhythm. Note: These rhythm strips include sinus, atrial, junctional, and ventricular rhythms, and heart blocks.

35. This rhythm strip is from a 66-year-old woman with abdominal pain and weakness that began suddenly while eating breakfast. Her blood pressure is 102/62 mm Hg. Identify the rhythm (lead II).

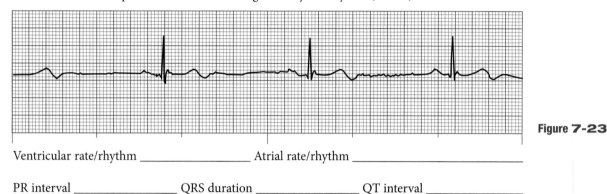

Figure 7-23

Ventricular rate/rhythm _____ Atrial rate/rhythm _____

PR interval _____ QRS duration _____ QT interval _____

Identification _____

36. Identify the rhythm (lead II).

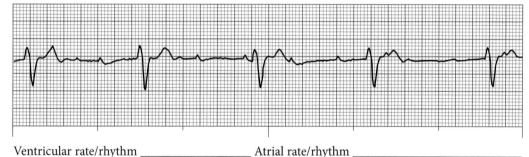

Figure 7-24

Ventricular rate/rhythm _____ Atrial rate/rhythm _____

PR interval _____ QRS duration _____ QT interval _____

Identification _____

37. This rhythm strip is from an 80-year-old woman who states, "The room is spinning." Her blood pressure is 180/90 mm Hg. Identify the rhythm (lead II).

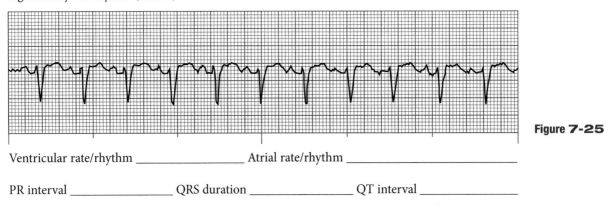

Figure 7-25

Ventricular rate/rhythm _____ Atrial rate/rhythm _____

PR interval _____ QRS duration _____ QT interval _____

Identification _____

38. Identify the rhythm.

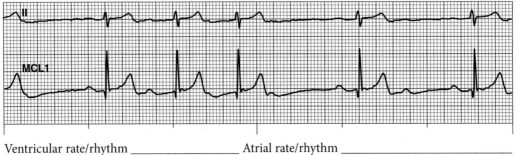

Figure 7-26

Ventricular rate/rhythm _____ Atrial rate/rhythm _____

PR interval _____ QRS duration _____ QT interval _____

Identification _____

39. Identify the rhythm (lead II).

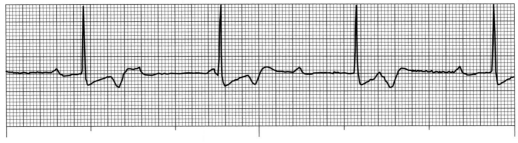

Figure 7-27

Ventricular rate/rhythm _____ Atrial rate/rhythm _____

PR interval _____ QRS duration _____ QT interval _____

Identification _____

40. Identify the rhythm (lead II).

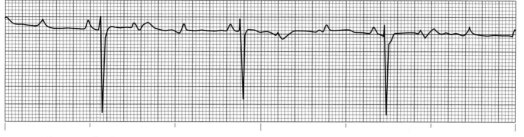

Figure 7-28

Ventricular rate/rhythm _____ Atrial rate/rhythm _____

PR interval _____ QRS duration _____ QT interval _____

Identification _____

41. Identify the rhythm (lead II).

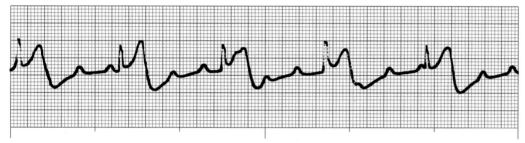

Figure 7-29

Ventricular rate/rhythm _____ Atrial rate/rhythm _____

PR interval _____ QRS duration _____ QT interval _____

Identification _____

42. This rhythm strip is from a 77-year-old woman who stated that she felt fine. She stopped at a blood pressure machine in Walmart and the machine would not read her pulse rate. She later went to her physician's office and then to the emergency department. Identify the rhythm (lead II).

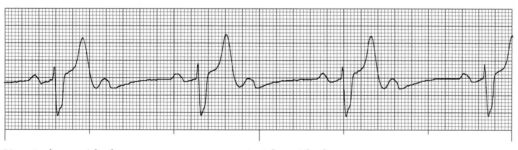

Figure 7-30

Ventricular rate/rhythm _____ Atrial rate/rhythm _____

PR interval _____ QRS duration _____ QT interval _____

Identification _____

43. Identify the rhythm (lead II).

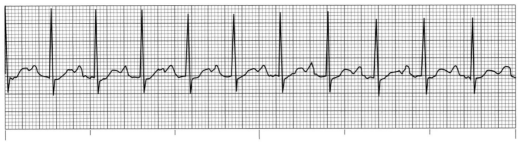

Figure **7-31**

Ventricular rate/rhythm _____ Atrial rate/rhythm _____

PR interval _____ QRS duration _____ QT interval _____

Identification _____

44. Identify the rhythm (lead II).

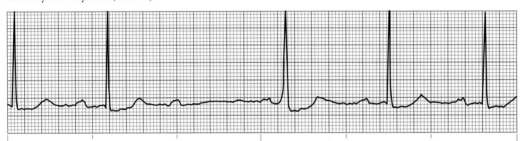

Figure **7-32**

Ventricular rate/rhythm _____ Atrial rate/rhythm _____

PR interval _____ QRS duration _____ QT interval _____

Identification _____

45. Identify the rhythm (lead II).

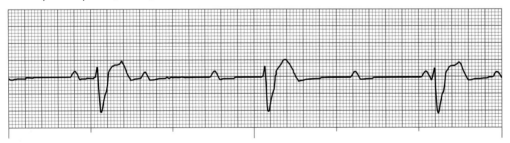

Figure **7-33**

Ventricular rate/rhythm _____ Atrial rate/rhythm _____

PR interval _____ QRS duration _____ QT interval _____

Identification _____

46. This rhythm strip is from an 81-year-old woman who is complaining of chest pain. Identify the rhythm.

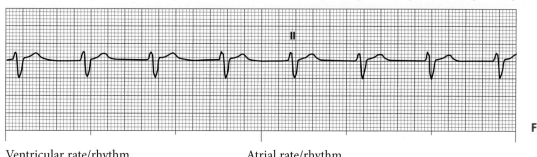

Figure 7-34

Ventricular rate/rhythm _____ Atrial rate/rhythm _____

PR interval _____ QRS duration _____ QT interval _____

Identification _____

47. Identify the rhythm (lead II).

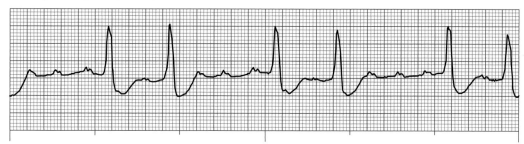

Figure 7-35

Ventricular rate/rhythm _____ Atrial rate/rhythm _____

PR interval _____ QRS duration _____ QT interval _____

Identification _____

48. Identify the rhythm.

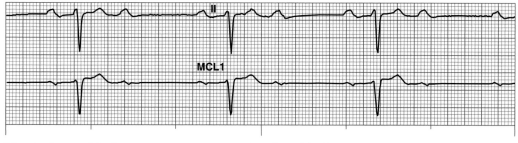

Figure 7-36

Ventricular rate/rhythm _____ Atrial rate/rhythm _____

PR interval _____ QRS duration _____ QT interval _____

Identification _____

49. Identify the rhythm.

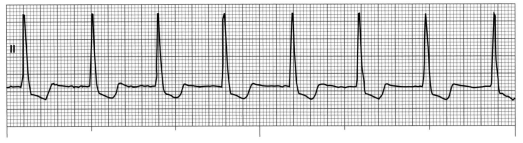

Figure 7-37

Ventricular rate/rhythm _____ Atrial rate/rhythm _____

PR interval _____ QRS duration _____ QT interval _____

Identification _____

50. Identify the rhythm (lead II).

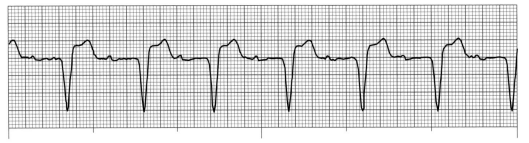

Figure 7-38

Ventricular rate/rhythm _____ Atrial rate/rhythm _____

PR interval _____ QRS duration _____ QT interval _____

Identification _____

51. Identify the rhythm (lead II).

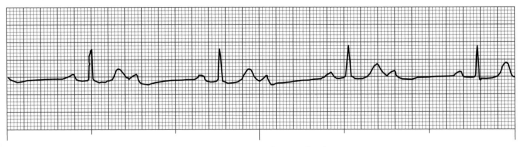

Figure 7-39

Ventricular rate/rhythm _____ Atrial rate/rhythm _____

PR interval _____ QRS duration _____ QT interval _____

Identification _____

52. This rhythm strip is from a 42-year-old man with chest pain. Identify the rhythm (lead II).

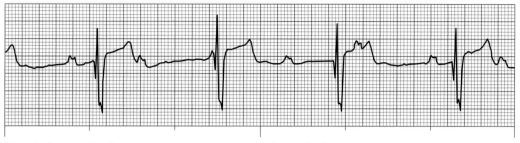

Figure 7-40

Ventricular rate/rhythm _____ Atrial rate/rhythm _____

PR interval _____ QRS duration _____ QT interval _____

Identification _____

53. Identify the rhythm (lead II).

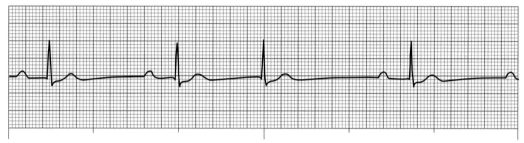

Figure 7-41

Ventricular rate/rhythm _____ Atrial rate/rhythm _____

PR interval _____ QRS duration _____ QT interval _____

Identification _____

54. Identify the rhythm (lead II).

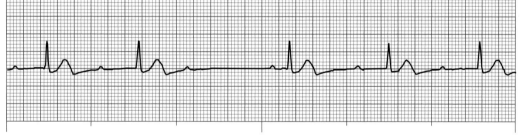

Figure 7-42

Ventricular rate/rhythm _____ Atrial rate/rhythm _____

PR interval _____ QRS duration _____ QT interval _____

Identification _____

STOP & REVIEW ANSWERS

True/False

1. ANS: F

With a first-degree atrioventricular (AV) block, there is a 1:1 relationship between P waves and QRS complexes. The PR intervals are prolonged (i.e., more than 0.20 second) but constant.

OBJ: Describe the ECG characteristics, possible causes, signs and symptoms, and emergency management for first-degree AV block.

2. ANS: F

A bundle branch block is a disruption in impulse conduction from the bundle of His through either the right or left bundle branch to the Purkinje fibers. A delay or interruption in impulse conduction from the atria to the ventricles that occurs because of a transient or permanent anatomic or functional impairment describes an atrioventricular block.

OBJ: Describe the ECG characteristics, possible causes, signs and symptoms, and emergency management for first-degree AV block.

3. ANS: T

Second-degree AV blocks are types of *incomplete* blocks because at least some of the impulses from the sinoatrial (SA) node are conducted to the ventricles. With third-degree AV block, there is a *complete* block in conduction of impulses between the atria and the ventricles.

OBJ: Describe the ECG characteristics, possible causes, signs and symptoms, and emergency management for third-degree AV block.

Multiple Choice

6. ANS: B

First-degree AV block may be a normal finding in individuals with no history of cardiac disease, especially in athletes. In some people, mild prolongation of the PR interval may be a normal variant, especially with sinus bradycardia during rest or sleep. Second-degree AV block type I can also occur in athletes, probably related to an increase in resting vagal tone, and in healthy individuals during sleep.

OBJ: Describe the ECG characteristics, possible causes, signs and symptoms, and emergency management for first-degree AV block.

7. ANS: C

A sinus tachycardia is present when there is a 1:1 relationship between P waves and QRS complexes and the ventricular rate is faster than 100 beats/min. A first-degree AV block is present when there is a 1:1 relationship between P waves and QRS complexes and the PR interval is prolonged (i.e., more than 0.20 second) and constant.

OBJ: Describe the ECG characteristics, possible causes, signs and symptoms, and emergency management for first-degree AV block.

4. ANS: F

The conduction delay in second-degree AV block type II occurs below the AV node, within the His-Purkinje system. About 70% of the time, the block occurs below the bundle of His, which usually produces a wide QRS (i.e., more than 0.11 second in duration). About 30% of the time, the block occurs in the bundle of His, which is associated with a narrow QRS.

OBJ: Describe the ECG characteristics, possible causes, signs and symptoms, and emergency management for second-degree AV block, type II.

5. ANS: T

With second-degree AV block type II, the PR intervals are within normal limits or prolonged but constant for the conducted beats and the PR intervals before and after a blocked sinus impulse (i.e., P wave) are constant.

OBJ: Describe the ECG characteristics, possible causes, signs and symptoms, and emergency management for second-degree AV block, type II.

8. ANS: C

Third-degree AV block is characterized by regular P to P intervals (i.e., a regular atrial rhythm) and regular R to R intervals (i.e., a regular ventricular rhythm); however, there is no relationship between the atrial and ventricular rhythms.

OBJ: Describe the ECG characteristics, possible causes, signs and symptoms, and emergency management for third-degree AV block.

9. ANS: D

Second-degree 2:1 AV block is characterized by P waves that are normal in size and shape, but every other P wave is not followed by a QRS. The atrial rate is twice the ventricular rate. Because there are no two PQRST cycles in a row from which to compare PR intervals, 2:1 AV block cannot be conclusively classified as type I or type II. To determine the type of block with certainty, it is necessary to continue close ECG monitoring of the patient until the conduction ratio of P waves to QRS complexes changes to 3:2, 4:3, and so on, which would enable PR interval comparison.

OBJ: Describe 2:1 AV block and advanced second-degree AV block.

10. ANS: C

Second-degree AV block type I is also known as *type I block*, *Mobitz I*, or *Wenckebach*.

OBJ: Describe the ECG characteristics, possible causes, signs and symptoms, and emergency management for second-degree AV block type I.

11. ANS: B

Remember that the right coronary artery (RCA) supplies the AV node in 90% of the population. The RCA also supplies the inferior wall of the left ventricle and the right ventricle in most individuals. Blockage of the RCA, resulting in an inferior myocardial infarction or right ventricular infarction, can also result in conduction delays such as first-degree AV block and second-degree AV block type I.

OBJ: Describe the ECG characteristics, possible causes, signs and symptoms, and emergency management for second-degree AV block type I.

12. ANS: D

With second-degree AV block type II the ventricular rhythm is irregular. There are more P waves than QRS complexes and the P-P interval is regular. P waves are normal in size and shape, but some P waves are not followed by a QRS complex. The PR interval may be within normal limits or prolonged, but it is constant for the conducted beats; the PR intervals before and after a blocked P wave are constant. The QRS duration is within normal limits if the block occurs above or within the bundle of His; it is greater than 0.11 second if the block occurs below the bundle of His. QRS complexes are periodically absent after P waves.

OBJ: Describe the ECG characteristics, possible causes, signs and symptoms, and emergency management for second-degree AV block type II.

13. ANS: B

The criteria for bundle branch block recognition may be found in any lead of the ECG. However, when differentiating right bundle branch block (RBBB) from left bundle branch block (LBBB), pay particular attention to the QRS morphology (i.e., shape) in specific leads. Lead V_1 is probably the single best lead to use when differentiating between RBBB and LBBB.

OBJ: Describe the appearance of right and left bundle branch block as seen in lead V1.

Matching

18. ANS: I
19. ANS: N
20. ANS: K
21. ANS: C
22. ANS: A
23. ANS: E
24. ANS: O
25. ANS: H

14. ANS: D

Although second-degree AV block type II is less common than second-degree AV block type I, type II is more serious and is a cause for concern because it has a greater potential to progress to a third-degree AV block.

OBJ: Describe the ECG characteristics, possible causes, signs and symptoms, and emergency management for second-degree AV block type II.

15. ANS: D

With both second-degree type I and type II AV blocks, P waves occur regularly and the ventricular rhythm is irregular. With second-degree type II, the QRS duration is within normal limits if the block occurs above or within the bundle of His and it is greater than 0.11 second if the block occurs below the bundle of His. QRS complexes are periodically absent after P waves. With second-degree AV block type II the PR intervals before and after a blocked P wave are constant; with second-degree AV block type I, the PR interval after a nonconducted P wave is shorter than the interval preceding the nonconducted beat.

OBJ: Describe the ECG characteristics, possible causes, signs and symptoms, and emergency management for second-degree AV block type II.

16. ANS: B

Third-degree AV block is characterized by regular P to P intervals (i.e., a regular atrial rhythm) and regular R to R intervals (i.e., a regular ventricular rhythm); however, because there is no relationship between the atrial and ventricular rhythms, there is no true PR interval.

OBJ: Describe the ECG characteristics, possible causes, signs and symptoms, and emergency management for third-degree AV block.

17. ANS: C

With second-degree AV block type I, the ventricular rhythm is irregular. There are more P waves than QRS complexes and the P-P interval is regular. P waves are normal in size and shape, but some P waves are not followed by a QRS complex. The PR intervals are inconstant. The PRI after a nonconducted P wave is shorter than the interval preceding the nonconducted beat. The QRS duration is usually 0.11 second or less and QRS complexes are periodically dropped.

OBJ: Describe the ECG characteristics, possible causes, signs and symptoms, and emergency management for second-degree AV block type I.

26. ANS: M
27. ANS: J
28. ANS: B
29. ANS: F
30. ANS: L
31. ANS: G
32. ANS: D

Short Answer

33. ANS:

	Second-Degree AV Block Type I	Third-Degree AV Block
Ventricular Rhythm	Irregular	Regular
PR Interval	Inconstant; generally progressive	None
QRS Width	Usually narrow	Narrow or wide

OBJ: Describe the ECG characteristics, possible causes, signs and symptoms, and emergency management for second-degree AV block type I.

34. ANS:

	Second-Degree AV Block Type II	2:1 AV Block
Ventricular Rhythm	Irregular	Regular
PR Interval	Constant	Constant
QRS Width	Narrow or wide	Narrow or wide

OBJ: Describe 2:1 AV block and advanced second-degree AV block.

35. Figure 7-23 answer

Ventricular rate/rhythm	37 beats/min; regular
Atrial rate/rhythm	37 beats/min; regular
PR interval	0.22 to 0.24 sec
QRS duration	0.06 to 0.08 sec
QT interval	0.48 sec
Identification	Sinus bradycardia at 37 beats/min with first-degree atrioventricular (AV) block

36. Figure 7-24 answer

Ventricular rate/rhythm	46 beats/min; regular
Atrial rate/rhythm	107 beats/min; regular
PR interval	None
QRS duration	0.14 sec
QT interval	0.44 sec
Identification	Third-degree atrioventricular (AV) block at 46 beats/min

37. Figure 7-25 answer

Ventricular rate/rhythm	107 beats/min; regular
Atrial rate/rhythm	107 beats/min; regular
PR interval	0.16 sec
QRS duration	0.12 sec
QT interval	0.32 sec
Identification	Sinus tachycardia at 107 beats/min with a wide QRS and ST-segment elevation

38. Figure 7-26 answer

Ventricular rate/rhythm	42 to 81 beats/min; irregular
Atrial rate/rhythm	75 beats/min; regular
PR interval	Inconstant
QRS duration	0.08 sec
QT interval	0.32 sec
Identification	Second-degree atrioventricular (AV) block type I at 42 to 81 beats/min; although the complexes on the right side of the rhythm strip show 2:1 conduction, comparison of the PR intervals of beats 1 through 3 enable a diagnosis of second-degree type I AV block

39. Figure 7-27 answer

Ventricular rate/rhythm	38 beats/min; regular
Atrial rate/rhythm	68 beats/min; regular
PR interval	None
QRS duration	0.06 sec
QT interval	0.52 sec (prolonged)
Identification	Third-degree atrioventricular (AV) block at 38 beats/min with ST-segment depression, inverted T waves, and a prolonged QT interval

40. Figure 7-28 answer

Ventricular rate/rhythm	36 beats/min; regular
Atrial rate/rhythm	108 beats/min; regular
PR interval	0.16 sec
QRS duration	0.08 to 0.10 sec
QT interval	Unable to determine
Identification	Advanced second-degree atrioventricular (AV) block with 3:1 conduction at 36 beats/min

41. Figure 7-29 answer

Ventricular rate/rhythm	50 beats/min; regular
Atrial rate/rhythm	167 beats/min; regular
PR interval	None
QRS duration	0.06 sec
QT interval	0.32 sec
Identification	Third-degree atrioventricular (AV) block at 50 beats/min with ST-segment elevation

42. Figure 7-30 answer

Ventricular rate/rhythm	30 beats/min; regular
Atrial rate/rhythm	68 beats/min; regular
PR interval	0.28 sec
QRS duration	0.16 sec
QT interval	0.44 sec
Identification	2:1 atrioventricular (AV) block at 30 beats/min

43. Figure 7-31 answer

Ventricular rate/rhythm	107 beats/min; regular
Atrial rate/rhythm	107 beats/min; regular
PR interval	0.24 sec
QRS duration	0.08 sec
QT interval	0.32 sec
Identification	Sinus tachycardia at 107 beats/min with first-degree atrioventricular (AV) block

44. Figure 7-32 answer

Ventricular rate/rhythm	28 to 58 beats/min; irregular
Atrial rate/rhythm	58 beats/min; regular
PR interval	Inconstant; the PR intervals after the nonconducted P waves are shorter than the interval preceding the nonconducted beat
QRS duration	0.06 to 0.08 sec
QT interval	0.48 sec
Identification	Second-degree atrioventricular (AV) block type I at 28 to 58 beats/min with ST-segment depression

45. Figure 7-33 answer

Ventricular rate/rhythm	29 beats/min; regular
Atrial rate/rhythm	71 beats/min; regular
PR interval	None
QRS duration	0.16 sec
QT interval	0.40 sec
Identification	Third-degree atrioventricular (AV) block at 29 beats/min

46. Figure 7-34 answer

Ventricular rate/rhythm	76 beats/min; regular
Atrial rate/rhythm	None
PR interval	None
QRS duration	0.12 to 0.14 sec
QT interval	0.32 sec
Identification	Accelerated idioventricular rhythm (AIVR) at 76 beats/min

47. Figure 7-35 answer

Ventricular rate/rhythm	48 to 83 beats/min; irregular
Atrial rate/rhythm	167 beats/min; regular
PR interval	0.26 sec; the PR intervals before and after the nonconducted P waves are constant
QRS duration	0.12 to 0.14 sec
QT interval	Unable to determine
Identification	Second-degree atrioventricular (AV) block type II at 48 to 83 beats/min with ST-segment depression

48. Figure 7-36 answer

Ventricular rate/rhythm	36 beats/min; regular
Atrial rate/rhythm	72 beats/min; regular
PR interval	0.32 sec
QRS duration	0.12 to 0.14 sec
QT interval	0.40 sec
Identification	2:1 atrioventricular (AV) block at 36 beats/min

49. Figure 7-37 answer

Ventricular rate/rhythm	75 beats/min; regular
Atrial rate/rhythm	None
PR interval	None
QRS duration	0.08 sec
QT interval	0.32 sec
Identification	Accelerated junctional rhythm at 75 beats/min with ST-segment depression

50. Figure 7-38 answer

Ventricular rate/rhythm	75 beats/min; regular
Atrial rate/rhythm	75 beats/min; regular
PR interval	0.36 sec
QRS duration	0.10 to 0.11 sec
QT interval	0.40 to 0.44 sec
Identification	Sinus rhythm at 75 beats/min with first-degree atrioventricular (AV) block and ST-segment elevation

51. Figure 7-39 answer

Ventricular rate/rhythm	37 beats/min; regular
Atrial rate/rhythm	75 beats/min; regular
PR interval	0.28 sec
QRS duration	0.06 sec
QT interval	0.48 sec
Identification	2:1 atrioventricular (AV) block at 37 beats/min

52. Figure 7-40 answer

Ventricular rate/rhythm	42 beats/min; regular
Atrial rate/rhythm	71 beats/min; regular
PR interval	None
QRS duration	0.12 sec
QT interval	0.48 sec
Identification	Third-degree atrioventricular (AV) block at 42 beats/min

53. Figure 7-41 answer

Ventricular rate/rhythm	34 to 60 beats/min; irregular
Atrial rate/rhythm	39 beats/min; irregular (sinus beats)
PR interval	0.36 sec
QRS duration	0.06 sec
QT interval	0.40 sec
Identification	Sinus bradycardia at 34 to 60 beats/min with first-degree atrioventricular (AV) block and a premature junctional complex

54. Figure 7-42 answer

Ventricular rate/rhythm	34 to 52 beats/min; irregular
Atrial rate/rhythm	60 beats/min; regular
PR interval	Inconstant; the PR intervals after the nonconducted P waves are shorter than the interval preceding the nonconducted beat
QRS duration	0.06 to 0.08 sec
QT interval	0.32 sec
Identification	Second-degree atrioventricular (AV) block type I at 34 to 52 beats/min

Pacemaker Rhythms

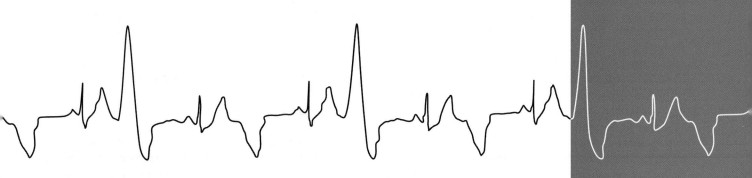

LEARNING OBJECTIVES

After reading this chapter, you should be able to:

1. Identify the components of a pacemaker system.
2. Discuss the terms *triggering, inhibition, pacing, capture, electrical capture, mechanical capture,* and *sensitivity.*
3. Describe the appearance of a typical pacemaker spike on the electrocardiogram (ECG).
4. Describe the appearance of the waveform on the ECG produced as a result of atrial pacing and ventricular pacing.

5. Explain the differences between single-chamber and dual-chamber pacemakers, and between fixed-rate and demand pacemakers.
6. List three types of pacemaker malfunction.
7. Describe how to analyze pacemaker function on the ECG.

KEY TERMS

Atrioventricular (AV) interval: In dual-chamber pacing, the length of time between an atrial sensed or atrial paced event and the delivery of a ventricular pacing stimulus; analogous to the PR interval of intrinsic waveforms; also called the *artificial* or *electronic PR interval*

Base rate: Rate at which the pacemaker's pulse generator initiates impulses when no intrinsic activity is detected; expressed in pulses/minute (ppm)

Capture: The successful conduction of an artificial pacemaker's impulse through the myocardium, resulting in depolarization

Demand pacemaker: Pacemaker that discharges only when the patient's heart rate drops below the preset rate for the pacemaker; also known as a *synchronous* or *noncompetitive pacemaker*

Dual-chamber pacemaker: Pacemaker that stimulates the atrium and ventricle; dual-chamber pacing is also called *physiologic pacing*

Escape interval: Time measured between a sensed cardiac event and the next pacemaker output

Failure to capture: A pacemaker malfunction that occurs when the artificial pacemaker stimulus is unable to depolarize the myocardium

Failure to pace: A pacemaker malfunction that occurs when the pacemaker fails to deliver an electrical stimulus at its programmed time; also referred to as failure to fire or failure of pulse generation

Fixed-rate pacemaker: Pacemaker that continuously discharges at a preset rate regardless of the patient's intrinsic activity; also known as an *asynchronous pacemaker*

Inhibition: Pacemaker response in which the output pulse is suppressed when an intrinsic event is sensed

Oversensing: A pacemaker malfunction that results from inappropriate sensing of extraneous electrical signals

Paced interval: Period between two consecutive paced events in the same cardiac chamber; also known as the *automatic interval*

Pacemaker: A battery-powered device that delivers an electrical current to the heart to stimulate depolarization

Sensitivity: The extent to which an artificial pacemaker recognizes intrinsic cardiac electrical activity

Threshold: The minimum amount of voltage (i.e., milliamperes) needed to obtain consistent capture

Undersensing: A pacemaker malfunction that occurs when the artificial pacemaker fails to recognize spontaneous myocardial depolarization

PACEMAKER SYSTEMS

[Objectives 1, 2]

A cardiac **pacemaker** is a battery-powered device that delivers an electrical current to the heart to stimulate depolarization. A pacemaker system consists of a *pulse generator* (i.e., the power source) and pacing leads. The pulse generator houses a battery and electronic circuitry. The circuitry works like a computer, converting energy from the battery into electrical pulses. A lithium battery is usually the power source for implanted pacemakers and implantable cardioverter-defibrillators (ICDs), whereas a 9-volt alkaline battery is usually used to power a temporary external pulse generator. A *pacing lead* is an insulated wire that is used to carry an electrical impulse from the pulse generator to the patient's heart. It also carries information about the heart's electrical activity back to the pacemaker. The pacemaker responds to the information received either by sending a pacing impulse to the heart (i.e., *triggering*) or by not sending a pacing impulse to the heart (i.e., *inhibition*).

An artificial pacemaker can be external (a temporary intervention) or implanted. An external pacemaker may be used to control transient disturbances in heart rate or conduction that result from drug toxicity or that occurs during a myocardial infarction (MI), or following cardiac surgery when increased vagal tone is often present. Patients who have chronic dysrhythmias that are unresponsive to medication therapy and that result in decreased cardiac output may require the surgical implantation of a permanent pacemaker or an ICD.

Permanent Pacemakers and Implantable Cardioverter-Defibrillators

A permanent pacemaker is used to treat disorders of the sinoatrial (SA) node (e.g., bradycardias), disorders of the AV conduction pathways (e.g., second-degree AV block type II, third-degree AV block), or both, that produce signs and symptoms as a result of inadequate cardiac output (Box 8-1, Figure 8-1). The pacemaker's pulse generator is usually implanted under local anesthesia into the subcutaneous tissue of the anterior chest just below the right or left clavicle (Figure 8-2). The patient's handedness, occupation, and hobbies determine whether the pacemaker is implanted on the right or left side.

Box **8-1**	Symptoms That May Result from a Decrease in Cardiac Output
Acutely altered mental status	Lightheadedness
Dizziness	Palpitations
Exercise intolerance	Pulsations in the neck
Fainting	Seizures
Fatigue	Shortness of breath
Heart failure	Tightness in the chest

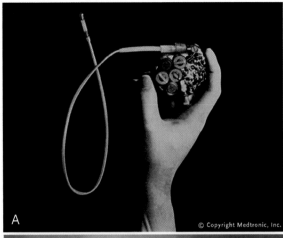
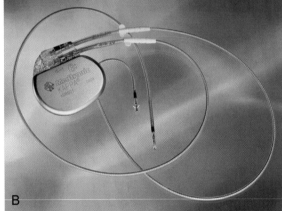

Figure 8-1   Permanent pacemakers. **A,** Early pacemaker with attached lead. **B,** An example of a pacemaker in use today.

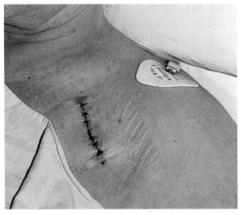

Figure 8-2   Site of implantation of a permanent pacemaker or implantable cardioverter-defibrillator. The pacemaker is usually implanted in the left pectoral region, but it may be placed elsewhere if necessary.

An ICD is a programmable device that can deliver a range of therapies (also called *tiered-therapy*) including defibrillation, antitachycardia pacing (i.e., *overdrive pacing*), synchronized cardioversion, and bradycardia pacing, depending on the dysrhythmia detected and how the device is programmed (Figure 8-3). A physician determines the appropriate therapies for each patient. When ICDs were initially introduced, they were surgically placed subcutaneously in the left upper

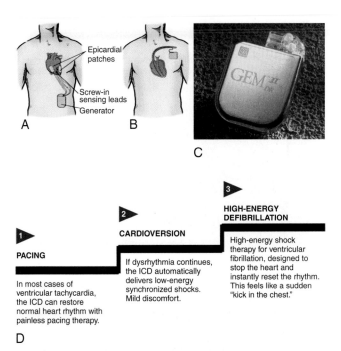

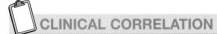

Figure 8-3 **A,** Placement of an implantable cardioverter-defibrillator (ICD) and epicardial lead system. The generator is placed in a subcutaneous "pocket" in the left upper abdominal quadrant. The epicardial screw-in sensing leads monitor the heart rhythm and connect to the generator. If a life-threatening dysrhythmia is sensed, the generator can pace-terminate the dysrhythmia or deliver electrical cardioversion or defibrillation through the epicardial patches. With this system, the leads and patches must be placed during an open chest procedure (sternal surgery or thoracotomy). **B,** In the transvenous lead system, open chest surgery is not required. The pacing, cardioversion, and defibrillation functions are all contained in a lead (or leads) inserted into the right atrium and ventricle. New generators are small enough to place in the pectoral region. **C,** An example of a dual-chamber ICD (Medtronic Gem II DR) with tiered therapy and pacing capabilities. **D,** Tiered therapy is designed to use increasing levels of intensity to terminate ventricular dysrhythmias.

quadrant of the patient's abdomen (Figure 8-4). With improvements in technology, ICDs are now small enough to be surgically placed in the pectoral area. ICDs were initially used for patients with one or more sudden cardiac arrests or drug-refractory ventricular fibrillation or sustained ventricular tachycardia. Today, ICDs are also used for patients who have experienced an extensive MI resulting in decreased cardiac output, patients who have a history of MI with recurrent episodes of unexplained syncope, and children with congenital long-QT syndrome, among other conditions.

CLINICAL CORRELATION

During overdrive pacing, the pacemaker is set to pace at a rate faster than the rate of the tachycardia. After a few seconds, the pacemaker is stopped to allow the return of the heart's intrinsic pacemaker.

The circuitry of pacemakers and ICDs is housed in a hermetically sealed case made of titanium that is airtight and impermeable to fluid. Pacemakers and ICDs store information about the activities of the patient's heart, as well

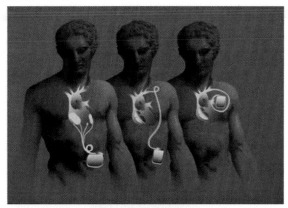

Figure 8-4 Evolution of the implantable cardioverter-defibrillator.

as information about the device itself (e.g., number of dysrhythmia episodes; provoking rhythm; dates of pacing, defibrillation, or both). The stored information is periodically retrieved and reviewed by the patient's physician and, if necessary, changes in the device's settings are made. Lithium batteries are almost exclusively used in modern pacemakers and ICDs. Battery life depends on the number of times therapies are delivered, the frequency of pacing, and the number of cardiac chambers paced.

Complications of permanent pacing associated with the implantation procedure include bleeding, local tissue reaction, pneumothorax, cardiac dysrhythmias, air embolism, and thrombosis. Long-term complications of permanent pacing may include infection, electrode displacement, heart failure, fracture of the pacing lead, pacemaker-induced dysrhythmias, externalization of the pacemaker generator, and perforation of the right ventricle with or without pericardial tamponade.

Temporary Pacemakers

The pulse generator of a temporary pacemaker is located externally (Figure 8-5). Temporary pacing can be accomplished through transvenous, epicardial, or transcutaneous means.

Transvenous pacemakers stimulate the endocardium of the right atrium or ventricle (or both) by means of an electrode introduced into a central vein, such as the subclavian, femoral, brachial, internal jugular, or external jugular vein. Epicardial pacing is the placement of pacing leads directly onto or through the epicardium. Epicardial leads may be used when a patient is undergoing cardiac surgery and the outer surface of the heart is easy to reach. Transcutaneous pacing delivers pacing impulses to the heart using large electrodes that are placed on the patient's chest. Transcutaneous pacing is also called *temporary external pacing* or *noninvasive pacing* and is discussed later in this chapter.

Complications of temporary transvenous pacing include bleeding, infection, pneumothorax, cardiac dysrhythmias, MI, lead displacement, fracture of the pacing lead, hematoma at the insertion site, perforation of the right ventricle with or without pericardial tamponade, and perforation of

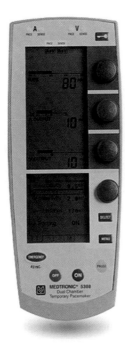

Figure 8-5 The pulse generator of a temporary pacemaker is located externally.

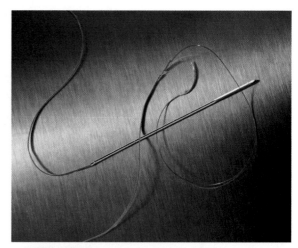

Figure 8-6 Example of a temporary unipolar pacing lead.

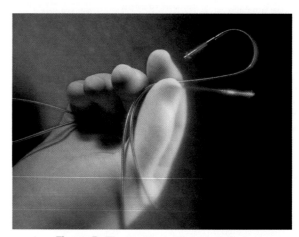

Figure 8-7 Example of a bipolar pacing lead.

the inferior vena cava, pulmonary artery, or coronary arteries because of improper placement of the pacing lead.

Pacing Lead Systems

[Objectives 2, 3]

Pacemaker lead systems may consist of single, double, or multiple leads. The exposed portion of the pacing lead is called an *electrode*, which is placed in direct contact with the heart. Pacing, which is also called *pacemaker firing*, occurs when the pacemaker's pulse generator delivers energy (milliamperes [mA]) through the pacing electrode to the myocardium. Evidence of pacing can be seen as a vertical line or spike on the ECG. **Capture** is the successful conduction of an artificial pacemaker's impulse through the myocardium, resulting in depolarization. Capture is obtained after the pacemaker electrode is properly positioned in the heart; with one-to-one capture, each pacing stimulus results in depolarization of the appropriate chamber. On the ECG, evidence of *electrical capture* can be seen as a pacemaker spike followed by an atrial or a ventricular complex, depending on the cardiac chamber that is being paced. *Mechanical capture* is assessed by palpating the patient's pulse or by observing right atrial pressure, left atrial pressure, or pulmonary artery or arterial pressure waveforms.

A unipolar electrode has one pacing electrode that is located at its distal tip (Figure 8-6). The negative electrode is in contact with the cardiac tissue, and the pulse generator (located outside the heart) functions as the positive electrode. The pacemaker spike produced by a unipolar lead system is often large because of the distance between the positive and negative electrode. Unipolar leads are less commonly used than bipolar lead systems because of the potential for pacing

the chest wall muscles and the susceptibility of the unipolar leads to electromagnetic interference.

A bipolar lead system contains a positive and negative electrode at the distal tip of the pacing lead wire (Figure 8-7). Most temporary transvenous pacemakers use a bipolar lead system. A permanent pacemaker may have either a bipolar or a unipolar lead system. The pacemaker spike produced by a bipolar lead system is smaller than that of a unipolar system because of the shorter distance between the positive and negative electrodes (Figure 8-8).

PACING CHAMBERS AND MODES

A pacemaker system may be single or dual chamber.

Single-Chamber Pacemakers

[Objectives 4, 5]

A pacemaker that paces a single heart chamber, either the atrium or ventricle, has one lead placed in the heart. Atrial

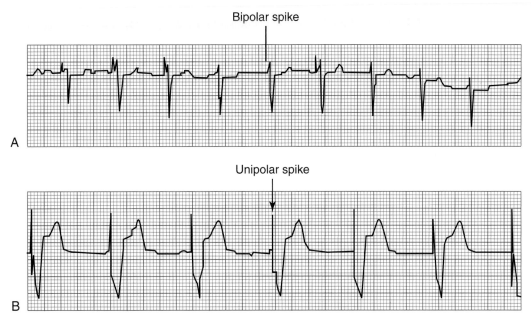

Figure 8-8   Bipolar and unipolar pacing. **A,** Pacemaker spike produced by a bipolar lead system. **B,** Pacemaker spike produced by a unipolar lead system.

pacing is achieved by placing the pacing electrode in the right atrium. Stimulation of the atria produces a pacemaker spike on the ECG, followed by a P wave (Figure 8-9). Atrial pacing may be used when the SA node is diseased or damaged, but conduction through the AV junction and ventricles is normal. This type of pacemaker is ineffective if an AV block develops because it cannot pace the ventricles.

Ventricular pacing is accomplished by placing the pacing electrode in the right ventricle. Stimulation of the ventricles produces a pacemaker spike on the ECG followed by a wide QRS, resembling a ventricular ectopic beat (Figure 8-10). The QRS complex is wide because a paced impulse does not follow the normal conduction pathway in the heart. A single-chamber ventricular pacemaker can pace the ventricles but it cannot coordinate pacing with the patient's intrinsic atrial rate. This results in asynchronous contraction of the atrium and ventricle (i.e., AV asynchrony). Because of this loss of AV synchrony, a ventricular demand pacemaker is rarely used in a patient with an intact SA node. Conversely, a ventricular demand pacemaker may be used for the patient with chronic atrial fibrillation.

Dual-Chamber Pacemakers

[Objectives 4, 5]

A **dual-chamber pacemaker** uses two leads: One lead is placed in the right atrium and the other in the right ventricle (Figure 8-11). Dual-chamber pacing is also called *physiologic pacing.* A dual-chamber pacemaker stimulates the right atrium and right ventricle sequentially (stimulating first the atrium, then the ventricle), mimicking normal cardiac physiology and thus preserving the atrial contribution to ventricular filling (i.e., atrial kick) (Figure 8-12).

When spontaneous atrial depolarization does not occur within a preset interval, the atrial pulse generator fires and stimulates atrial depolarization at a preset rate. The pacemaker is programmed to wait—simulating the normal delay in conduction through the AV node (i.e., the PR interval). The artificial or electronic PR interval is referred to as an **AV interval**. If spontaneous ventricular depolarization does not occur within a preset interval, the pacemaker fires and stimulates ventricular depolarization at a preset rate.

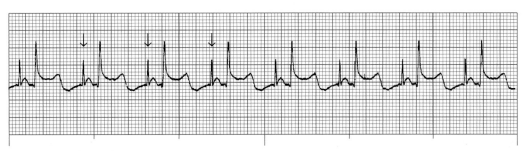

Figure 8-9   Electrocardiogram of a single-chamber pacemaker with atrial pacing spikes (arrows).

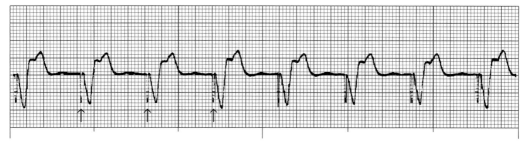

Figure 8-10   Electrocardiogram of a single-chamber pacemaker with ventricular pacing spikes (arrows).

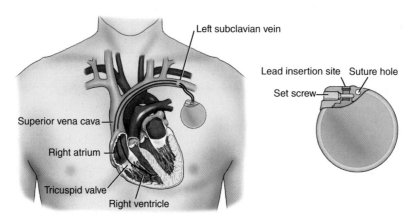

Left subclavian vein

Lead insertion site   Suture hole

Set screw

Superior vena cava

Right atrium

Tricuspid valve

Right ventricle

Figure 8-11   Dual-chamber pacemaker.

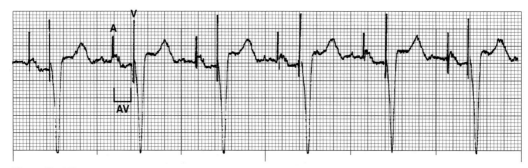

Figure 8-12   Electrocardiogram of a dual-chamber pacemaker with atrial pacing spikes (A), ventricular pacing spikes (V). AV, AV interval.

Biventricular Pacemakers

A *biventricular pacemaker* has three leads; one lead for each ventricle and one lead for the right atrium. This device uses cardiac resynchronization therapy to restore normal simultaneous ventricular contraction for patients with heart failure, thereby improving cardiac output and exercise tolerance.

Fixed-Rate Pacemakers

[Objective 5]

A **fixed-rate pacemaker**, which is also known as an *asynchronous* pacemaker, continuously discharges at a preset rate (usually 70 to 80 impulses/min) regardless of the patient's heart rate or metabolic demands. An advantage of the fixed-rate

pacemaker is its simple circuitry, reducing the risk of pacemaker failure; however, this type of pacemaker does not sense the patient's own cardiac rhythm. This may result in competition between the patient's cardiac rhythm and that of the pacemaker. Ventricular tachycardia or ventricular fibrillation may be induced if the pacemaker were to fire during the T wave (i.e., the vulnerable period) of a preceding patient beat. Fixed-rate pacemakers are not often used today.

Demand Pacemakers

[Objective 5]

A **demand pacemaker**, which is also known as a *synchronous* or *noncompetitive* pacemaker, discharges only when the patient's heart rate drops below the pacemaker's **base rate**.

Position	I	II	III	IV	V
Category	Chamber(s) Paced	Chamber(s) Sensed	Response to Sensing	Rate Modulation	Multisite Pacing
	O = None	O = None	O = None	O = None	O = None
	A = Atrium	A = Atrium	T = Triggered	R = Rate Modulation	A = Atrium
	V = Ventricle	V = Ventricle	I = Inhibited		V = Ventricle
	D = Dual (A + V)	D = Dual (A + V)	D = Dual (T + I)		D = Dual (A + V)
Manufacturer's Designation Only	S = Single (A or V)	S = Single (A or V)			

Table 8-1   Revised NASPE/BPEG* Generic Code for Antibradycardia Pacing

From Bernstein A, Daubert J, Fletcher R, et al: The revised NASPE/BPEG generic code for antibradycardia, adaptive-rate, and multisite pacing, *Pacing Clin Electrophysiol* 25(2):260–264, 2002.
*NASPE/BPEG, North American Society of Pacing and Electrophysiology/British Pacing and Electrophysiology Group.

For example, if the demand pacemaker was preset at a base rate of 70 impulses/min, it would sense the patient's heart rate and allow electrical impulses to flow from the pacemaker through the pacing lead to stimulate the heart only when the rate fell below 70 beats/min. Demand pacemakers can be programmable or nonprogrammable. The voltage level and impulse rate are preset at the time of manufacture in nonprogrammable pacemakers.

Pacemaker Codes

[Objective 5]

Pacemaker codes are used to assist in identifying a pacemaker's preprogrammed pacing, sensing, and response functions (Table 8-1). The *first letter* of the code identifies the heart chamber (or chambers) paced (stimulated). A pacemaker used to pace only a single chamber is represented by either A (atrial) or V (ventricular). A pacemaker capable of pacing in both chambers is represented by D (dual). The *second letter* identifies the chamber of the heart where patient-initiated (i.e., intrinsic) electrical activity is sensed by the pacemaker. The *third letter* indicates how the pacemaker will respond when it senses patient-initiated electrical activity. The *fourth letter* identifies the availability of rate modulation (i.e., the pacemaker's ability to adapt its rate to meet the body's needs caused by increased physical activity and then increase or decrease the pacing rate accordingly). A pacemaker's rate modulation capability may also be referred to as *rate responsiveness* or *rate adaptation*. The *fifth letter* denotes multisite pacing.

The ventricular demand (VVI) pacemaker is a common type of pacemaker. With this device, the pacemaker electrode is placed in the right ventricle (V); the ventricle is sensed (V), and the pacemaker is inhibited (I) when spontaneous ventricular depolarization occurs within a preset interval. When spontaneous ventricular depolarization does not occur within this preset interval, the pacemaker fires and stimulates ventricular depolarization at a preset rate (Figure 8-13). P waves can appear anywhere in the cardiac cycle and have

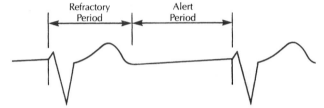

Figure 8-13   During the refractory period, a ventricular demand pacemaker does not sense any electrical activity. The refractory period is followed by the alert period. If no QRS complex is sensed by the end of the alert period, the pacemaker fires and stimulates ventricular depolarization at a preset rate.

no relationship with the QRS complexes because a ventricular demand pacemaker does not sense or pace atrial activity. A disadvantage of ventricular demand pacing is its fixed rate, regardless of the patient's level of physical activity.

A dual-chamber pacemaker may also be called a *DDD pacemaker*, indicating that both the atrium and ventricle are paced (D), both chambers are sensed (D), and the pacemaker has both a triggered and inhibited mode of response (D) (Figure 8-14). The presence of a DDD pacemaker does not necessarily mean that the pacemaker is in DDD mode. DDD pacemakers can be programmed to VVI mode, depending on patient need (e.g., the development of chronic atrial fibrillation).

A defibrillator code was developed in 1993 and it is used to describe the capabilities and operation of ICDs (Table 8-2).

TRANSCUTANEOUS PACING

[Objective 2]

Transcutaneous pacing (TCP) is the use of electrical stimulation through pacing pads positioned on a patient's torso to stimulate contraction of the heart. TCP is indicated for significant bradycardias that are unresponsive to atropine therapy or when atropine is not immediately available or indicated. It may also be used as a bridge until

Dual-Chamber (DDD) Pacemaker Functions

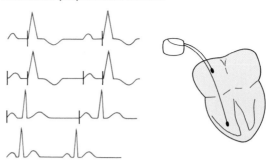

A. Atrial sensing
Ventricular pacing

B. Atrial pacing
Ventricular pacing

C. Atrial pacing
Ventricular sensing

D. Atrial and ventricular
sensing

Figure 8-14   A dual-chamber (DDD) pacemaker senses and paces in both the atria and ventricles. The pacemaker emits a stimulus (spike) whenever an intrinsic P wave or QRS complex is not sensed within some programmed time interval.

Table **8-2**	NASPE/BPEG* Defibrillator Codes		
Position I	**Position II**	**Position III**	**Position IV**
Shock Chamber	Antitachycardia Pacing Chamber	Tachycardia Detection	Antibradycardia Pacing Chamber
O = None	O = None	E = Electrogram	O = None
A = Atrium	A = Atrium	H = Hemodynamic	A = Atrium
V = Ventricle	V = Ventricle		V = Ventricle
D = Dual (A + V)	D = Dual (A + V)		D = Dual (A + V)

From Bernstein AD, Camm AJ, Fisher JD, et al: North American Society of Pacing and Electrophysiology policy statement: The NASPE/BPEG defibrillator code, *Pacing Clin Electrophysiol* 16:1776–1780, 1993.
*NASPE/BPEG, North American Society of Pacing and Electrophysiology/British Pacing and Electrophysiology Group.

transvenous pacing can be accomplished or the cause of the bradycardia is reversed (e.g., drug overdose, hyperkalemia). *Standby pacing* refers to the application of the pacing pads to the patient's chest in anticipation of possible use, but pacing is not yet needed. For example, standby pacing is often warranted when second-degree AV block type II or third-degree AV block are present in the setting of acute MI.

TCP requires attaching two pacing electrodes to the skin surface of the patient's outer chest wall. The pacing pads used during TCP function as a bipolar pacing system. The electrical signal exits from the negative terminal on the machine (and subsequently the negative electrode) and passes through the chest wall to the heart. The range of output current of a transcutaneous pacemaker varies depending on the manufacturer (Figure 8-15). You must be familiar with your equipment before you need to use it. The steps to perform TCP are shown in Skill 8-1.

The primary limitation of TCP is patient discomfort that is proportional to the intensity of skeletal muscle contraction and the direct electrical stimulation of cutaneous nerves. The degree of discomfort varies with the device used and the stimulating current required to achieve capture. Because TCP is uncomfortable, the administration of sedatives or analgesics is usually necessary in responsive patients. Temporary transvenous pacing is indicated when prolonged TCP is needed.

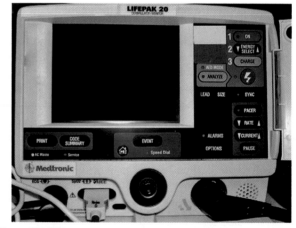

Figure 8-15   An example of a monitor/defibrillator that provides cardiac monitoring, defibrillation, cardioversion, and transcutaneous pacing.

Complications of TCP include the following:
- Coughing
- Failure to recognize that the pacemaker is not capturing
- Interference with sensing from patient agitation or muscle contractions
- Pain from electrical stimulation of the skin and muscles
- Skin burns
- Tissue damage, including third-degree burns
- When pacing is prolonged, pacing **threshold** changes, leading to capture failure

SKILL 8-1   Transcutaneous Pacing

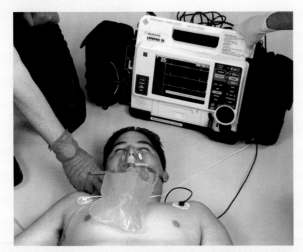

Step 1 Take appropriate standard precautions and verify that the procedure is indicated. Place the patient on oxygen, assess the patient's vital signs, establish intravenous (IV) access, and apply electrocardiogram (ECG) electrodes. Identify the rhythm on the cardiac monitor. Record a rhythm strip and verify the presence of a paceable rhythm. Continuous monitoring of the patient's ECG is *essential* throughout the procedure.

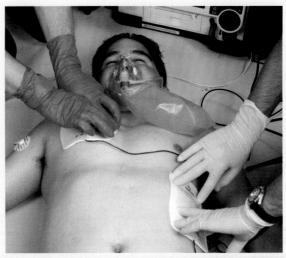

Step 2 Apply adhesive pacing pads to the patient according to the manufacturer's recommendations. Do not place the pads over open cuts, sores, or metal objects. The pacing pads should fit completely on the patient's chest; have a minimum of 1 to 2 inches of space between electrodes (pads); and not overlap bony areas of the sternum, spine, or scapula.

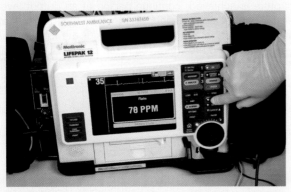

Step 3 Connect the pacing cable to the pacemaker and to the adhesive pads on the patient. Turn the power on to the pacemaker. Set the pacing rate to the desired number of paced pulses per minute (ppm). In an adult, set the initial rate at a nonbradycardic rate between 60 and 80 ppm.

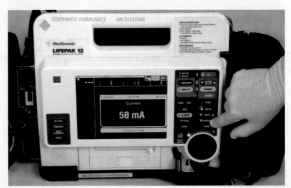

Step 4 After the rate has been regulated, start the pacemaker. Increase the stimulating current (output or milliamperes) until pacer spikes are visible before each QRS complex. Increase the current slowly but steadily until capture is achieved. Sedation or analgesia may be needed to minimize the discomfort associated with this procedure (common with currents of 50 mA or more). Give medications according to local protocol or physician instructions.

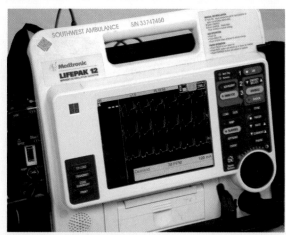

Step 5 Watch the cardiac monitor closely for *electrical* capture. This usually is seen by a wide QRS and broad T wave. In some patients electrical capture is less obvious and is indicated only as a change in the shape of the QRS. Skeletal muscle twitching is common at lower mA settings until capture occurs and may make ECG interpretation difficult.

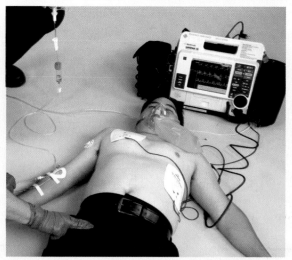

Step 6 Assess *mechanical* capture. Mechanical capture occurs when pacing produces a response that can be measured, such as a palpable pulse and blood pressure. Assess mechanical capture by assessing the patient's right upper extremity or right femoral pulses. Because the electrical stimulation from the pacemaker may mimic a pulse, the carotid pulses usually are not palpated. Once capture is achieved, continue pacing at an output level slightly higher (approximately 2 mA) than the threshold of initial electrical capture. For example, if the monitor reveals 100% capture when you reached 80 mA, your final setting would be 82 mA.

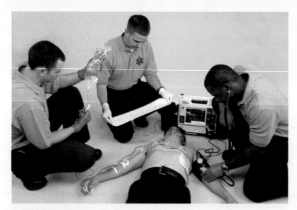

Step 7 Assess the patient's level of responsiveness, vital signs, and oxygen saturation as measured by pulse oximetry (SpO_2). Closely monitor the patient, including assessment of the skin for irritation where the pacing pads have been applied. Reevaluate pacemaker function with any change in the patient's condition or vital signs. Document and record the ECG rhythm. Documentation should include the date and time pacing was initiated (including baseline and pacing rhythm strips), the current required to obtain capture, the pacing rate selected, the patient's responses to electrical and mechanical capture, medications administered during the procedure, and the date and time pacing was terminated (if applicable).

PACEMAKER MALFUNCTION

Problems that can occur with pacing include failure to pace, failure to capture, failure to sense (e.g., undersensing, oversensing).

Failure to Pace

[Objective 6]

Failure to pace, which is also referred to as *failure to fire* or *failure of pulse generation*, is a pacemaker malfunction that occurs when the pacemaker fails to deliver an electrical stimulus at its programmed time. Failure to pace is recognized on the ECG as an absence of pacemaker spikes, even though the patient's intrinsic rate is less than that of the pacemaker, and a return of the underlying rhythm for which pacing was initiated (Figure 8-16). Patient signs and symptoms may include bradycardia, chest discomfort, hypotension, and syncope.

Causes of failure to pace include battery failure, fracture of the pacing lead wire, displacement of the electrode tip, pulse generator failure, a broken or loose connection between the pacing lead and the pulse generator, electromagnetic interference, or the sensitivity setting set too high. Treatment may include adjusting the sensitivity setting, replacing the pulse generator battery, replacing the pacing lead, replacing the pulse generator unit, tightening connections between the pacing lead and pulse generator, or removing the source of electromagnetic interference.

Failure to Capture

[Objective 6]

Failure to capture is the inability of the artificial pacemaker stimulus to depolarize the myocardium and is recognized on the ECG by visible pacemaker spikes not followed by P waves (if the electrode is located in the atrium) or QRS complexes (if the electrode is located in the right ventricle) (Figure 8-17). Patient signs and symptoms may include bradycardia, fatigue, and hypotension.

Causes of failure to capture include displacement of pacing lead wire (common cause), output energy (i.e., mA) set too low (common cause), battery failure, fracture of the pacing lead wire, edema or scar tissue formation at the electrode tip, or increased stimulation threshold as a result of medications or electrolyte imbalance. If the problem is a result of low output energy, slowly increasing the output setting (mA) until capture occurs may resolve the problem. With transvenous pacing, repositioning the patient to the left side may promote the contact of a transvenous pacing lead with the endocardium and septum.

Failure to Sense

[Objective 6]

Sensitivity is the extent to which an artificial pacemaker recognizes intrinsic cardiac electrical activity. **Undersensing** occurs when the artificial pacemaker fails to recognize spontaneous myocardial depolarization and it is recognized on the ECG by pacemaker spikes that occur within P waves, pacemaker spikes that follow too closely

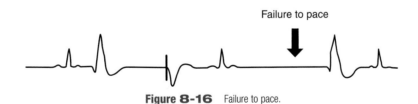

Failure to pace

Figure 8-16   Failure to pace.

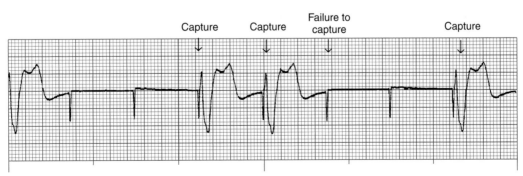

Capture   Capture   Failure to capture   Capture

Figure 8-17   Failure to capture.

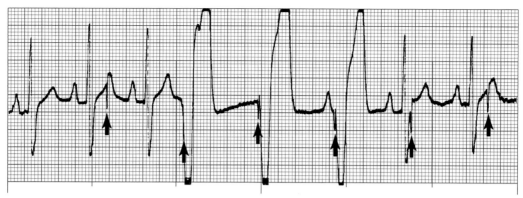

Figure 8-18   Undersensing.

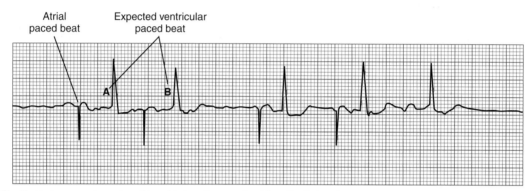

Figure 8-19   Ventricular oversensing and possibly ventricular pulse generation failure. Ventricular spike expected at 150 milliseconds. Ventricular spike and corresponding ventricular depolarization did not occur at points A and B. Also, atrial timing reset by oversensed ventricular activity resulted in erratic atrial pacing (suspicious for fracture of ventricular lead).

behind the patient's QRS complexes, or pacemaker spikes that appear within T waves (Figure 8-18). Because pacemaker spikes occur when they should not, this type of pacemaker malfunction may result in pacemaker spikes that fall on T waves (i.e., R-on-T phenomenon), competition between the pacemaker and the patient's own cardiac rhythm, or both. The patient may complain of palpitations or skipped beats.

Causes of failure to sense include displacement of the electrode tip (most common cause), battery failure, fracture of the pacing lead wire, decreased P wave or QRS voltage, circuitry dysfunction (e.g., pulse generator unable to process the QRS signal), increased sensing threshold from antiarrhythmic medications, severe electrolyte disturbances, and myocardial perforation. Treatment may include increasing the sensitivity setting, replacing the pulse generator battery, or replacing or repositioning the pacing lead.

Oversensing is a pacemaker malfunction that results from inappropriate sensing of extraneous electrical signals. Atrial sensing pacemakers may inappropriately sense ventricular activity; ventricular sensing pacemakers may misidentify a tall, peaked intrinsic T wave as a QRS complex.

Oversensing is recognized on the ECG as pacemaker spikes at a rate slower than the pacemaker's preset rate or no paced beats even though the pacemaker's preset rate is greater than the patient's intrinsic rate (Figure 8-19). Treatment includes adjustment of the pacemaker's sensitivity setting or possible insertion of a bipolar lead if oversensing is caused by unipolar lead dysfunction.

ANALYZING PACEMAKER FUNCTION ON THE ELECTROCARDIOGRAM

[Objective 7]

To practice analyzing pacemaker function on the ECG, let's look at Figure 8-20. The first step in our analysis of this rhythm strip should include identification of the patient's underlying rhythm and its rate, if possible. Figure 8-20 provides a look at the patient's rhythm from two leads, and six QRS complexes are visible in each lead. Each QRS complex is preceded by one upright P wave. Based on this information, we know that the underlying rhythm is sinus in origin. The atrial and ventricular rates are regular at 65 beats/min.

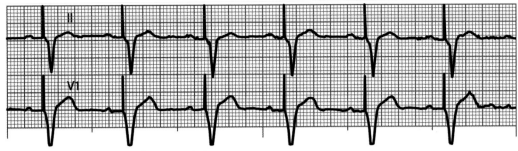

Figure 8-20   Practice strip, analyzing pacemaker function.

Next, let's look for evidence of paced activity (i.e., atrial pacer spikes, ventricular pacer spikes, or both) and evaluate the paced interval. The **paced interval**, which is also called the *automatic interval*, is the period between two consecutive paced events in the same cardiac chamber. Measure the distance between two consecutively paced atrial beats using calipers or paper when atrial pacer spikes are present. Because there is no pacemaker spike before any of the P waves in this rhythm strip, there is no evidence of paced atrial activity; however, a pacer spike is clearly visible before each QRS complex. Because paced ventricular activity is present, we must evaluate the rate and regularity of the ventricular paced interval by measuring the distance between two consecutively paced ventricular beats. The ventricular paced interval is regular at 65 pulses/min. If both atrial and ventricular pacemaker spikes were present, you would know that this patient had a dual-chamber pacemaker. Because only wide-QRS complexes are present and each QRS is preceded by a pacemaker spike, it is reasonable to conclude that this patient has a ventricular pacemaker. Next, compare the escape interval to the paced interval measured earlier. The **escape interval** is the time measured between a sensed cardiac event and the next pacemaker output. The paced interval and escape interval should measure the same. In Figure 8-20, the paced interval and the escape interval are the same.

Next, analyze the rhythm strip for failure to pace, failure to capture, and failure to sense. Remember that with failure to pace, the ECG will reveal an absence of pacemaker spikes at their programmed time. Because the pacer spikes in Figure 8-20 occur regularly, we know that failure to pace is not present. When failure to capture occurs, pacer spikes appear regularly but waveforms are periodically absent following them (i.e., P waves are periodically absent if the pacing electrode is in the atrium, QRS complexes are periodically absent if the pacing electrode is in the ventricle). Because there is a 1:1 relationship between pacemaker spikes and QRS complexes in this rhythm strip, we know that 100% ventricular capture is present. When failure to sense exists, unexpected paced beats or unexpected pacer spikes are present (i.e., undersensing), or prolonged pauses are present (i.e., oversensing). Evaluation of the waveforms and pacer spikes in

Figure 8-20 reveals that there are no unexpected beats, there are no unexpected pacer spikes, and there are no prolonged pauses; thus, failure to sense is not present.

Before we complete our identification, we should briefly discuss what looks like ST-segment elevation in this rhythm strip. The QRS complexes are negatively deflected (i.e., a QS configuration) and the ST segments and T waves are in the opposite direction of the last portion of the QRS complex. As you have learned, these findings are common in ventricular rhythms and in left bundle branch block (LBBB). A ventricular paced beat can be thought of as a manmade LBBB. Consider that when LBBB occurs, the electrical impulse travels down the right bundle branch, depolarizes the right ventricle, and the impulse spreads through the myocardium to depolarize the left ventricle. Pacemakers are most often introduced into the right ventricle. When a pacemaker fires, it sends its impulse into the right ventricle, which depolarizes, and the impulse is spread through the myocardium to depolarize the left ventricle. The similarity between LBBB and a ventricular paced beat is shown in Figure 8-21. Therefore, just

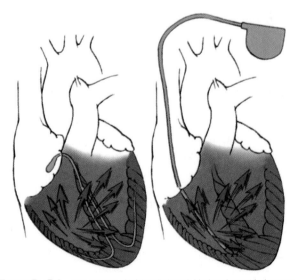

Figure 8-21   The patterns of left bundle branch block and a ventricular pacemaker are similar because in both cases the ventricular impulse begins in the right ventricle and conducts throughout the myocardium to depolarize the left ventricle.

as with LBBB, ventricular paced rhythms may exhibit ST-segment elevation that is not the result of any infarct-related causes because ventricular depolarization is abnormal. Careful correlation of the patient's ECG, his or her clinical presentation, and the results of other diagnostic studies is essential.

In summary, we will identify the rhythm strip in Figure 8-20 as a sinus rhythm with a ventricular pacemaker and 100% capture, and a paced interval of 65 pulses/min. If the patient's intrinsic rate were different from that of the pacemaker, we would include the paced rate in pulses/min and the patient's heart rate in beats/min in our rhythm description.

STOP & REVIEW—CHAPTER 8

Matching

Match the key terms with their definitions by placing the letter of each correct answer in the space provided.

a. AV interval
b. Oversensing
c. Dual-chamber
d. Inhibition
e. Demand
f. Failure to capture
g. Base rate
h. Pacemaker spike

i. Failure to pace
j. Rate modulation
k. Pulse generator
l. Undersensing
m. Threshold
n. Paced interval
o. Fixed-rate

_____ **1.** A vertical line on the ECG that indicates the pacemaker has discharged

_____ **2.** A pacemaker malfunction that occurs when the artificial pacemaker fails to recognize spontaneous myocardial depolarization

_____ **3.** A pacemaker malfunction that occurs when the artificial pacemaker stimulus is unable to depolarize the myocardium

_____ **4.** The period between two consecutive paced events in the same cardiac chamber

_____ **5.** This type of pacemaker stimulates the atrium and ventricle.

_____ **6.** In dual-chamber pacing, the length of time between an atrial sensed or atrial paced event and the delivery of a ventricular pacing stimulus; an artificial or electronic PR interval

_____ **7.** This type of pacemaker discharges only when the patient's heart rate drops below the preset rate for the pacemaker.

_____ **8.** Ability of a pacemaker to increase the pacing rate in response to physical activity or metabolic demand

_____ **9.** This type of pacemaker continuously discharges at a preset rate regardless of the patient's intrinsic activity.

_____ **10.** A pacemaker malfunction that results from inappropriate sensing of extraneous electrical signals

_____ **11.** Power source that houses the battery and circuitry for regulating a pacemaker

_____ **12.** The rate at which the pacemaker's pulse generator initiates impulses when no intrinsic activity is detected; expressed in pulses per minute

_____ **13.** The minimum amount of voltage (i.e., milliamperes) needed to obtain consistent capture

_____ **14.** Pacemaker response in which the output pulse is suppressed when an intrinsic event is sensed

_____ **15.** A pacemaker malfunction that occurs when the pacemaker fails to deliver an electrical stimulus at its programmed time

PACEMAKER RHYTHMS—*PRACTICE RHYTHM STRIPS*

For each of the following rhythm strips, identify the patient's underlying rhythm (if possible); determine the presence of atrial paced activity, ventricular paced activity, or both; and then analyze the rhythm strip for pacemaker malfunction. All rhythm strips were recorded in lead II unless otherwise noted.

16. Identify the rhythm.

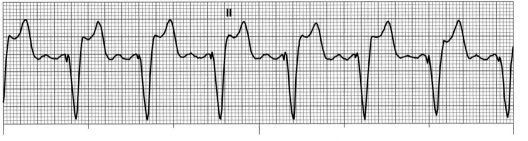

Figure 8-22

Atrial paced activity? _____ Ventricular paced activity? _____

Pacemaker malfunction? _____ Identification: _____

17. Identify the rhythm (lead II).

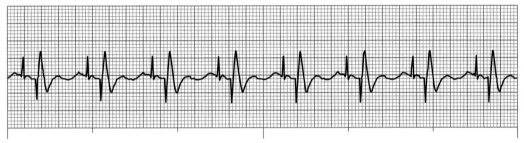

Figure 8-23

Atrial paced activity? _____ Ventricular paced activity? _____

Pacemaker malfunction? _____ Identification: _____

18. Identify the rhythm (lead II).

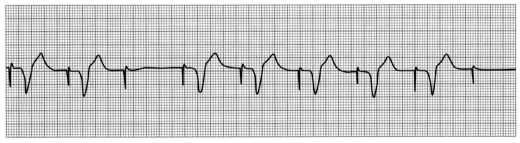

Figure 8-24

Atrial paced activity? _____ Ventricular paced activity? _____

Pacemaker malfunction? _____ Identification: _____

19. This rhythm strip is from a 71-year-old woman with vomitus that looks like coffee grounds. She has a history of esophageal cancer. Her blood pressure is 130/60 mm Hg. Identify the rhythm (lead II).

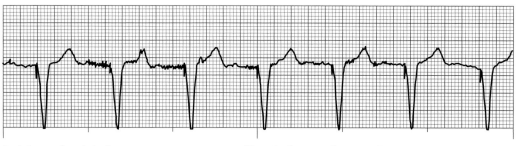

Figure **8-25**

Atrial paced activity? _____ Ventricular paced activity? _____

Pacemaker malfunction? _____ Identification: _____

20. These rhythm strips are from a 52-year-old man with syncope. Identify the rhythm.

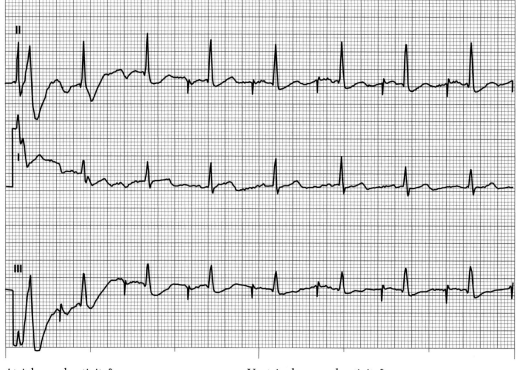

Figure **8-26**

Atrial paced activity? _____ Ventricular paced activity? _____

Pacemaker malfunction? _____ Identification: _____

21. Identify the rhythm.

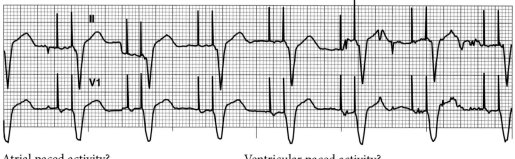

Figure **8-27**

Atrial paced activity? _____ Ventricular paced activity? _____

Pacemaker malfunction? _____ Identification: _____

22. Identify the rhythm (lead II).

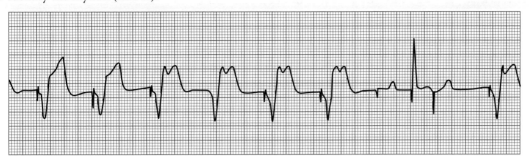

Figure **8-28**

Atrial paced activity? _____   Ventricular paced activity? _____

Pacemaker malfunction? _____   Identification: _____

23. This rhythm strip is from an 80-year-old woman with chest pain. Her blood pressure is 140/78 mm Hg. She states she had a new pacemaker "installed" 13 days ago. Identify the rhythm (lead II).

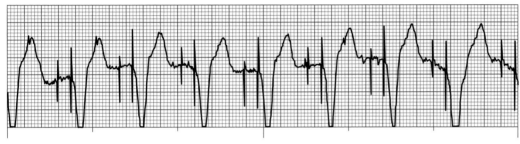

Figure **8-29**

Atrial paced activity? _____   Ventricular paced activity? _____

Pacemaker malfunction? _____   Identification: _____

24. Identify the rhythm (lead II).

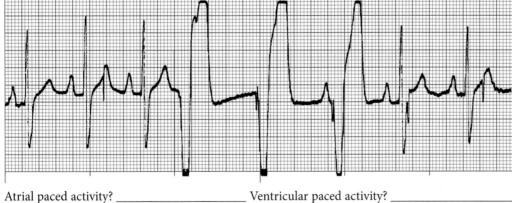

Figure **8-30**

Atrial paced activity? _____   Ventricular paced activity? _____

Pacemaker malfunction? _____   Identification: _____

STOP & REVIEW ANSWERS

Matching

1. ANS: H
2. ANS: L
3. ANS: F
4. ANS: N
5. ANS: C
6. ANS: A
7. ANS: E
8. ANS: J

9. ANS: O
10. ANS: B
11. ANS: K
12. ANS: G
13. ANS: M
14. ANS: D
15. ANS: I

16. **Figure 8-22 answer**

Atrial paced activity?	No
Ventricular paced activity?	Yes
Pacemaker malfunction?	No
Identification:	Sinus rhythm with a ventricular pacemaker and 100% ventricular capture at 68 pulses/min

17. **Figure 8-23 answer**

Atrial paced activity?	Yes
Ventricular paced activity?	Yes
Pacemaker malfunction?	No
Identification:	Dual-chamber pacemaker rhythm with 100% capture at 79 pulses/min

18. **Figure 8-24 answer**

Atrial paced activity?	No
Ventricular paced activity?	Yes
Pacemaker malfunction?	Yes—failure to capture; 7 of 9 pacer spikes captured
Identification:	Ventricular paced rhythm at 65 pulses/min with failure to capture

19. **Figure 8-25 answer**

Atrial paced activity?	No
Ventricular paced activity?	Yes
Pacemaker malfunction?	No
Identification:	Ventricular paced rhythm with 100% capture at 72 pulses/min

20. **Figure 8-26 answer**

Atrial paced activity?	Yes
Ventricular paced activity?	No
Pacemaker malfunction?	No
Identification:	Atrial paced rhythm with 100% capture at 79 pulses/min

21. **Figure 8-27 answer**

Atrial paced activity?	Yes
Ventricular paced activity?	Yes
Pacemaker malfunction?	No
Identification:	Dual-chamber pacemaker rhythm with 100% capture at 71 pulses/min

22. **Figure 8-28 answer**

Atrial paced activity?	Yes
Ventricular paced activity?	Yes
Pacemaker malfunction?	Yes—failure to capture and failure to sense (undersensing)
Identification:	Ventricular paced rhythm with failure to capture (seventh spike) and failure to sense (eighth spike) at 71 pulses/min

23. **Figure 8-29 answer**

Atrial paced activity?	Yes
Ventricular paced activity?	Yes
Pacemaker malfunction?	No
Identification:	Dual-chamber pacemaker rhythm with 100% capture at 83 pulses/min

24. **Figure 8-30 answer**

Atrial paced activity?	No
Ventricular paced activity?	Yes
Pacemaker malfunction?	Yes—failure to sense (undersensing)
Identification:	Sinus rhythm at 88 beats/min with a ventricular pacemaker and pacemaker malfunction (undersensing); note the pacer spikes in the T waves of the second and eighth beats from the left

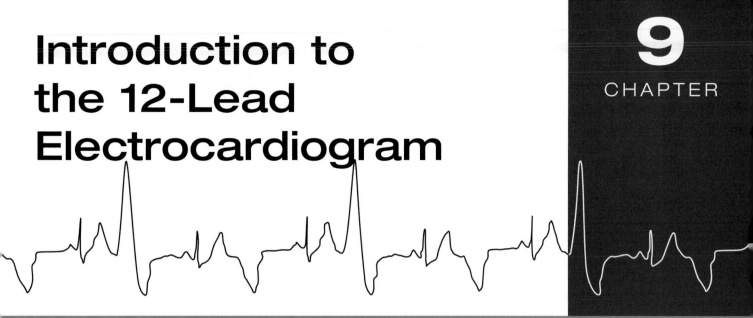

Introduction to the 12-Lead Electrocardiogram

LEARNING OBJECTIVES

After reading this chapter, you should be able to:

1. Give examples of indications for using a 12-lead electrocardiogram (ECG).
2. Explain the term *electrical axis* and its significance.
3. Discuss the determination of electrical axis using leads I and aVF.
4. Recognize the changes on the ECG that may reflect evidence of myocardial ischemia, injury, or infarction.

5. Distinguish patterns of normal and abnormal R-wave progression.
6. Explain what is meant by the terms *dilatation*, *hypertrophy*, and *enlargement*.
7. Describe a systematic method for analyzing a 12-lead ECG.

KEY TERMS

Dilatation: Increase in the diameter of a chamber of the heart caused by volume overload

Electrical axis: Direction, or angle in degrees, in which the main vector of depolarization is pointed

Enlargement: Implies the presence of dilatation or hypertrophy or both

Hypertrophy: An increase in the thickness of a heart chamber caused by chronic pressure overload

Indeterminate axis deviation: Current flow in the direction opposite of normal (−91 to −179 degrees)

Vector: Quantity having direction and magnitude, usually depicted by a straight arrow whose length represents magnitude and whose head represents direction

INTRODUCTION

[Objective 1]

A standard 12-lead ECG provides views of the heart in both the frontal and horizontal planes and views the surfaces of the left ventricle from 12 different angles. Multiple views of the heart can provide useful information including the following:

- Identification of ST-segment and T-wave changes associated with myocardial ischemia, injury, and infarction
- Identification of ECG changes associated with certain medications and electrolyte imbalances
- Recognition of bundle branch blocks

Indications for using a 12-lead ECG include the following:

- Assisting in dysrhythmia interpretation
- Chest pain or discomfort
- Electrical injuries

- Known or suspected electrolyte imbalances
- Known or suspected medication overdoses
- Right or left ventricular failure
- Status before and after electrical therapy (e.g., defibrillation, cardioversion, pacing)
- Stroke
- Syncope or near syncope
- Unstable patient, unknown etiology

LAYOUT OF THE 12-LEAD ELECTROCARDIOGRAM

Most 12-lead monitors record all 12 leads simultaneously but display them in a conventional three-row by four-column format. The standard limb leads are recorded in the first column, the augmented limb leads in the second

Table **9-1**	Layout of the Four-Column 12-Lead Electrocardiogram		
LIMB LEADS		**CHEST LEADS**	
Standard Leads	Augmented Leads	V₁-V₃	V₄-V₆
Column I	Column II	Column III	Column IV
I: Lateral	aVR: None	V₁: Septum	V₄: Anterior
II: Inferior	aVL: Lateral	V₂: Septum	V₅: Lateral
III: Inferior	aVF: Inferior	V₃: Anterior	V₆: Lateral

column, and the chest leads in the third and fourth columns (Table 9-1).

All of the QRS complexes in a row are consecutive, while QRS complexes that are aligned vertically represent a simultaneous recording of the same beat. The 12-lead ECG provides a 2.5-second view of each lead because it is assumed that 2.5 seconds is long enough to capture at least one representative complex. However, a 2.5-second view is not long enough to properly assess rate and rhythm, so at least one continuous rhythm strip is usually included at the bottom of the tracing. Because the leads are obtained simultaneously, only 10 seconds of sampling time is required to record all 12 leads. The 12-lead computer's interpretive program provides measurements of intervals and duration in milliseconds (ms). Seconds can be easily converted to milliseconds by moving the decimal point three places to the right. A 12-lead ECG is shown in Figure 9-1.

ECG Pearl

When viewing a 12-lead, keep in mind that leads that line up vertically are simultaneous recordings of the same beat. When you read the 12-lead from left to right, the ECG tracing is continuous. As you switch from one lead to the next, it is still continuous.

VECTORS

[Objective 2]

Leads have a negative (−) and positive (+) electrode pole that senses the magnitude and direction of the electrical force caused by the spread of waves of depolarization and repolarization throughout the myocardium. A **vector** (arrow) is a symbol representing this force. A vector points in the direction of depolarization. Leads that face the tip or

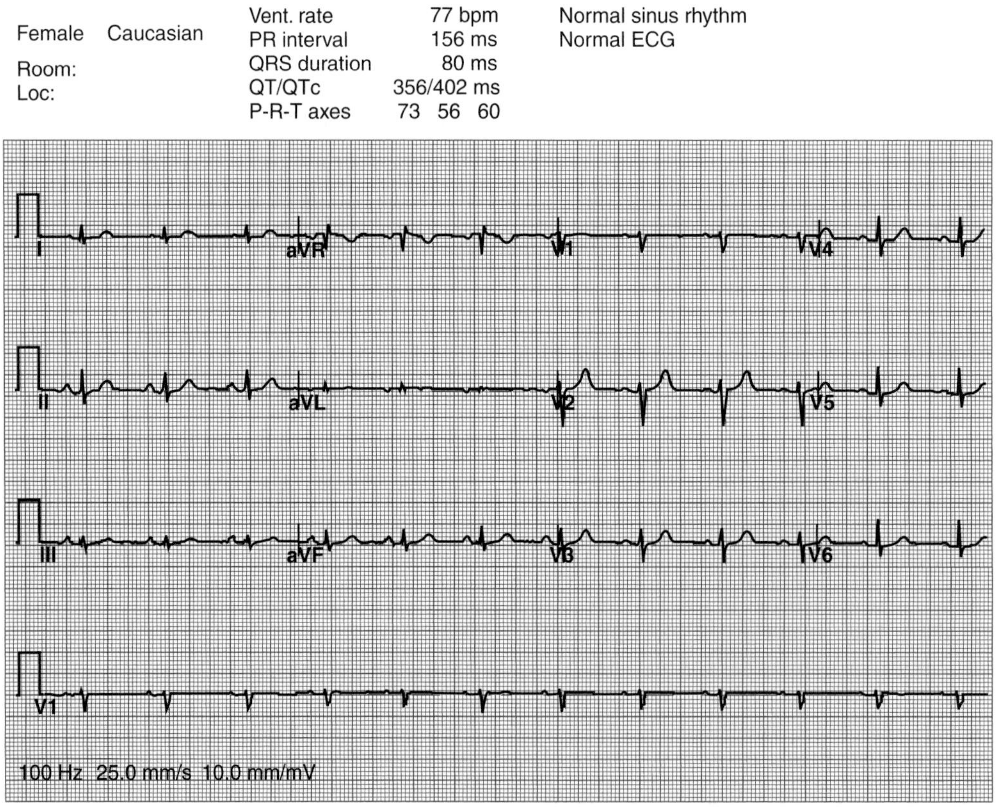

Female   Caucasian

Room:
Loc:

Vent. rate	77 bpm
PR interval	156 ms
QRS duration	80 ms
QT/QTc	356/402 ms
P-R-T axes	73 56 60

Normal sinus rhythm
Normal ECG

100 Hz 25.0 mm/s 10.0 mm/mV

Figure 9-1   An example of a 12-lead electrocardiogram (ECG). Note the four-column format used on the majority of the page. A continuous recording of lead V₁ is shown at the bottom of the page.

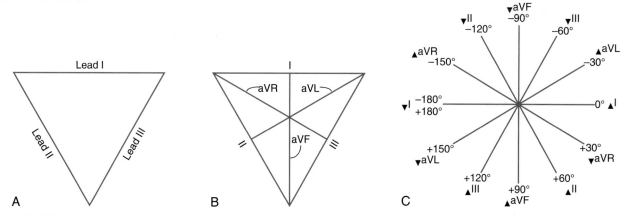

Figure 9-2 **A,** Einthoven's equilateral triangle formed by leads I, II, and III. **B,** The augmented leads are added to the equilateral triangle. **C,** The hexaxial reference system derived from B.

point of a vector record a positive deflection on ECG paper. A *mean vector* identifies the average of depolarization waves in one portion of the heart. The *mean P vector* represents the average magnitude and direction of both right and left atrial depolarization. The *mean QRS vector* represents the average magnitude and direction of both right and left ventricular depolarization. The average direction of a mean vector is called the *mean axis* and is only identified in the frontal plane. An imaginary line joining the positive and negative electrodes of a lead is called the *axis* of the lead. **Electrical axis** refers to determining the direction, or angle in degrees, in which the main vector of depolarization is pointed. When *axis* is used by itself, it refers to the QRS axis.

Axis

[Objectives 2, 3]
During normal ventricular depolarization, the left side of the interventricular septum is stimulated first. The electrical impulse then traverses the septum to stimulate the right side. The left and right ventricles are then depolarized simultaneously. Because the left ventricle is considerably larger than the right, right ventricular depolarization forces are overshadowed on the ECG. As a result, the mean QRS vector points down (i.e., inferior) and to the left.

The axes of leads I, II, and III form an equilateral triangle with the heart at the center (i.e., Einthoven's triangle) (Figure 9-2, A). Einthoven's law states that the sum of the electrical currents recorded in leads I and III equals the sum of the electrical current recorded in lead II. This can be expressed as lead I + lead III = lead II.

If the augmented limb leads are added to the equilateral triangle and the axes of the six leads moved in a way in which they bisect each other, the result is the *hexaxial reference system* (Figure 9-2, B). The hexaxial reference system represents all of the frontal plane (limb) leads with the heart in the center and is the means used to express the location of the frontal plane axis. This system forms a 360-degree circle

surrounding the heart. The positive end of lead I is designated at 0 degrees. The six frontal plane leads divide the circle into segments, each representing 30 degrees. All degrees in the upper hemisphere are labeled as negative degrees, and all degrees in the lower hemisphere are labeled as positive degrees (Figure 9-2, C).

In the hexaxial reference system, the axes of some leads are perpendicular to each other. Lead I is perpendicular to lead aVF. Lead II is perpendicular to aVL, and lead III is perpendicular to aVR. If the electrical force moves toward a positive electrode, a positive (i.e., upright) deflection will be recorded. If the electrical force moves away from a positive electrode, a negative (i.e., downward) deflection will be recorded. If the electrical force is parallel to a given lead, the largest deflection in that lead will be recorded. If the electrical force is perpendicular to a lead axis, the resulting ECG complex will be isoelectric, equiphasic, or both, in that lead. Notice that leads III and aVL are positioned on opposite (i.e., reciprocal) sides of the hexaxial reference system (Figure 9-3). Axis determination can provide clues in the

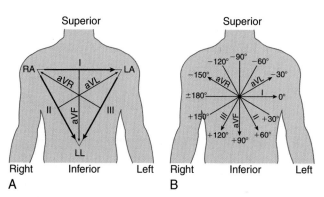

Figure 9-3   Axis of electrical activation. **A,** Vectors for the limb leads in the frontal plane. **B,** Hexaxial reference for determining the frontal plane axis. Note that the vectors for leads I, II, and III are in the same direction as in A, but now, like the augmented limb leads, these standard limb lead vectors have been moved so that they emanate from the center of the figure. *LA,* left arm; *LL,* left leg; *RA,* right arm.

differential diagnosis of wide QRS tachycardia and localization of accessory pathways.

To determine electrical axis, look at the 12-lead ECG in Figure 9-1. Because the hexaxial reference system is derived from the limb leads, we will be focusing the leads shown in the two columns on the left side of the figure (leads I, II, III, aVR, aVL, and aVF). Look for the most equiphasic or isoelectric QRS complexes in these leads. Lead aVL shows QRS complexes that most closely reflect our criteria. The patient's QRS axis is perpendicular to the positive electrode in lead aVL. Look at the hexaxial reference system diagram (see Figure 9-3) to determine which ECG lead is perpendicular to lead aVL. Lead II is perpendicular to lead aVL. Now we know that the patient's QRS axis is moving along the same vector as lead II. Note that the values associated with lead II in the hexaxial reference system diagram are −120 degrees and +60 degrees. To determine if the QRS axis is moving in a positive or negative direction, look at lead II in Figure 9-1 and determine if the QRS complex is primarily positive or negative in this lead. You will see that the QRS is primarily positive in lead II; therefore this patient's QRS axis is approximately +60 degrees. At the top of Figure 9-1, you will see the computer's calculation of the patient's P-QRS-T axes. The computer calculated the patient's QRS axis at +56 degrees. Our estimate of +60 degrees was very close!

In adults, the normal QRS axis is considered to be between −30 and +90 degrees in the frontal plane. Current flow to the right of normal is called *right axis deviation* (between +90 and ±180 degrees). Current flow in the direction opposite of normal is called **indeterminate**, "no man's land," *northwest* or *extreme right axis deviation* (between −90 and ±180 degrees). Current flow to the left of normal is called *left axis deviation* (between −30 and −90 degrees).

Shortcuts exist to determine axis deviation. Leads I and aVF divide the heart into four quadrants. These two leads can be used to quickly estimate electrical axis. In leads I and aVF, the QRS complex is normally positive. If the QRS complex in either or both of these leads is negative, axis deviation is present (Figure 9-4).

Right axis deviation may be a normal variant, particularly in the young and in thin individuals. Other causes of right axis deviation include mechanical shifts associated with inspiration or emphysema, right ventricular hypertrophy,

chronic obstructive pulmonary disease, Wolff-Parkinson-White syndrome, and pulmonary embolism.

Left axis deviation may be a normal variant, particularly in older individuals and obesity. Other causes of left axis deviation include mechanical shifts associated with expiration; a high diaphragm caused by pregnancy, ascites, or abdominal tumors; hyperkalemia; emphysema; left atrial hypertrophy; and dextrocardia.

ACUTE CORONARY SYNDROMES

You will recall from Chapter 1 that acute coronary syndromes (ACSs) are conditions that are caused by a similar sequence of pathologic events and that involve a temporary or permanent blockage of a coronary artery. ACSs include unstable angina, non-ST (segment) elevation myocardial infarction (NSTEMI), and ST (segment) elevation myocardial infarction (STEMI). Sudden cardiac death can occur with any of these conditions.

CLINICAL CORRELATION

Distinguishing patients with unstable angina from those with acute myocardial infarction (MI) may be impossible during their initial presentation because their signs, symptoms, and ECG findings may be identical. The diagnosis of infarction is made based on the patient's signs and symptoms, ECG findings, history, cardiac biomarkers, and other test results that confirm the presence of an infarction.

ST-Elevation Myocardial Infarction

[Objective 4]

Recognition of infarction on the ECG relies on the detection of morphologic changes (i.e., changes in shape) of the QRS complex, the T wave, and the ST segment. These changes occur in relation to certain events during the infarction. Figure 9-5 shows the ECG changes attributable to STEMI that often occur in a predictable pattern. The ECG changes

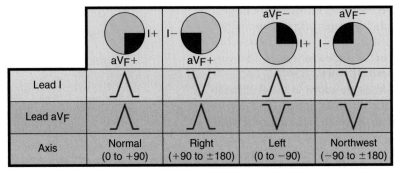

Figure 9-4 Determination of QRS axis quadrant by noting predominant QRS polarity in leads I and aVF. Normal axis: If the QRS is primarily positive in both I and aVF, the axis falls within the normal quadrant from 0 to 90 degrees. Right axis deviation: If the QRS complex is primarily negative in I and positive in aVF, right axis deviation is present. Left axis deviation: If the QRS complex is predominantly positive in I and negative in aVF, left axis deviation is present. Indeterminate axis: If the QRS is primarily negative in both I and aVF, a markedly abnormal "indeterminate" or "northwest" axis is present.

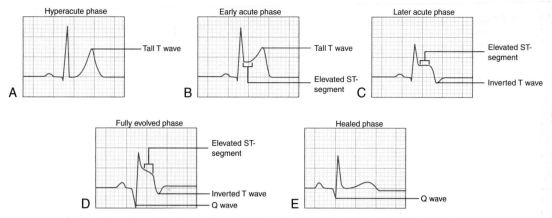

Figure 9-5   The evolving pattern of ST-segment elevation myocardial infarction on the electrocardiogram.

described below appear in leads looking at the area fed by the blocked (i.e., culprit) vessel.

- *Hyperacute phase.* The first change you might notice in the ECG is the development of a tall T wave. Hyperacute T waves are sometimes called "tombstone" T waves and typically measure more than 50% of the preceding R wave. In addition to an increase in height, the T wave becomes more symmetric and may become pointed (Figure 9-5, A). These changes are often not recorded on the ECG because they have typically resolved by the time the patient seeks medical assistance.

- *Early acute phase.* Over time, ST-segment elevation may develop, indicating myocardial injury in progress (Figure 9-5, B). ST-segment elevation may occur within the first hour or first few hours of infarction.

- *Later acute phase.* In the later acute phase of the infarction, you may see the presence of T-wave inversion, suggesting the presence of ischemia (Figure 9-5, C). In fact, T-wave inversion may precede the development of ST-segment elevation, or they may occur at the same time.

- *Fully evolved phase.* A few hours later, the ECG may show the first signs that tissue death has occurred. That evidence comes with the development of abnormal (i.e., pathologic) Q waves (Figure 9-5, D). An abnormal Q wave indicates the presence of dead myocardial tissue and, subsequently, a loss of electrical activity. They can appear within hours after blockage of a coronary artery, but more commonly appear several hours or days after the onset of signs and symptoms of an acute MI. However, when combined with ST-segment or T-wave changes, the presence of abnormal Q waves suggests an acute MI.

- *Healed phase.* In time, the T wave regains its normal shape and the ST segment returns to the baseline. The Q wave, however, often remains as evidence that tissue death has occurred (Figure 9-5, E). When this pattern is seen, establishing the time of the infarction is impossible. It is only possible to recognize the presence of a previous MI.

Non–ST-Elevation Myocardial Infarction

As its name implies, patients experiencing a NSTEMI do not show signs of myocardial injury (ST-segment elevation) on their ECG. The diagnosis of NSTEMI is made based on the patient's signs and symptoms, history, and cardiac biomarker test results that confirm the presence of an infarction. If serum biomarkers are not present in the patient's circulation based on two or more samples collected at least 6 hours apart, the diagnosis is unstable angina. If elevated biomarker levels are present, the diagnosis is NSTEMI.

Localization of Infarctions[1]

ECG changes of myocardial ischemia, injury, or infarction are considered significant if they are viewed in two or more anatomically contiguous leads. If these ECG findings are seen in leads that look directly at the affected area, they are called *indicative changes*. If findings are seen in leads opposite the affected area, they are called *reciprocal changes* (Figure 9-6).

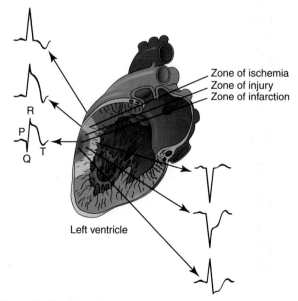

Figure 9-6   Zones of ischemia, injury, and infarction showing indicative electrocardiogram changes and reciprocal changes corresponding to each zone.

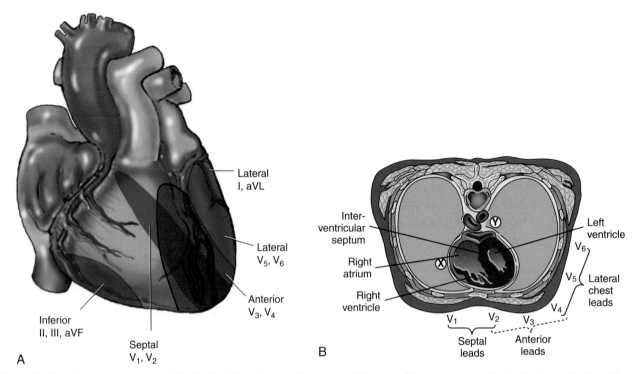

Figure 9-7   A, The surfaces of the heart. The inferobasal (posterior) surface is not shown. **B,** The areas of the heart as seen by the chest leads. Leads V_1, V_2, and V_3 are contiguous. Leads V_3, V_4, and V_5 are contiguous as well as V_4, V_5, and V_6. Note that neither the right ventricular wall (X) nor the inferobasal surface of the left ventricle (Y) is well visualized by any of the usual six chest leads.

To better understand contiguous leads, let's look at Figure 9-7 and Table 9-2. The colors in the table were added so that you can quickly see the areas of the heart viewed by the same leads. For example, leads II, III, and aVF appear the same color in the table because they view the inferior wall of the left ventricle. Because these leads "see" the same part of the heart, they are considered contiguous leads. Leads I, aVL, V_5, and V_6 are contiguous because they all look at adjoining tissue in the lateral wall of the left ventricle. Leads V_1 and V_2 are contiguous because both leads look at the septum. Leads V_3 and V_4 are contiguous because both leads look at the anterior wall of the left ventricle. If right chest leads such as V_4R, V_5R, and V_6R are used, they are contiguous because they view the right ventricle. Leads V_7, V_8, and V_9 are contiguous because they look at the posterior surface of the heart.

Are leads II and V_2 contiguous? No. Leads II and V_2 are not contiguous. Remember: Two leads are contiguous if they look at the same or adjacent areas of the heart or they are numerically consecutive *chest* leads. Lead II is a *limb* lead that looks at the inferior wall. V_2 is a *chest* lead that looks at the septum.

Now look at Figure 9-7. We have already determined that V_1 and V_2 are contiguous leads. Are leads V_2 and V_3 con-

tiguous? Yes. V_2 and V_3 are right next to each other on the patient's chest. When each of these positive electrodes "looks in" at tissue, they see adjoining tissue in the heart as well. Leads V_3, V_4, and V_5 are contiguous, as well as V_4, V_5, and V_6.

Predicting the Site of Coronary Artery Occlusion[1]

[Objective 4]

To recognize ECG signs of ischemia, injury, and infarction, you need to be able to recognize changes in the shape of the QRS complex, ST segment, and T wave. To localize the site of infarction, note which leads are displaying that evidence, and consider which part of the heart that those leads "see." Because an MI is the result of a blocked coronary artery, it is useful to know which arteries supply the heart. Once the infarction has been recognized and localized, an understanding of coronary artery anatomy makes it possible to predict which coronary artery is affected.

In the standard 12-lead ECG, leads II, III, and aVF "look" at tissue supplied by the right coronary artery. Eight leads "look" at tissue supplied by the left coronary artery: leads I, aVL, V_1, V_2, V_3, V_4, V_5, and V_6. When evaluating the extent of infarction produced by a left coronary artery occlusion, decide how many of these leads are showing indicative changes. The more of these eight leads that show indicative changes, the larger the infarction is presumed to be.

The left ventricle has been divided into regions where an MI may occur: septal, anterior, lateral, inferior, and inferobasal (i.e., posterior) (Figure 9-7, A). If an ECG shows changes in

Table **9-2**	Localizing Electrocardiogram Changes		
I: Lateral	aVR: ———	V_1: Septum	V_4: Anterior
II: Inferior	aVL: Lateral	V_2: Septum	V_5: Lateral
III: Inferior	aVF: Inferior	V_3: Anterior	V_6: Lateral

leads II, III, and aVF, the inferior wall is affected. Because the inferior wall of the left ventricle is supplied by the right coronary artery (RCA) in most people, it is reasonable to suppose that these ECG changes are caused by partial or complete blockage of the RCA. When indicative changes are seen in the leads viewing the septal, anterior, and/or lateral walls of the left ventricle (i.e., V_1-V_6, I, and aVL), it is reasonable to suspect that these ECG changes are caused by partial or complete blockage of the left coronary artery.

One way to gauge the relative extent or size of an infarction is to evaluate how many leads are showing indicative changes. An ECG showing changes in only a few leads suggests a smaller infarction than one that produces changes in many leads. In general, the more proximal the blockage in the vessel, the larger the infarction and the greater the number of leads showing indicative changes.

CLINICAL CORRELATION

It is important to remember that some areas of the heart are not shown on a standard 12-lead ECG. It is also essential to recall that some infarctions do not show changes on the 12-lead ECG. Therefore, if infarct changes are seen on the 12-lead ECG, the greater the number of leads showing indicative changes, the larger the infarction. But, if the patient presents with signs and symptoms suggestive of an acute coronary syndrome and the 12-lead ECG does not show indicative changes, a myocardial infarction cannot be ruled out based solely on the ECG findings.

Although ECG localization of the infarct site is possible, it is not perfect. For example, what appears to be a lateral wall infarction on the ECG may actually be an anterior wall infarction. This can occur with any location of infarction and reflects the fact that the ECG is simply a measurement of current flow on the patient's skin. Factors including anatomic variations, patient position, and other underlying conditions may affect the perceived infarct location versus the actual location. The patient's unique pattern of coronary artery distribution is one anatomic variation that can affect the location of an infarction and so can the presence of collateral circulation. For these reasons, you may occasionally encounter infarctions that are difficult to localize into the previously mentioned areas.

An MI may not be limited to one area. For example, if the chest leads indicate ECG changes in leads V_3 and V_4, suggestive of an anterior wall MI, and indicative changes are also present in V_5 and V_6, the infarction would be called an *anterolateral infarction* or an *anterior infarction with lateral extension*.

With an understanding of coronary anatomy, it is possible to predict which coronary artery is occluded. Table 9-3 summarizes the pattern in which coronary arteries most commonly supply the myocardium.

Septal Infarction
[Objective 4]

The left main coronary artery supplies the left anterior descending (LAD) artery and the circumflex artery. Blockage of the left main coronary artery (i.e., the "widow maker") often leads to cardiogenic shock and death without prompt

Table 9-3	Localization of a Myocardial Infarction		
Location of MI	Indicative Changes (Leads facing affected area)	Reciprocal Changes (Leads opposite affected area)	Affected (Culprit) Coronary Artery
Anterior	V_3, V_4	V_7, V_8, V_9	Left coronary artery • LAD—diagonal branch
Anteroseptal	V_1, V_2, V_3, V_4	V_7, V_8, V_9	Left coronary artery • LAD—diagonal branch • LAD—septal branch
Anterolateral	I, aVL, V_3, V_4, V_5, V_6	II, III, aVF, V_7, V_8, V_9	Left coronary artery • LAD—diagonal branch and/or • Circumflex branch
Inferior	II, III, aVF	I, aVL	Right coronary artery (most common)—posterior descending branch or circumflex branch of left coronary artery
Lateral	I, aVL, V_5, V_6	II, III, aVF	Left coronary artery • LAD—diagonal branch and/or • Circumflex branch Right coronary artery
Septum	V_1, V_2	V_7, V_8, V_9	Left coronary artery • LAD—septal branch
Posterior	V_7, V_8, V_9	V_1, V_2, V_3	Right coronary or circumflex artery
Right ventricle	V_1R-V_6R	I, aVL	Right coronary artery • Proximal branches

LAD, left anterior descending; MI, myocardial infarction.

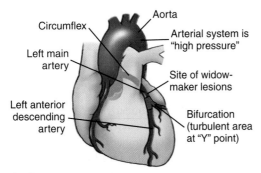

Figure 9-8   The left main coronary artery supplies the left anterior descending artery and the circumflex artery. Blockage of the left main coronary artery (the "widow maker") often leads to cardiogenic shock and death without prompt reperfusion.

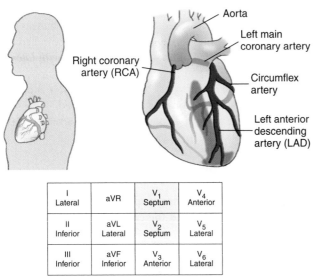

I Lateral	aVR	V_1 Septum	V_4 Anterior
II Inferior	aVL Lateral	V_2 Septum	V_5 Lateral
III Inferior	aVF Inferior	V_3 Anterior	V_6 Lateral

Figure 9-9   Septal infarction.

reperfusion (Figure 9-8). Because the LAD artery supplies approximately 40% of the heart's blood and a critical section of the left ventricle, a blockage in this area can lead to left ventricular dysfunction, including heart failure and cardiogenic shock.

The septum, which contains the bundle of His and bundle branches, is normally supplied by the LAD artery (Figure 9-9). Because leads V_1 and V_2 face the septum, ECG changes of infarction are seen in these leads if the site of infarction is limited to the septum. A blockage in this area may result in both right and left bundle branch blocks (BBBs) (left BBB is more common), second-degree atrioventricular (AV) block type II, and third-degree AV block.

Anterior Infarction
[Objective 4]

Leads V_3 and V_4 face the anterior wall of the left ventricle (Figure 9-10). ECG changes of infarction will be visible in V_1, V_2, V_3, and V_4 if the entire anterior wall is involved. Increased sympathetic nervous system activity is common with anterior MIs with resulting sinus tachycardia, hypertension, or both. An anterior wall MI may cause dysrhythmias including premature ventricular complexes (PVCs), atrial flutter, or atrial fibrillation (AFib). Although some portions of the bundle branches are supplied by the RCA, the left coronary artery supplies most of the bundle branch tissue. Thus BBBs may occur if the left coronary artery is blocked. An example of an anterior wall infarction is shown in Figure 9-11.

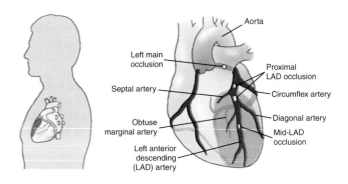

I Lateral	aVR	V_1 Septum	V_4 Anterior
II Inferior	aVL Lateral	V_2 Septum	V_5 Lateral
III Inferior	aVF Inferior	V_3 Anterior	V_6 Lateral

Figure 9-10   Anterior infarction. Occlusion of the midportion of the left anterior descending (LAD) artery results in an anterior infarction. Proximal occlusion of the LAD may become an anteroseptal infarction if the septal branch is involved or an anterolateral infarction if the marginal branch is involved. If the occlusion occurs proximal to both the septal and diagonal branches, an extensive anterior infarction (anteroseptal-lateral myocardial infarction) will result.

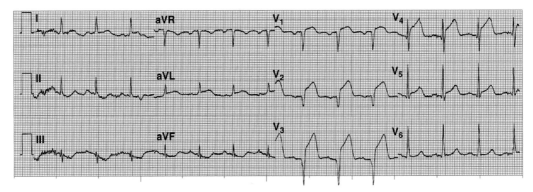

Figure 9-11   Anteroseptal infarction. Note the ST-segment elevation in leads V_1 through V_4.

Inferior Infarction
[Objective 4]

Leads II, III, and aVF view the inferior surface of the left ventricle. In most individuals the inferior wall of the left ventricle is supplied by the posterior descending branch of the RCA (Figure 9-12). Increased parasympathetic nervous system activity is common with inferior MIs, resulting in bradydysrhythmias. Conduction delays (e.g., first-degree AV block, second-degree AV block type I) are common and are usually transient. An example of an infarction involving the inferior wall is shown in Figure 9-13.

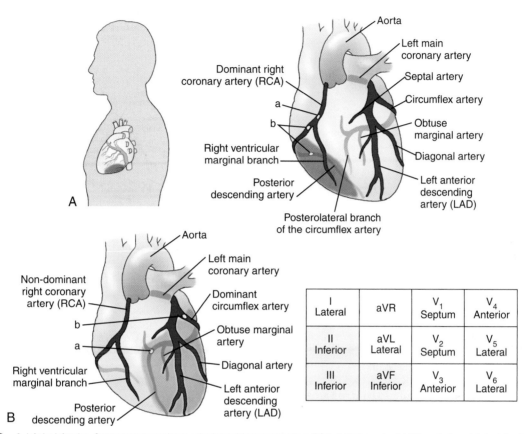

I Lateral	aVR	V$_1$ Septum	V$_4$ Anterior
II Inferior	aVL Lateral	V$_2$ Septum	V$_5$ Lateral
III Inferior	aVF Inferior	V$_3$ Anterior	V$_6$ Lateral

Figure 9-12   **A,** Inferior infarction. Coronary anatomy shows a dominant right coronary artery (RCA). A blockage at point "A" results in an inferior infarction and right ventricular infarction. A blockage at point "B" involves only the inferior wall, sparing the right ventricle. **B,** Inferior infarction. Coronary anatomy shows a dominant circumflex artery. A blockage at point "A" results in an inferior infarction. A blockage at point "B" may result in a lateral and inferobasal infarction.

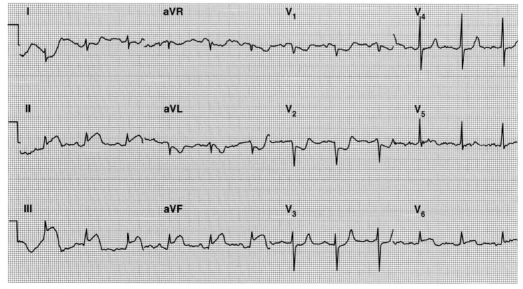

Figure 9-13   Inferior infarction. Note the ST-segment elevation in leads II, III, and aVF, and the reciprocal ST depression in leads I and aVL.

Lateral Infarction

[Objective 4]

Leads I, aVL, V₅, and V₆ view the lateral wall of the left ventricle. The lateral wall of the left ventricle may be supplied by the circumflex artery, the LAD artery, or a branch of the RCA (Figure 9-14). An example of an infarction involving the lateral wall is shown in Figure 9-15.

Inferobasal Infarction

[Objective 4]

Inferobasal (i.e., posterior) infarctions usually occur in conjunction with an inferior or lateral infarction. The inferobasal

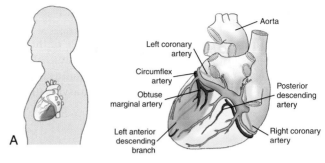

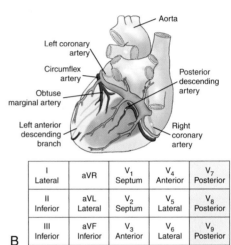

I Lateral	aVR	V₁ Septum	V₄ Anterior	V₇ Posterior
II Inferior	aVL Lateral	V₂ Septum	V₅ Lateral	V₈ Posterior
III Inferior	aVF Inferior	V₃ Anterior	V₆ Lateral	V₉ Posterior

Figure 9-16   Inferobasal infarction. **A,** Coronary anatomy shows a dominant right coronary artery (RCA). Occlusion of the RCA commonly results in an inferior and inferobasal infarction. **B,** Coronary anatomy shows a dominant circumflex artery. Occlusion of a marginal branch is the cause of most isolated inferobasal infarctions.

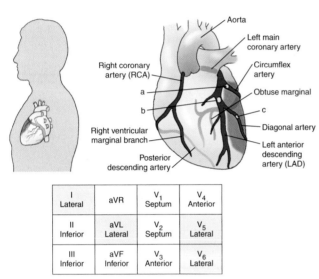

I Lateral	aVR	V₁ Septum	V₄ Anterior
II Inferior	aVL Lateral	V₂ Septum	V₅ Lateral
III Inferior	aVF Inferior	V₃ Anterior	V₆ Lateral

Figure 9-14   Lateral infarction. Coronary artery anatomy shows a occlusion of the circumflex, b occlusion of the proximal LAD artery, and c occlusion of the diagonal artery.

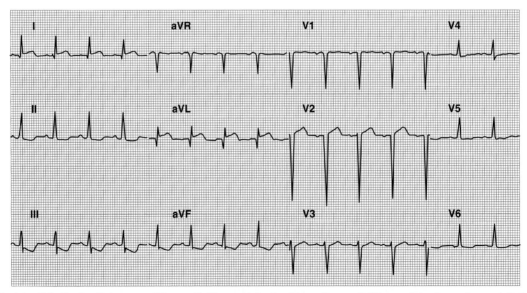

Figure 9-15   Lateral infarction. Lead I shows a small Q wave with ST-segment elevation. A larger Q wave with ST-segment elevation can be seen in lead aVL. This patient had an anterior non-ST-elevation infarction 4 days earlier with ST-segment elevation and T-wave inversion in leads V₂ through V₆. A coronary arteriogram at that time showed a blocked left anterior descending artery distal to its first large septal perforator. The ST-segment elevation evolved and the T waves in all of the chest leads had become upright the day before this tracing was recorded. The patient then had another episode of chest pain associated with the appearance of signs of acute lateral infarction as shown in this tracing. A repeat coronary arteriogram showed new blockage of the obtuse marginal branch of the circumflex artery.

wall of the left ventricle is supplied by the circumflex artery in most patients; however, in some patients it is supplied by the RCA (Figure 9-16). Because no leads of a standard 12-lead ECG directly view the posterior wall of the left ventricle, additional chest leads (V_7 to V_9) may be used to view the heart's posterior surface. Indicative changes of a posterior wall infarction include ST-segment elevation in these leads.

If placement of posterior chest leads is not feasible, changes in the opposite (anterior) wall of the heart can be viewed as reciprocal changes. An inferobasal MI usually produces tall R waves and ST-segment depression in leads V_1, V_2, and to a lesser extent in lead V_3. The "mirror test" is helpful in the recognition of ECG changes suggesting an inferobasal MI (Figure 9-17).

Complications of a posterior wall MI may include left ventricular dysfunction. If the posterior wall is supplied by the RCA, complications may include dysrhythmias involving the sinoatrial (SA) node, AV node, and bundle of His. An example of an inferobasal MI is shown in Figure 9-18.

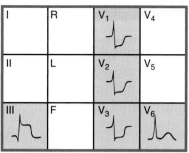

Figure 9-17   Application of the mirror test. This test is most helpful in assessing a patient with an acute inferior infarction, in whom you suspect an acute inferobasal infarction. **A,** Schematic 12-lead ECG with indicative changes of inferior infarction in lead III. Note the tall R wave in lead V_1 and the ST-segment depression in leads V_1, V_2, and V_3. **B,** The tracing in A is now flipped over. Looking through the paper (as it is held up to the light), you now see Q waves and ST-segment elevation in leads V_1, V_2, and V_3. This is a positive mirror test and suggests that the lead changes observed in A may reflect associated acute inferobasal infarction.

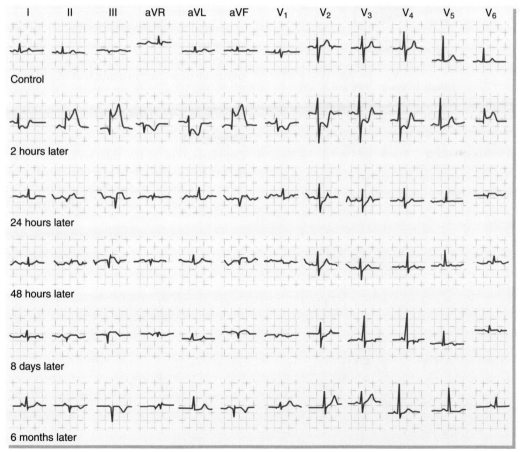

Figure 9-18   Evolutionary changes in a posteroinferior myocardial infarction. Control tracing is normal. The tracing recorded 2 hours after onset of chest pain demonstrated development of early Q waves, marked ST-segment elevation, and hyperacute T waves in leads II, III, and aVF. In addition, a larger R wave, ST-segment depression, and negative T waves have developed in leads V_1 and V_2. These are early changes indicating acute posteroinferior myocardial infarction. The 24-hour tracing demaonstrates evolutionary changes. In leads II, III, and aVF, the Q wave is larger, the ST segments have almost returned to baseline, and the T wave has begun to invert. In leads V_1 to V_2, the duration of the R wave now exceeds 0.04 second, the ST segment is depressed, and the T wave is upright. (In this example, ECG changes of true posterior involvement extend past lead V_2; ordinarily, only leads V_1 and V_2 may be involved.) Only minor further changes occur through the 8-day tracing. Finally, 6 months later, the ECG illustrates large Q waves, isoelectric ST segments, and inverted T waves in leads II, III, and aVF and large R waves, isoelectric ST segment, and upright T waves in leads V_1 and V_2, indicative of an *old* posteroinferior myocardial infarction.

Right Ventricular Infarction[1]
[Objective 4]

The right ventricle is supplied by the right ventricular marginal branch of the RCA (Figure 9-19). An occlusion of the right ventricular marginal branch results in an isolated right ventricular infarction (RVI). Occlusion of the RCA proximal to the right ventricular marginal branch results in an inferior and RVI. Although a RVI may occur by itself, it is more commonly associated with an inferior MI and it should be suspected when ECG changes suggesting an inferior infarction are seen. An example of an infarction involving the right ventricle is shown in Figure 9-20.

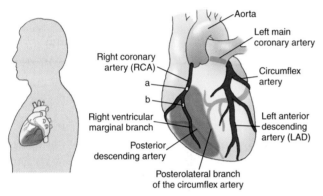

I Lateral	aVR	V₁ Septum	V₄ Anterior	V₄R Rt vent
II Inferior	aVL Lateral	V₂ Septum	V₅ Lateral	V₅R Rt vent
III Inferior	aVF Inferior	V₃ Anterior	V₆ Lateral	V₆R Rt vent

Figure 9-19   Right ventricular infarction (RVI). Occlusion of the right coronary artery (RCA) proximal to the right ventricular marginal branch results in an inferior and RVI. An occlusion of the right ventricular marginal branch results in an isolated RVI.

In addition to ECG evidence, certain clinical signs also support the suspicion of RVI. The clinical evidence of RVI involves three main areas: hypotension, jugular venous distention, and clear breath sounds. This triad of signs is estimated to be present in only 10% to 15% of patients with RVI.[2]

In the setting of RVI, the right ventricle may lose some of its ability to pump blood into the pulmonary circuit. When this happens, blood stalls in the right ventricle and may begin to back up. (Technically, the blood does not back up; the venous return exceeds ventricular output and blood begins to build up.) This stalling and backing up produce the hypotension, jugular venous distention, and absence of pulmonary edema (i.e., clear lung sounds) considered the clinical triad of RVI. As blood backs up from the right ventricle, the jugular veins become enlarged. Hypotension results from the decrease in blood volume moving into the lungs and left ventricle. The left ventricle can only pump as much blood as it receives, and if less blood reaches the left ventricle, less blood is pumped into the systemic circulation. The net effect of this reduction in left ventricular output is a decrease in blood pressure and engorgement of the central venous system.

Complications associated with RVI include hypotension, cardiogenic shock, AV blocks, atrial flutter or fibrillation, and premature atrial complexes. AV blocks are particularly common, occurring in about half of patients with RVI.

R-Wave Progression

[Objective 5]

Depolarization of the interventricular septum normally occurs from left to right and posteriorly to anteriorly. The wave of ventricular depolarization in the major portions of the ventricles is normally from right to left and in an

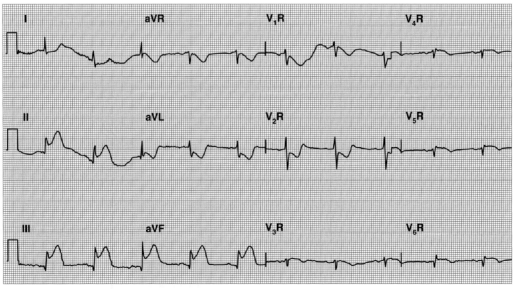

Figure 9-20   Inferior infarction, right ventricular infarction.

anterior to posterior direction. When viewing the chest leads in a normal heart, the R wave becomes taller and the S wave becomes smaller as the electrode is moved from right to left. This pattern is called *R-wave progression* (Figure 9-21). In V_1 and V_2, the QRS deflection is predominantly negative (i.e., moving away from the positive chest electrode), reflecting depolarization of the septum and right ventricle (small R wave) and the left ventricle (large S wave). As the chest electrode is placed further left, the wave of depolarization is moving toward the positive electrode. V_3 and V_4 normally record an equiphasic (i.e., equally positive and negative) RS complex. The area in which this equiphasic complex occurs is called the *transitional zone*. V_5 and V_6 normally record a QR complex in which the Q wave is small, reflecting depolarization of the septum, and the R wave is tall, reflecting ventricular depolarization.

Poor R-wave progression (Figure 9-22) is a phrase used to describe R waves that decrease in size from V_1 to V_4. This is often seen in an anteroseptal infarction but may be a normal variant in young persons, particularly in young women. Other causes of poor R-wave progression include left BBB, left ventricular hypertrophy, and severe chronic obstructive pulmonary disease (particularly emphysema).

CHAMBER ENLARGEMENT

[Objective 6]

Enlargement of the atrial chambers, ventricular chambers, or both, may occur if there is a volume or pressure overload in the heart. **Dilatation** is an increase in the diameter of a chamber of the heart caused by volume overload. Dilatation may be acute or chronic. **Hypertrophy** is an increase in the thickness of a heart chamber because of chronic pressure overload. Hypertrophy is commonly accompanied by dilatation. **Enlargement** is a term that implies the presence of dilatation or hypertrophy or both.

ECG Pearl

When evaluating the ECG for the presence of chamber enlargement, it is particularly important to check the calibration marker to ensure that it is 10-mm tall.

Atrial Abnormalities

The first half of the P wave is recorded when the electrical impulse that originated in the SA node stimulates the right atrium and reaches the AV node. The downslope of the P wave reflects stimulation of the left atrium. The appearance of abnormal P waves on the ECG may be caused by delayed intraatrial conduction, elevated atrial pressure, atrial dilatation, and atrial muscular hypertrophy, among other causes. In the past, terms used to describe atrial abnormalities have included *P-mitrale, P-pulmonale, left atrial enlargement, right atrial enlargement, atrial hypertrophy,* and *atrial overload,* among others. Today, experts recommend that the terms *left atrial abnormality* and *right atrial abnormality* be used because a combination of several factors that may not be distinguishable can result in abnormal P waves.[3]

Enlargement of the right atrium produces an abnormally tall initial part of the P wave. The P wave is tall (more than 2.5 mm in height in leads II, III, and aVF), peaked, and usually of normal duration (Figure 9-23). The P wave may be biphasic in lead V_1 with a more prominent positive portion. Examples of conditions that may cause right atrial abnormality include chronic obstructive pulmonary disease with or without pulmonary hypertension, congenital heart disease, or right ventricular failure of any cause.

The latter part of the P wave is prominent in left atrial abnormality. This is because the impulse starts in the right

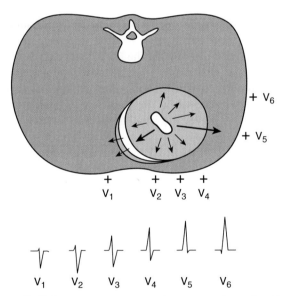

Figure 9-21 Ventricular activation and R-wave progression as viewed in the chest leads. In normal R-wave progression, the QRS complex is negative in V_1, positive in V_6 and switches from negative to positive in the V_3 to V_4 transition zone.

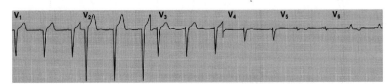

Figure 9-22 Poor R-wave progression in V_1 through V_4; QRS greater than 0.12 second; and left bundle branch block.

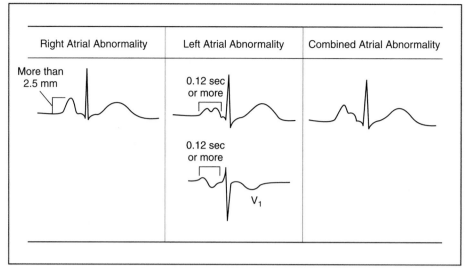

Figure 9-23 Criteria for atrial abnormalities.

atrium where the SA node is located and chamber size is normal. The electrical impulse then travels to the left to depolarize the left atrium. The P wave inscribed on the ECG is generally 0.12 second in duration or more because it takes longer to depolarize an enlarged muscle (see Figure 9-23). The P wave is often notched in leads I, II, aVL, and V_4, V_5, and V_6. The P wave may be biphasic in lead V_1 with a more prominent negative portion. Left atrial enlargement occurs because of conditions that increase left atrial pressure, volume overload, or both (e.g., mitral regurgitation, mitral stenosis, left ventricular failure, systemic hypertension).

When the ECG reflects features of both right atrial and left atrial abnormality, the term *combined atrial abnormality* is used.

Ventricular Hypertrophy

Ventricular muscle thickens (i.e., hypertrophies) when it sustains a persistent pressure overload. Dilatation occurs because of persistent volume overload. The two often go hand in hand. Hypertrophy increases the QRS amplitude

and is often associated with ST-segment depression and asymmetric T-wave inversion.

The amplitude (i.e., voltage) of the QRS complex can be affected by various factors, including age, body weight, and lung disease. Increased QRS amplitude may occur normally in thin-chested individuals or young adults because the chest electrodes are closer to the heart in these patients.

Because the right ventricle is normally considerably smaller than the left, it must become extremely enlarged before changes are visible on the ECG. Right axis deviation is one of the earliest and most reliable findings of right ventricular hypertrophy (RVH). Further, normal R-wave progression is reversed in the chest leads, revealing taller than normal R waves and small S waves in V_1 and V_2 and deeper than normal S waves and small R waves in V_5 and V_6 (Figure 9-24). Causes of RVH include pulmonary hypertension and chronic pulmonary diseases, valvular heart disease, and congenital heart disease.

Left ventricular hypertrophy (LVH) is recognized on the ECG by increased QRS amplitude. However, recognition of LVH on the ECG is not always obvious and several formulas

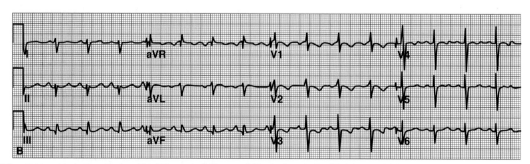

Figure 9-24 Right ventricular hypertrophy with tall R wave in right precordial leads, downsloping ST depression in the chest leads, right axis deviation, and evidence of right atrial enlargement.

exist to assist in its recognition. The formula presented here was selected because it is easy to remember and may be used to quickly check for the presence of LVH.[1]

- Step 1. Look at V_1 and determine the depth of the S wave by counting in millimeters the amount of negative deflection measuring from the baseline to the most negative point in V_1 (count the small boxes—one box equals 1 mm).
- Step 2. Look at V_5 and V_6 and determine which lead has the tallest R wave. Determine the height of the taller R wave in millimeters (count the small boxes).
- Step 3. Add the height of the taller R wave and the deeper S wave. If the number is equal to or greater than 35, suspect LVH.

Causes of LVH include systemic hypertension, hypertrophic cardiomyopathy, aortic stenosis, and aortic insufficiency. LVH may be accompanied by left axis deviation.

Examples of LVH are shown in Figures 9-25 and 9-26. Note that the ST segment in Figure 9-25 is elevated in leads V_1, V_2, and V_3. Also note the ST-segment depression shown in leads V_5 and V_6. Recall that when the QRS complexes of left BBBs, ventricular rhythms, and ventricular paced rhythms are negatively deflected (i.e., a QS configuration), the ST segments and T waves are in the opposite direction of the last portion of the QRS complex. Similarly, when the QRS complex of LVH is negatively deflected, these ECG findings are shared by LVH (as shown in Figure 9-25), making the identification of ECG changes associated with acute MI difficult. Careful correlation

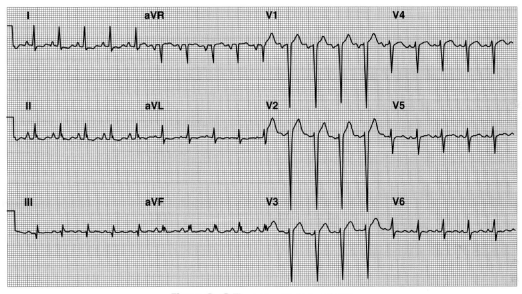

Figure 9-25   Left ventricular hypertrophy.

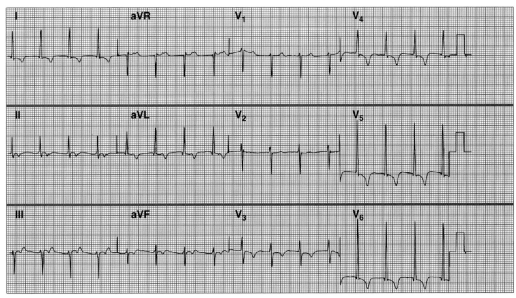

Figure 9-26   Left ventricular hypertrophy with first-degree atrioventricular (AV) block, ST-segment depression, and T-wave inversion.

of the patient's ECG, his or her clinical presentation, and the results of other diagnostic studies is essential.

ECG Pearl

A 12-lead ECG's interpretive algorithm checks for the presence of LVH using preprogrammed criteria, including formulas, to measure voltage. If the 12-lead machine determines that an ECG meets the criteria for LVH, a message is displayed such as, "Meets voltage criteria for left ventricular hypertrophy."[1]

ANALYZING THE 12-LEAD ELECTROCARDIOGRAM

[Objective 7]

The following five-step approach is recommended when reviewing a 12-lead ECG:[1]

1. *Identify the rate and underlying rhythm.* Determining rate and rhythm is the first priority when interpreting the ECG. Remember, the treatment of life-threatening dysrhythmias initially takes precedence over the acquisition and interpretation of the 12-lead ECG. If baseline wander or artifact is present to any significant degree, note it. If the presence of either of these conditions interferes with the assessment of any lead, use a modifier such as "possible" or "apparent" in your interpretation.

2. *Analyze waveforms.* Examine each lead, selecting one good representative waveform or complex in each lead. Examine each lead for the presence of a wide Q wave. If a Q wave is present, express the duration in milliseconds. Next, look for the presence of ST-segment displacement (i.e., elevation or depression). Elevation of the ST segment is the most reliable marker during the first hours of infarction, and may be recognizable before significant tissue loss has occurred. Therefore, each lead, with the exception of aVR, should be examined for the presence of indicative changes with special emphasis on ST-segment elevation and pathologic Q waves. Evidence must be found in at least two anatomically contiguous leads. If ST-segment elevation is present, express it in millimeters. Examine the T waves for any changes in orientation, shape, and size. Note the presence of tall, peaked T waves or T-wave inversion.

3. *Examine for evidence of infarction.* Is a STEMI suspected? What is the location? If ST-segment displacement is present, assess the areas of ischemia or injury by assessing lead groupings. If acute MI is suspected, mentally picture the cardiac anatomy to localize the infarction and predict which coronary artery is occluded. The relative extent of the infarction can be gauged by the number of

leads showing ST-segment elevation. Remember that in suspected RCA occlusions, right-sided chest leads should be obtained to help gauge the extent of the infarct and identify possible RVI.

ECG Pearl

Please note that more advanced 12-lead interpretation generally includes a careful analysis of R-wave progression and axis deviation, among other factors. In this text, our focus is on the identification of ECG findings suggestive of acute MI.

4. *Ascertain if STEMI imposters are present that may account for ECG changes.* When changes indicative of an acute infarction are noted on the ECG, ascertain if other conditions are present that might also account for the changes. In cases where these conditions are present, do not rule out infarction, but recognize that these ECG changes may be a result of infarction or one of the infarct impostors (e.g., LVH, left BBB, ventricular rhythm, ventricular paced rhythm). Remember, infarction can still occur in the presence of each of these conditions. Therefore, when you are screening potential infarct patients, recognition of indicative changes in the presence of one of the infarct impostors warrants an immediate physician over-read (i.e., careful physician review and interpretation of the 12-lead ECG).

5. *Make a STEMI decision.* On the basis of your ECG findings, decide if clear evidence is present that a STEMI exists: (1) a STEMI is definitely not present, (2) a suspected STEMI is present, and (3) possible STEMI (i.e., a STEMI imposter is present, making interpretation difficult).

REFERENCES

1. Phalen T, Aehlert B: *The 12-Lead ECG in acute coronary syndromes*, ed 3, St. Louis, 2012, Mosby, pp 75–161.
2. Anderson JL: ST segment elevation acute myocardial infarction and complications of myocardial infarction. In Goldman L, Ausiello D, editors: *Cecil medicine*, ed 23, Philadelphia, 2007, Saunders, pp 500–517.
3. Hancock EW, Deal BJ, Mirvis DM, et al: American Heart Association/American College of Cardiology Foundation/Heart Rhythm Society recommendations for the standardization and interpretation of the electrocardiogram: part V: electrocardiogram changes associated with cardiac chamber hypertrophy: a scientific statement from the American Heart Association Electrocardiography and Arrhythmias Committee, Council on Clinical Cardiology; the American College of Cardiology Foundation; and the Heart Rhythm Society. *J Am Coll Cardiol* 53:992–1002, 2009.

STOP & REVIEW—CHAPTER 9

True/False

Indicate whether the statement is true or false.

____ 1. In a patient experiencing an acute coronary syndrome, ST-segment elevation in the shape of a "smiley" face (i.e., upward concavity) is usually associated with an acute injury pattern.

____ 2. *Poor R-wave progression* is a phrase used to describe R waves that decrease in size from V_1 to V_4.

____ 3. Placement of right chest leads is identical to the standard chest leads except on the right side of the chest.

____ 4. In most patients, the posterior wall of the left ventricle is supplied by the right coronary artery.

____ 5. When you read a 12-lead ECG from left to right, the ECG tracing is continuous.

____ 6. The six limb leads view the heart in the frontal plane as if the body were flat.

____ 7. In a patient presenting with an acute coronary syndrome, the presence of ST-segment elevation on the ECG suggests that myocardial injury in progress.

Multiple Choice

Identify the choice that best completes the statement or answers the question.

____ 8. Which of the following leads view the heart in the frontal plane?
   a. II, III, V_1, V_2
   b. I, aVL, V_5, V_6
   c. V_1, V_2, V_3, V_4, V_5, V_6
   d. I, II, III, aVR, aVL, aVF

____ 9. Although a right ventricular infarction may occur by itself, it is more commonly associated with a(n) _____ wall myocardial infarction.
   a. Anterior
   b. Lateral
   c. Septal
   d. Inferior

____ 10. Patients experiencing _____ infarctions are most likely to develop bundle branch block.
   a. Inferior and lateral
   b. Anterior and inferobasal
   c. Septal and anteroseptal
   d. Inferior and septal

____ 11. Which of the following statements is true regarding ventricular hypertrophy?
   a. Hypertrophy increases the QRS amplitude.
   b. Hypertrophy increases the duration of the QRS complex.
   c. Leads I, aVL, V_5, and V_6 are the best leads to use when looking for ECG evidence of hypertrophy.
   d. ECG evidence of right ventricular hypertrophy is usually more readily evident than left ventricular hypertrophy.

____ 12. When correctly positioned, lead V_1 lies:
   a. In the midaxillary line, fifth intercostal space.
   b. In the anterior axillary line, third intercostal space.
   c. In the fourth intercostal space, just to the left of the sternum.
   d. In the fourth intercostal space, just to the right of the sternum.

____ 13. If time does not permit obtaining an entire right-sided 12-lead ECG to view the right ventricle, the lead of choice is:
   a. V_1R.
   b. V_4R.
   c. V_9.
   d. V_6R.

____ 14. When leads I and aVF are used to determine electrical axis, left axis deviation is present if:
   a. The QRS is positive in lead I and positive in lead aVF.
   b. The QRS is positive in lead I and negative in lead aVF.
   c. The QRS is negative in lead I and negative in lead aVF.
   d. The QRS is negative in lead I and positive in lead aVF.

____ 15. Which of the following leads are anatomically contiguous?
   a. II, V_2
   b. II, III, V_3
   c. V_2, V_3, V_4
   d. I, V_3, V_4

____**16.** In a patient experiencing an acute coronary syndrome, T-wave inversion suggests the presence of:
  a. Injury.
  b. Ischemia.
  c. Infarction.
  d. Cardiogenic shock.

____**17.** Indicative ECG changes observed in leads I, aVL, V_3, V_4, V_5, and V_6 suggest that the _____ is affected.
  a. Septum
  b. Anterolateral wall of the left ventricle
  c. Inferolateral wall of the left ventricle
  d. Anteroseptal wall of the right ventricle

Matching

Match the key terms with their definitions by placing the letter of each correct answer in the space provided.

a. Fully evolved phase
b. Indicative changes
c. V_1R-V_6R
d. Hexaxial reference system
e. Right coronary artery
f. Dilatation
g. Left coronary artery
h. V_1-V_2
i. Injury
j. aVL

k. I, aVL, V_5, V_6
l. Hyperacute phase
m. Lead II
n. Hypertrophy
o. II, III, aVF
p. Reciprocal changes
q. Early acute phase
r. aVF
s. V_3-V_4
t. Ischemia

____**18.** A branch of this vessel supplies most of the bundle branch tissue and a critical section of the left ventricle.

____**19.** Lead II is perpendicular to this lead.

____**20.** Significant ECG findings that are seen in leads that are opposite the affected area of the heart

____**21.** ST-segment elevation in these leads suggest an anterior infarction.

____**22.** Tall T waves may be observed on the ECG during this phase of ST-elevation MI.

____**23.** An increase in the diameter of a chamber of the heart caused by volume overload

____**24.** Lead I + Lead III = _____

____**25.** The zone of _____ is typically characterized by ST-segment depression.

____**26.** An increase in the thickness of a heart chamber because of chronic pressure overload

____**27.** ST-segment elevation in these leads suggest an inferior infarction.

____**28.** This represents all of the frontal plane leads with the heart in the center.

____**29.** Pathologic Q waves may first appear on the ECG during this phase of ST-elevation MI.

____**30.** Lead I is perpendicular to this lead.

____**31.** ST-segment elevation in these leads suggest a septal infarction.

____**32.** Significant ECG findings that are seen in leads that look directly at the affected area of the heart

____**33.** ST-segment elevation may be observed on the ECG during this phase of ST-elevation MI.

____**34.** Occlusion of a branch of this vessel can result in an inferior or right ventricular infarction.

____**35.** ST-segment elevation in these leads suggest a lateral infarction.

____**36.** Leads used to view the right ventricle

____**37.** The zone of _____ is typically characterized by ST-segment elevation.

Short Answer

38. Explain what is meant by the phrase *anatomically contiguous leads.*

_____

_____

_____

39. Describe a systematic method for analyzing a 12-lead ECG.

_____

_____

_____

40. What causes the ST-segment elevation seen in acute myocardial infarction?

_____

_____

_____

41. When should you suspect a right ventricular infarction?

_____

_____

_____

42. List three conditions that can mimic myocardial infarction by producing ST-segment elevation.

1.

2.

3.

43. Briefly describe how to determine the presence of left ventricular hypertrophy using the 12-lead ECG.

_____

_____

_____

12-LEAD ELECTROCARDIOGRAMS PRACTICE

44. Analyze this 12-lead ECG and record your findings below.

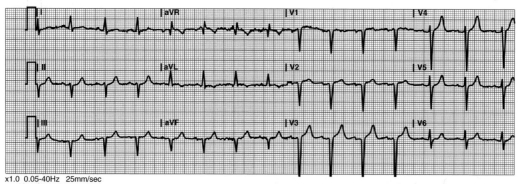

x1.0 0.05-40Hz 25mm/sec

Figure 9-27

I	Lateral	aVR	---------	V₁	Septum	V₄	Anterior
II	Inferior	aVL	Lateral	V₂	Septum	V₅	Lateral
III	Inferior	aVF	Inferior	V₃	Anterior	V₆	Lateral

Rate and rhythm _____ Pathologic Q waves _____

ST-segment elevation _____ ST-segment depression _____

T-wave changes _____ STEMI present? _____

Interpretation: _____

45. Analyze this 12-lead ECG and record your findings below.

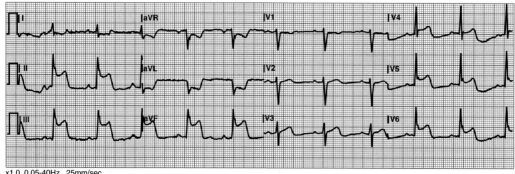

x1.0 0.05-40Hz 25mm/sec

Figure 9-28

I	Lateral	aVR	---------	V₁	Septum	V₄	Anterior
II	Inferior	aVL	Lateral	V₂	Septum	V₅	Lateral
III	Inferior	aVF	Inferior	V₃	Anterior	V₆	Lateral

Rate and rhythm _____ Pathologic Q waves _____

ST-segment elevation _____ ST-segment depression _____

T-wave changes _____ STEMI present? _____

Interpretation: _____

46. Analyze this 12-lead ECG and record your findings below.

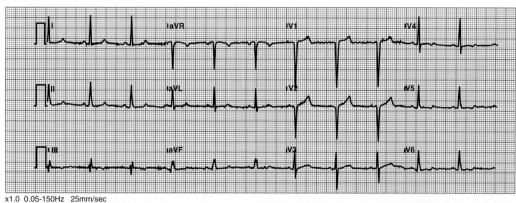

x1.0 0.05-150Hz 25mm/sec

Figure **9-29**

I	Lateral	aVR	---------	V₁	Septum	V₄	Anterior
II	Inferior	aVL	Lateral	V₂	Septum	V₅	Lateral
III	Inferior	aVF	Inferior	V₃	Anterior	V₆	Lateral

Rate and rhythm _____ Pathologic Q waves _____

ST-segment elevation _____ ST-segment depression _____

T-wave changes _____ STEMI present? _____

Interpretation: _____

47. Analyze this 12-lead ECG and record your findings below.

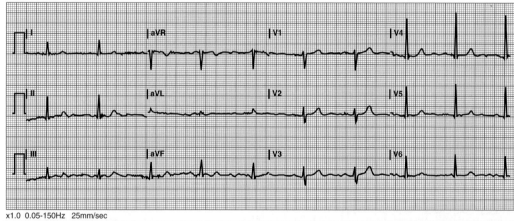

x1.0 0.05-150Hz 25mm/sec

Figure **9-30**

I	Lateral	aVR	---------	V₁	Septum	V₄	Anterior
II	Inferior	aVL	Lateral	V₂	Septum	V₅	Lateral
III	Inferior	aVF	Inferior	V₃	Anterior	V₆	Lateral

Rate and rhythm _____ Pathologic Q waves _____

ST-segment elevation _____ ST-segment depression _____

T-wave changes _____ STEMI present? _____

Interpretation: _____

48. Analyze this 12-lead ECG and record your findings below.

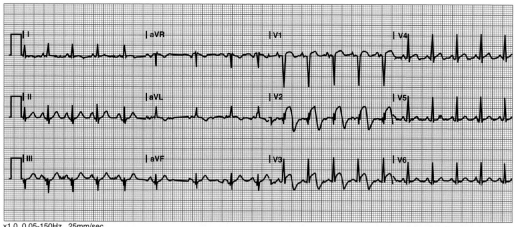

x1.0 0.05-150Hz 25mm/sec

I	Lateral	aVR	---------	V₁	Septum	V₄	Anterior
II	Inferior	aVL	Lateral	V₂	Septum	V₅	Lateral
III	Inferior	aVF	Inferior	V₃	Anterior	V₆	Lateral

Figure 9-31

Rate and rhythm _____   Pathologic Q waves _____

ST-segment elevation _____   ST-segment depression _____

T-wave changes _____   STEMI present? _____

Interpretation: _____

49. Analyze this 12-lead ECG and record your findings below.

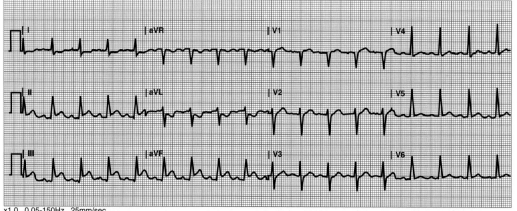

x1.0 0.05-150Hz 25mm/sec

I	Lateral	aVR	---------	V₁	Septum	V₄	Anterior
II	Inferior	aVL	Lateral	V₂	Septum	V₅	Lateral
III	Inferior	aVF	Inferior	V₃	Anterior	V₆	Lateral

Figure 9-32

Rate and rhythm _____   Pathologic Q waves _____

ST-segment elevation _____   ST-segment depression _____

T-wave changes _____   STEMI present? _____

Interpretation: _____

50. Analyze this 12-lead ECG and record your findings below.

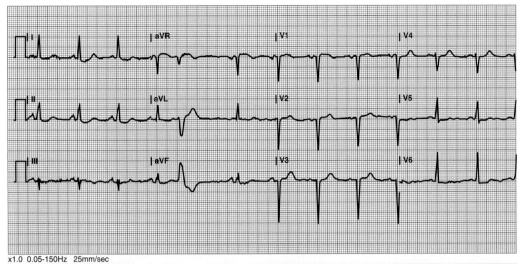

x1.0 0.05-150Hz 25mm/sec

I	Lateral	aVR	---------	V₁	Septum	V₄	Anterior
II	Inferior	aVL	Lateral	V₂	Septum	V₅	Lateral
III	Inferior	aVF	Inferior	V₃	Anterior	V₆	Lateral

Figure 9-33

Rate and rhythm _____ Pathologic Q waves _____

ST-segment elevation _____ ST-segment depression _____

T-wave changes _____ STEMI present? _____

Interpretation: _____

51. Analyze this 12-lead ECG and record your findings below.

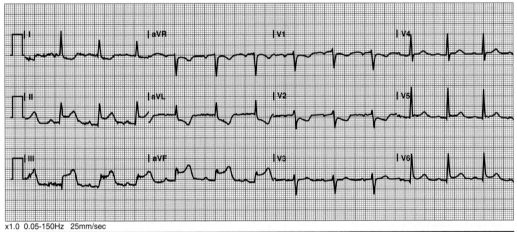

x1.0 0.05-150Hz 25mm/sec

I	Lateral	aVR	---------	V₁	Septum	V₄	Anterior
II	Inferior	aVL	Lateral	V₂	Septum	V₅	Lateral
III	Inferior	aVF	Inferior	V₃	Anterior	V₆	Lateral

Figure 9-34

Rate and rhythm _____ Pathologic Q waves _____

ST-segment elevation _____ ST-segment depression _____

T-wave changes _____ STEMI present? _____

Interpretation: _____

52. Analyze this 12-lead ECG and record your findings below.

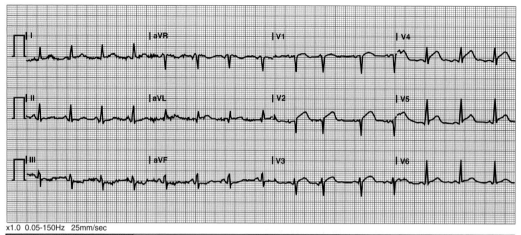

x1.0 0.05-150Hz 25mm/sec

I	Lateral	aVR	----------	V₁	Septum	V₄	Anterior
II	Inferior	aVL	Lateral	V₂	Septum	V₅	Lateral
III	Inferior	aVF	Inferior	V₃	Anterior	V₆	Lateral

Figure 9-35

Rate and rhythm _____ Pathologic Q waves _____

ST-segment elevation _____ ST-segment depression _____

T-wave changes _____ STEMI present? _____

Interpretation: _____

53. Analyze this 12-lead ECG and record your findings below.

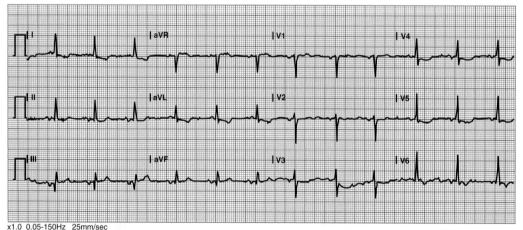

x1.0 0.05-150Hz 25mm/sec

I	Lateral	aVR	----------	V₁	Septum	V₄	Anterior
II	Inferior	aVL	Lateral	V₂	Septum	V₅	Lateral
III	Inferior	aVF	Inferior	V₃	Anterior	V₆	Lateral

Figure 9-36

Rate and rhythm _____ Pathologic Q waves _____

ST-segment elevation _____ ST-segment depression _____

T-wave changes _____ STEMI present? _____

Interpretation: _____

54. Analyze this 12-lead ECG and record your findings below.

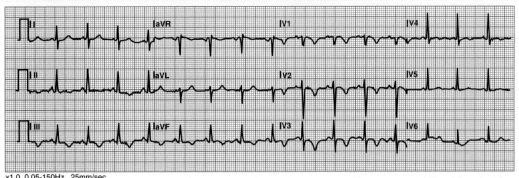

x1.0 0.05-150Hz 25mm/sec

I	Lateral	aVR	---------	V₁	Septum	V₄	Anterior
II	Inferior	aVL	Lateral	V₂	Septum	V₅	Lateral
III	Inferior	aVF	Inferior	V₃	Anterior	V₆	Lateral

Figure 9-37

Rate and rhythm _____ Pathologic Q waves _____

ST-segment elevation _____ ST-segment depression _____

T-wave changes _____ STEMI present? _____

Interpretation: _____

55. Analyze this 12-lead ECG and record your findings below.

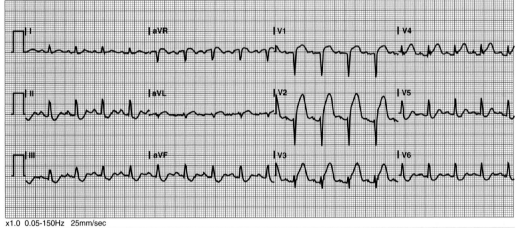

x1.0 0.05-150Hz 25mm/sec

I	Lateral	aVR	---------	V₁	Septum	V₄	Anterior
II	Inferior	aVL	Lateral	V₂	Septum	V₅	Lateral
III	Inferior	aVF	Inferior	V₃	Anterior	V₆	Lateral

Figure 9-38

Rate and rhythm _____ Pathologic Q waves _____

ST-segment elevation _____ ST-segment depression _____

T-wave changes _____ STEMI present? _____

Interpretation: _____

STOP & REVIEW ANSWERS

True/False

1. ANS: F

Myocardial ischemia, injury, and infarction are among the causes of ST-segment deviation. ST-segment elevation in the shape of a "smiley" face (i.e., upward concavity) is usually benign, particularly when it occurs in an otherwise healthy, asymptomatic patient. The appearance of coved (i.e., "frowny face") ST-segment elevation is called an *acute injury pattern*. Other causes of ST-segment elevation may represent a normal variant, pericarditis, or ventricular aneurysm, among other causes.

OBJ: Recognize the changes on the ECG that may reflect evidence of myocardial ischemia, injury, or infarction.

2. ANS: T

When viewing the chest leads in a normal heart, the R wave becomes taller and the S wave becomes smaller as the electrode is moved from right to left. This pattern is called *R-wave progression*. *Poor R-wave progression* is a phrase used to describe R waves that decrease in size from V_1 to V_4.

OBJ: Distinguish patterns of normal and abnormal R-wave progression.

3. ANS: T

Right chest leads are used to evaluate the right ventricle. The placement of right chest leads is identical to the placement of the standard chest leads except that it is done on the right side of the chest. A standard 12-lead ECG should be obtained first; the cables for the standard chest leads are then moved to the electrodes repositioned on the right chest for the additional leads.

OBJ: Describe correct anatomic placement of the standard limb leads, the augmented leads, and the chest leads.

Multiple Choice

8. ANS: D

Frontal plane leads view the heart from the front of the body as if it were flat. Directions in the frontal plane are superior, inferior, right, and left. Six leads view the heart in the frontal plane. Leads I, II, and III are called *standard limb leads*. Leads aVR, aVL, and aVF are called *augmented limb leads*.

OBJ: Differentiate between the frontal plane and the horizontal plane leads.

9. ANS: D

The right ventricle is supplied by the right ventricular marginal branch of the right coronary artery (RCA). An occlusion of the right ventricular marginal branch results in an isolated right ventricular infarction (RVI). Occlusion of the RCA proximal to the right ventricular marginal branch results in an inferior and right ventricular infarction. RVI should be suspected when ECG changes suggesting an inferior infarction are seen.

OBJ: Recognize the changes on the ECG that may reflect evidence of myocardial ischemia, injury, or infarction.

4. ANS: F

The posterior wall of the left ventricle is supplied by the circumflex coronary artery in most patients; however, in some patients it is supplied by the right coronary artery.

OBJ: Name the primary branches and areas of the heart supplied by the right and left coronary arteries.

5. ANS: T

When viewing a 12-lead, leads that line up vertically are simultaneous recordings of the same beat. When you read the 12-lead from left to right, the ECG tracing is continuous. As you switch from one lead to the next, it is still continuous.

OBJ: N/A

6. ANS: T

Frontal plane leads view the heart from the front of the body as if it were flat. Directions in the frontal plane are superior, inferior, right, and left. Six leads view the heart in the frontal plane. Leads I, II, and III are called *standard limb leads*. Leads aVR, aVL, and aVF are called *augmented limb leads*.

OBJ: Describe correct anatomic placement of the standard limb leads, the augmented leads, and the chest leads.

7. ANS: T

In a patient presenting with an acute coronary syndrome, ST-segment elevation may develop, indicating myocardial injury in progress. ST-segment elevation may occur within the first hour or first few hours of infarction.

OBJ: Recognize the changes on the ECG that may reflect evidence of myocardial ischemia, injury, or infarction.

10. ANS: C

The septum, which contains the bundle of His and bundle branches, is normally supplied by the left anterior descending coronary artery. ECG changes of infarction are seen in leads V_1 and V_2 if the site of infarction is limited to the septum. If the entire anterior wall is involved, ECG changes will be visible in V_1, V_2, V_3, and V_4. A blockage in this area may result in both right and left bundle branch blocks (BBBs) (left BBB is more common), second-degree atrioventricular (AV) block type II, and third-degree AV block.

OBJ: Recognize the changes on the ECG that may reflect evidence of myocardial ischemia, injury, or infarction.

11. ANS: A

Ventricular muscle thickens (i.e., hypertrophies) when it sustains a persistent pressure overload. Dilatation occurs because of persistent volume overload. The two often go hand in hand. Hypertrophy increases the QRS amplitude and is often associated with ST-segment depression and asymmetric T-wave inversion. Because the right ventricle is normally considerably smaller than the left, it must become extremely enlarged before changes are visible on the ECG. Leads V_1, V_5, and V_6 are used when looking for ECG evidence of hypertrophy.

OBJ: Explain what is meant by the terms *dilatation*, *hypertrophy*, and *enlargement*.

12. ANS: D

When correctly positioned, lead V_1 lies in the fourth intercostal space, just to the right of the sternum.

OBJ: Describe correct anatomic placement of the standard limb leads, the augmented leads, and the chest leads.

13. ANS: B

If time does not permit obtaining an entire right-sided 12-lead ECG to view the right ventricle, the lead of choice is V_4R.

OBJ: Relate the cardiac surfaces or areas represented by the ECG leads.

14. ANS: B

Current flow to the left of normal is called *left axis deviation* (between −30 and −90 degrees). If the QRS complex is predominantly positive in I and negative in aVF, left axis deviation is present.

OBJ: Discuss the determination of electrical axis using leads I and aVF.

15. ANS: C

Leads V_2, V_3, V_4 are anatomically contiguous leads because they view the same or adjacent areas of the heart and because they are numerically consecutive chest leads.

OBJ: Relate the cardiac surfaces or areas represented by the ECG leads.

16. ANS: B

In a patient experiencing an acute coronary syndrome, T-wave inversion suggests the presence of myocardial ischemia.

OBJ: Recognize the changes on the ECG that may reflect evidence of myocardial ischemia, injury, or infarction.

17. ANS: B

Leads V_3 and V_4 view the anterior wall of the left ventricle. Leads I, aVL, V_5, and V_6 view the lateral wall of the left ventricle; therefore, indicative ECG changes observed in these leads suggest that the anterolateral wall of the left ventricle is affected.

OBJ: Relate the cardiac surfaces or areas represented by the ECG leads.

Matching

18. ANS: G
19. ANS: J
20. ANS: P
21. ANS: S
22. ANS: L
23. ANS: F
24. ANS: M
25. ANS: T
26. ANS: N
27. ANS: O
28. ANS: D
29. ANS: A
30. ANS: R
31. ANS: H
32. ANS: B
33. ANS: Q
34. ANS: E
35. ANS: K
36. ANS: C
37. ANS: I

Short Answer

38. ANS:

Anatomically contiguous leads refers to those leads that "see" the same area of the heart. Two leads are contiguous if they look at the same or an adjacent area of the heart or they are numerically consecutive *chest* leads.
OBJ: Relate the cardiac surfaces or areas represented by the ECG leads.

39. ANS:

1. Identify the rate and underlying rhythm.
2. Analyze waveforms.
3. Examine for evidence of infarction.
4. Ascertain if ST-elevation myocardial infarction (STEMI) imposters are present that may account for ECG changes.
5. Make a STEMI decision (i.e., definitely not present, suspected STEMI, possible STEMI [i.e., a STEMI imposter is present, making interpretation difficult]).

OBJ: Describe a systematic method for analyzing a 12-lead ECG.

40. ANS:

ST-segment elevation is not caused by myocardial infarction per se. Although the theories are complex, suffice it to say that ST-segment elevation is caused by changes that affect ventricular repolarization, ventricular depolarization, or both; therefore, myocardial infarction produces ST-segment elevation because the infarction affects ventricular repolarization, ventricular depolarization, or both.
OBJ: Recognize the changes on the ECG that may reflect evidence of myocardial ischemia, injury, or infarction.

41. ANS:

Right ventricular infarction (RVI) should be suspected when ECG changes suggesting an inferior infarction (ST-segment elevation in leads II, III, and/or aVF) are observed.
OBJ: Relate the cardiac surfaces or areas represented by the ECG leads.

42. ANS:

Examples of conditions that can mimic myocardial infarction by producing ST-segment elevation include the following: left bundle branch block (LBBB), ventricular rhythms, ventricular paced rhythms, left ventricular hypertrophy (LVH), pericarditis, and benign early repolarization.
OBJ: Recognize the changes on the ECG that may reflect evidence of myocardial ischemia, injury, or infarction.

43. ANS:

- Step 1. Look at V_1 and determine the depth of the S wave by counting in millimeters the amount of negative deflection measuring from the baseline to the most negative point in V_1 (count the small boxes—one box equals 1 mm).
- Step 2. Look at V_5 and V_6 and determine which lead has the tallest R wave. Determine the height of the taller R wave in millimeters (count the small boxes).
- Step 3. Add the height of the taller R wave and the deeper S wave. If the number is equal to or greater than 35, suspect left ventricular hypertrophy.

OBJ: Explain what is meant by the terms *dilatation*, *hypertrophy*, and *enlargement*.

44. Figure 9-27 answer

Rate and rhythm	Sinus rhythm at 90 beats/min
Pathologic Q waves	V_1-V_3
ST-segment elevation	V_1-V_4
ST-segment depression	
T-wave changes	Inverted in aVL
STEMI present?	Possible STEMI
Interpretation	Possible ST-elevation myocardial infarction (STEMI): inferior, anteroseptal. Borderline ST elevation in III, aVF, V_1-V_4. As with all inferior STEMI, obtain V_4R to assess for right ventricular infarction. Poor R wave progression. Left axis deviation. Artifact in aVR, aVL, and V_1.

- PR interval 148 ms
- P-QRS-T axes 6, −61, 65
- QRS duration 98 ms
- QT/QTc 340/415 ms

45. Figure 9-28 answer

Rate and rhythm	Sinus rhythm at 65 beats/min
Pathologic Q waves	
ST-segment elevation	II, III, aVF, V_3, V_4, V_5, V_6
ST-segment depression	I, aVL
T-wave changes	
STEMI present?	Yes
Interpretation	Suspected ST-elevation myocardial infarction (STEMI), inferolateral. Obtain V_4R to assess for right ventricular infarction (RVI). Artifact in I, III.

- PR interval 192 ms
- P-QRS-T axes 66, 86, 92
- QRS duration 110 ms
- QT/QTc 392/407 ms

46. Figure 9-29 answer

Rate and rhythm	Sinus rhythm at 69 beats/min
Pathologic Q waves	
ST-segment elevation	V_1–V_2
ST-segment depression	
T-wave changes	Inverted V_4, V_5, V_6
STEMI present?	Possible STEMI
Interpretation	Possible ST-elevation myocardial infarction (STEMI), septal. May be normal variant. Baseline wander in III, aVF, V_1.

- PR interval 152 ms
- P-QRS-T axes 48, 27, 26
- QRS duration 92 ms
- QT/QTc 380/199 ms

47. Figure 9-30 answer

Rate and rhythm	Sinus bradycardia with first-degree atrioventricular (AV) block at 57 beats/min
Pathologic Q waves	
ST-segment elevation	
ST-segment depression	
T-wave changes	
STEMI present?	No
Interpretation	No ECG evidence of ST-elevation myocardial infarction (STEMI). Artifact in II, III, aVL, aVF.

- PR interval 224 ms
- P-QRS-T axes 61, 49, 53
- QRS duration 92 ms
- QT/QTc 436/430 ms

48. Figure 9-31 answer

Rate and rhythm	Sinus tachycardia at 111 beats/min with marked sinus arrhythmia
Pathologic Q waves	V_1
ST-segment elevation	V_1, V_2, V_3, V_4
ST-segment depression	
T-wave changes	Inverted V_2, V_3
STEMI present?	Yes
Interpretation	Suspected ST-elevation myocardial infarction (STEMI), anteroseptal.

- PR interval 136 ms
- P-QRS-T axes 64, −1, 92
- QRS duration 76 ms
- QT/QTc 320/386 ms

49. Figure 9-32 answer

Rate and rhythm	Sinus tachycardia at 107 beats/min
Pathologic Q waves	
ST-segment elevation	II, III, aVF
ST-segment depression	I, aVL
T-wave changes	Inverted in I
STEMI present?	Yes
Interpretation	Suspected ST-elevation myocardial infarction (STEMI), inferior. ST depression, T-wave inversion (presumed reciprocal change) in lead aVL. T-wave inversion and slight ST depression in I.

- PR interval 192 ms
- P-QRS-T axes 75, 82, 92
- QRS duration 100 ms
- QT/QTc 332/395 ms

50. Figure 9-33 answer

Rate and rhythm	Sinus rhythm at 75 beats/min with occasional premature ventricular complexes
Pathologic Q waves	
ST-segment elevation	
ST-segment depression	I, II, aVF, V_5, V_6
T-wave changes	
STEMI present?	No
Interpretation	No ECG evidence of ST-elevation myocardial infarction (STEMI). Artifact in III.

- PR interval 168 ms
- P-QRS-T axes 55, 19, 101
- QRS duration 92 ms
- QT/QTc 392/420 ms

51. Figure 9-34 answer

Rate and rhythm	Sinus rhythm with first-degree atrioventricular (AV) block at 77 beats/min
Pathologic Q waves	
ST-segment elevation	II, III, aVF, V_5, V_6
ST-segment depression	I, aVL, V_2
T-wave changes	Inverted aVL, V_1, V_2
STEMI present?	Yes
Interpretation	Suspected ST-elevation myocardial infarction (STEMI), inferior. Obtain V_4R to assess for right ventricular infarction (RVI). Poor R wave progression. Baseline wander in III.

- PR interval 224 ms
- P-QRS-T axes 62, 28, 101
- QRS duration 104 ms
- QT/QTc 404/436 ms

52. Figure 9-35 answer

Rate and rhythm	Sinus rhythm at 92 beats/min with occasional supraventricular premature complexes
Pathologic Q waves	V₁, V₂
ST-segment elevation	V₂—V₅
ST-segment depression	II, III, aVF
T-wave changes	Inverted in III
STEMI present?	Yes
Interpretation	Suspected ST-elevation myocardial infarction (STEMI), anteroseptal. ST elevation V₂—V₅, borderline in V₁ and V₅. Artifact in I, III, aVL, aVF.

- PR interval 140 ms
- P-QRS-T axes 65, 24, 17
- QRS duration 76 ms
- QT/QTc 344/394 ms

53. Figure 9-36 answer

Rate and rhythm	Sinus rhythm at 74 beats/min
Pathologic Q waves	III, borderline in aVF
ST-segment elevation	
ST-segment depression	I, aVL, V₄-V₆, slight in II
T-wave changes	Inverted in I, aVL, V₄-V₆
STEMI present?	No
Interpretation	No ECG evidence of ST-elevation myocardial infarction (STEMI). Inferolateral ischemia.

- PR interval 168 ms
- P-QRS-T axes −61, 22, 139
- QRS duration 80 ms
- QT/QTc 364/392 ms

54. Figure 9-37 answer

Rate and rhythm	Sinus rhythm at 97 beats/min
Pathologic Q waves	
ST-segment elevation	
ST-segment depression	
T-wave changes	Inverted in II, III, aVF, V₁ V₂, V₃
STEMI present?	No
Interpretation	T-wave abnormality, consider anterior ischemia

- PR interval 124 ms
- P-QRS-T axes 63, 79, −8
- QRS duration 76 ms
- QT/QTc 326/414 ms

55. Figure 9-38 answer

Rate and rhythm	Sinus tachycardia at 111 beats/min
Pathologic Q waves	
ST-segment elevation	V₁-V₄
ST-segment depression	II, III, aVF, V₅, V₆
T-wave changes	Tall in V₂
STEMI present?	Yes
Interpretation	Suspected ST-elevation myocardial infarction (STEMI), anteroseptal.

- PR interval 192 ms
- P-QRS-T axes 63, 66, 55
- QRS duration 92 ms
- QT/QTc 328/393 ms

Post-Test

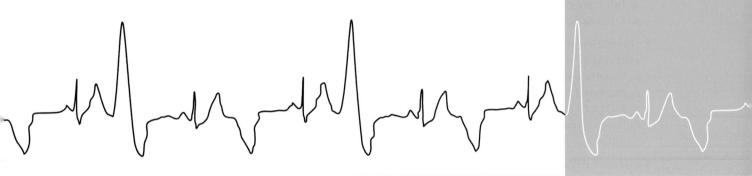

Multiple Choice

Identify the choice that best completes the statement or answers the question.

_____ 1. The _____ supplies the right atrium and right ventricle with blood.
   a. Circumflex artery
   b. Right coronary artery
   c. Left main coronary artery
   d. Left anterior descending artery

_____ 2. Stimulation of parasympathetic nerve fibers typically results in which of the following actions?
   a. Constriction of coronary blood vessels
   b. Increased strength of cardiac muscle contraction
   c. Increased rate of discharge of the sinoatrial node
   d. Slowed conduction through the atrioventricular node

_____ 3. The contribution of blood that is added to the ventricles and results from atrial contraction is called:
   a. Afterload.
   b. Atrial kick.
   c. Cardiac output.
   d. Peripheral resistance.

_____ 4. Which of the following are semilunar valves?
   a. Aortic and pulmonic
   b. Aortic and tricuspid
   c. Pulmonic and mitral
   d. Tricuspid and mitral

_____ 5. The left main coronary artery divides into the:
   a. Marginal and circumflex branches.
   b. Marginal and anterior descending branches.
   c. Anterior and posterior descending branches.
   d. Anterior descending and circumflex branches.

_____ 6. _____ cells are specialized cells of the electrical conduction system responsible for the spontaneous generation and conduction of electrical impulses.
   a. Working
   b. Pacemaker
   c. Mechanical
   d. Contractile

_____ 7. The absolute refractory period:
   a. Begins with the onset of the P wave and terminates with the end of the QRS complex.
   b. Begins with the onset of the QRS complex and terminates at approximately the apex of the T wave.
   c. Begins with the onset of the QRS complex and terminates with the end of the T wave.
   d. Begins with the onset of the P wave and terminates with the beginning of the QRS complex.

_____ 8. Which of the following statements is true regarding the QT interval?
   a. The QT interval represents atrial depolarization, followed immediately by atrial systole.
   b. The QT interval corresponds to atrial depolarization and impulse delay in the atrioventricular node.
   c. The QT interval represents ventricular depolarization, followed immediately by ventricular systole.
   d. The QT interval represents the time from initial depolarization of the ventricles to the end of ventricular repolarization.

_____ 9. How do you determine whether the atrial rhythm on an ECG tracing is regular or irregular?
   a. Compare QT intervals
   b. Compare PR intervals
   c. Compare R to R intervals
   d. Compare P to P intervals

_____ 10. Which of the following ECG leads use two distinct electrodes, one of which is positive and the other negative?
   a. Leads I, II, and III
   b. Leads V_1, V_2, and V_3
   c. Leads V_4, V_5, and V_6
   d. Leads aVR, aVL, and aVF

_____ 11. In sinus arrhythmia, a gradual decreasing of the heart rate is usually associated with:
   a. Expiration.
   b. Inspiration.
   c. Excessive caffeine intake.
   d. Early signs of heart failure.

_____ 12. An ECG rhythm strip shows a ventricular rate of 46, a regular rhythm, a PR interval of 0.14 second, a QRS duration of 0.06 second, and one upright P wave before each QRS. This rhythm is:
   a. Sinus arrest.
   b. Sinus rhythm.
   c. Sinoatrial block.
   d. Sinus bradycardia.

_____ 13. Sinoatrial block is a disorder of impulse _____ and sinus arrest is a disorder of impulse _____.
   a. formation, conduction
   b. conduction, formation

_____ 14. Signs and symptoms experienced during a tachydysrhythmia are usually primarily related to:
   a. Vasoconstriction.
   b. Atrial irritability.
   c. Slowed conduction through the atrioventricular node.
   d. Decreased ventricular filling time and stroke volume.

____15. Which of the following correctly reflects examples of ectopic (latent) pacemakers?
   a. The SA node and AV junction
   b. The AV junction and ventricles
   c. The SA node and right bundle branch
   d. The AV junction and left bundle branch

____16. A wandering atrial pacemaker rhythm with a ventricular rate of 60 to 100 beats/min may also be referred to as:
   a. Atrial flutter.
   b. Atrial fibrillation.
   c. Multiformed atrial rhythm.
   d. Multifocal atrial tachycardia.

____17. The most common type of supraventricular tachycardia is:
   a. Atrial flutter.
   b. Atrial tachycardia.
   c. AV reentrant tachycardia.
   d. AV nodal reentrant tachycardia.

____18. What is meant by the term "uncontrolled" atrial fibrillation?
   a. The atrial rate is less than 100 beats/min.
   b. The atrial rate is greater than 100 beats/min.
   c. The overall ventricular rate is less than 100 beats/min.
   d. The overall ventricular rate is greater than 100 beats/min.

____19. If the onset or end of paroxysmal atrial tachycardia or paroxysmal supraventricular tachycardia is not observed on the ECG, the dysrhythmia is called:
   a. Sinus tachycardia.
   b. Junctional tachycardia.
   c. Supraventricular tachycardia.
   d. Multifocal atrial tachycardia.

____20. Which of the following is the most common sustained dysrhythmia in adults?
   a. Atrial fibrillation
   b. Sinus bradycardia
   c. Junctional rhythm
   d. Ventricular tachycardia

____21. Which of the following statements is true regarding the differences between premature atrial complexes (PACs) and premature junctional complexes (PJCs) in leads II, III, and aVF?
   a. A PAC has a narrow QRS complex and a PJC has a wide QRS complex.
   b. A PAC has a negative P wave before the QRS complex and a PJC has a positive P wave before each QRS complex.
   c. A P wave may or may not be present with a PAC, whereas a PJC typically has a positive P wave before the QRS complex.
   d. A PAC typically has a positive P wave before the QRS complex, whereas a P wave may or may not be present with a PJC.

____22. Wolff-Parkinson-White syndrome is associated with a:
   a. Long PR interval, delta wave, and wide QRS complex.
   b. Short PR interval, delta wave, and wide QRS complex.
   c. Long PR interval, flutter waves, and narrow QRS complex.
   d. Short PR interval, flutter waves, and narrow QRS complex.

____23. Which of the following ECG characteristics distinguishes atrial flutter from other atrial dysrhythmias?
   a. The presence of fibrillatory waves
   b. The presence of delta waves before the QRS
   c. Clearly identifiable P waves of varying size and amplitude
   d. The "saw-tooth" or "picket-fence" appearance of waveforms before the QRS

____24. When a junctional rhythm is viewed in lead II, where is the location of the P wave on the ECG if atrial and ventricular depolarization occur simultaneously?
   a. Before the QRS complex
   b. Within the QRS complex
   c. After the QRS complex

____25. The usual rate of nonparoxysmal junctional tachycardia is:
   a. 50 to 80 beats/min.
   b. 80 to 120 beats/min.
   c. 101 to 140 beats/min.
   d. 150 to 300 beats/min.

____26. Junctional (or ventricular) complexes may come early (before the next expected sinus beat) or late (after the next expected sinus beat). If the complex is *early* it is called a(n) _____. If the complex is *late* it is called a(n) _____.
   a. Escape beat; premature complex
   b. Premature complex; escape beat

____27. Depending on the severity of the patient's signs and symptoms, management of slow rhythms may require therapeutic intervention including:
   a. Defibrillation.
   b. Administration of atropine.
   c. Synchronized cardioversion.
   d. Vagal maneuvers and administration of adenosine.

____28. The term for three or more premature ventricular complexes (PVCs) occurring in a row at a rate of more than 100/min is:
   a. Ventricular trigeminy.
   b. Ventricular fibrillation.
   c. A run of ventricular tachycardia.
   d. A run of ventricular escape beats.

____**29.** Premature ventricular complexes (PVCs) that look alike in the same lead and begin from the same anatomic site (i.e., focus) are called _____ PVCs.
    a. Uniform
    b. Isolated
    c. Multiform
    d. Interpolated

____**30.** Which of the following dysrhythmias has QRS complexes that vary in shape and amplitude from beat to beat and appear to twist from upright to negative or negative to upright and back, resembling a spindle?
    a. Atrial fibrillation
    b. Idioventricular rhythm
    c. Polymorphic ventricular tachycardia
    d. Monomorphic ventricular tachycardia

____**31.** When a delay or interruption in impulse conduction from the atria to the ventricles occurs as a result of a transient or permanent anatomic or functional impairment, the resulting dysrhythmia is called a(n):
    a. Sinus arrest.
    b. Sinoatrial block.
    c. Bundle branch block.
    d. Atrioventricular block.

____**32.** Whenever the criteria for bundle branch block have been met and lead V_1 displays an rSR′ pattern, you should suspect a:
    a. Left bundle branch block.
    b. Right bundle branch block.

____**33.** The PR interval of a first-degree AV block:
    a. Is constant and less than 0.12 second in duration.
    b. Is constant and more than 0.20 second in duration.
    c. Is generally progressive until a P wave appears without a QRS complex.
    d. Gradually decreases in duration until a P wave appears without a QRS complex.

____**34.** Which of the following is an example of a complete atrioventricular (AV) block?
    a. First-degree AV block
    b. Second-degree AV block type I
    c. Second-degree AV block type II
    d. Third-degree AV block

____**35.** Which of the following statements is correct regarding 2:1 AV block?
    a. The atrial rhythm is irregular.
    b. The PR interval remains constant.
    c. The ventricular rate is twice the atrial rate.
    d. The level of the block is located within the sinoatrial node.

____**36.** The terms *advanced* or *high-grade* second-degree AV block may be used to describe one or more consecutive P waves that are not conducted.
    a. True
    b. False

____**37.** Which lead is probably the best to use when differentiating between right and left bundle branch block?
    a. V_1
    b. V_4
    c. II
    d. aVR

____**38.** The term *capture*, as it pertains to pacing, refers to:
    a. A vertical line on the ECG that indicates the pacemaker has discharged.
    b. The extent to which an artificial pacemaker recognizes intrinsic cardiac electrical activity.
    c. A pacemaker response in which the output pulse is suppressed when an intrinsic event is sensed.
    d. The successful conduction of an artificial pacemaker's impulse through the myocardium, resulting in depolarization.

____**39.** The 12-lead ECG only provides a _____ -second view of each lead.
    a. 1
    b. 2.5
    c. 4
    d. 6

____**40.** Although a right ventricular infarction may occur by itself, it is more commonly associated with a(n) _____ wall myocardial infarction.
    a. Septal
    b. Lateral
    c. Inferior
    d. Anterior

____**41.** *Poor R-wave progression* is a phrase used to describe R waves that decrease in size from V_1 to V_4. This is often seen in an _____ infarction.
    a. Inferobasal
    b. Anteroseptal
    c. Anterolateral
    d. Inferoposterior

Completion

Complete each statement.

42. The right atrium receives deoxygenated blood from the _____ _____ _____ (which carries blood from the head and upper extremities), the _____ _____ _____ (which carries blood from the lower body), and the _____ _____ (which receives blood from the intracardiac circulation).

43. A beat originating from the AV junction that appears later than the next expected sinus beat is called a _____ _____ _____.

44. A rapid, wide-QRS rhythm associated with pulselessness, shock, or heart failure should be presumed to be _____ _____.

45. PACs associated with a wide QRS complex are called _____ _____ PACs, indicating that conduction through the ventricles is abnormal.

46. _____ is the period of relaxation during which a heart chamber is filling.

47. The thick, muscular middle layer of the heart wall that contains the atrial and ventricular muscle fibers necessary for contraction is the _____.

48. Delivery of an electrical current timed for delivery during the QRS complex is called _____ _____.

49. Sometimes, when a premature atrial complex (PAC) occurs very prematurely and close to the T wave of the preceding beat, only a P wave may be seen with no QRS after it (appearing as a pause). This type of PAC is termed a(n) _____ PAC.

50. If the AV junction paces the heart, the electrical impulse must travel in a(n) _____ direction to activate the atria.

51. A demand pacemaker is also known as a _____ pacemaker.

52. The axes of leads I, II, and III form an equilateral triangle with the heart at the center (Einthoven's triangle). If the augmented limb leads are added to this configuration and the axes of the six leads moved in a way in which they bisect each other, the result is the _____ _____ _____.

53. Indicate the heart surface viewed by each of the following.

    Leads II, III, aVF: _____

    Leads V_1, V_2:   _____

    Leads V_3, V_4:   _____

    Leads I, aVL, V_5, V_6:   _____

Short Answer

54. Beginning with the right atrium, describe blood flow through the normal heart and lungs to the systemic circulation.

    _____ Right atrium   _____ Left ventricle

    _____ Mitral valve   _____ Pulmonary arteries

    _____ Aorta   _____ Tricuspid valve

    _____ Right ventricle   _____ Pulmonary veins

    _____ Pulmonic valve   _____ Aortic valve

    _____ Left atrium   _____ Systemic circulation

55. List five (5) steps used in ECG rhythm analysis.

1.

2.

3.

4.

5.

56. Explain the benefits of a dual-chamber pacemaker.

_____

_____

_____

57. List three (3) uses for ECG monitoring.

1.

2.

3.

58. Describe the appearance of a pathologic Q wave.

_____

_____

_____

59. What is the most important difference between sinus rhythm and sinus tachycardia?

_____

_____

_____

60. List three (3) causes of artifact on an ECG tracing.

1.

2.

3.

61. How do coarse and fine ventricular fibrillation differ?

_____

_____

_____

62. List four (4) reasons why the AV junction may assume responsibility for pacing the heart.

1.

2.

3.

4.

63. Explain why patients who experience atrial fibrillation are at increased risk of having a stroke.

_____

_____

_____

64. On the ECG, what do the ST segment and T wave represent?

_____

_____

_____

65. Fill in the blank areas in the table below.

ECG Finding	Atrioventricular Nodal Reentrant Tachycardia (AVNRT)	Atrial Flutter	Atrial Fibrillation
Rhythm			
Rate (beats/min)			
P waves (lead II)			
PR interval			
QRS duration			

66. Explain the difference between "electrical capture" and "mechanical capture."

_____

_____

_____

67. List four (4) primary characteristics of cardiac cells.

1.

2.

3.

4.

68. Explain what is meant by the phrase "anatomically contiguous leads."

_____

_____

_____

69. Indicate the ECG criteria for the following dysrhythmias.

	Second-Degree Atrioventricular (AV) Block Type II	2:1 AV Block
Ventricular Rhythm	_____	_____
PR Interval	_____	_____
QRS Width	_____	_____

70. Fill in the blank areas in the table below.

ECG Finding	Idioventricular Rhythm	Accelerated Idioventricular Rhythm	Monomorphic Ventricular Tachycardia
Rhythm			
Rate (beats/min)			
P waves (lead II)			
PR interval			
QRS duration			

POST-TEST RHYTHM STRIPS

For each of the following rhythm strips, determine the atrial and ventricular rates, measure the PR interval, QRS duration, and QT interval, and then identify the rhythm.

71. This rhythm strip is from a 97-year-old woman after a fall. Identify the rhythm (lead II).

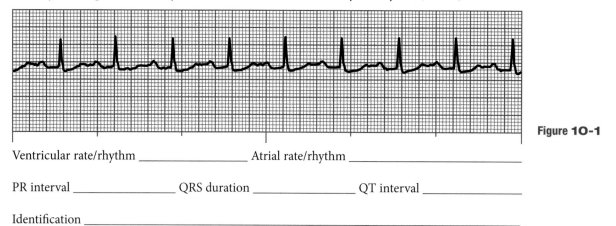

Figure 10-1

Ventricular rate/rhythm _____ Atrial rate/rhythm _____

PR interval _____ QRS duration _____ QT interval _____

Identification _____

72. This rhythm strip is from a 70-year-old man who is complaining of a sharp pain across his shoulders. His blood pressure is 218/86 mm Hg. Identify the rhythm (lead II).

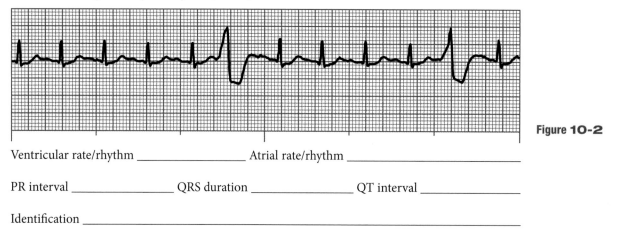

Figure 10-2

Ventricular rate/rhythm _____ Atrial rate/rhythm _____

PR interval _____ QRS duration _____ QT interval _____

Identification _____

73. This rhythm strip is a 71-year-old man who is complaining of abdominal pain. Identify the rhythm (lead II).

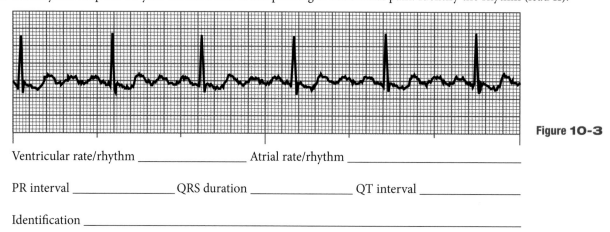

Figure 10-3

Ventricular rate/rhythm _____ Atrial rate/rhythm _____

PR interval _____ QRS duration _____ QT interval _____

Identification _____

74. Identify the rhythm.

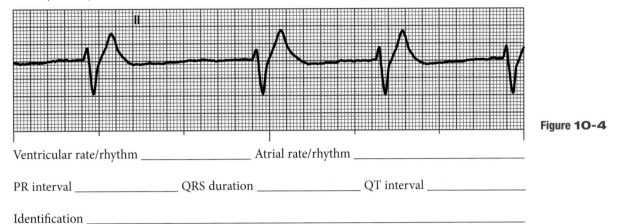

Figure 10-4

Ventricular rate/rhythm _____ Atrial rate/rhythm _____

PR interval _____ QRS duration _____ QT interval _____

Identification _____

75. This rhythm strip is from an 89-year-old man with chest pain. He had a myocardial infarction 15 years ago and a coronary artery bypass graft 5 years ago. His blood pressure is 140/90 mm Hg. Identify the rhythm (lead II).

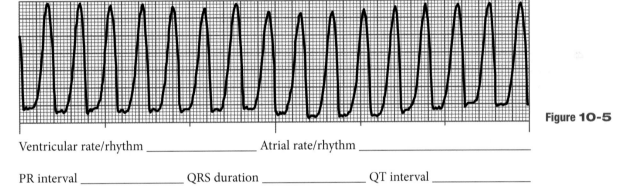

Figure 10-5

Ventricular rate/rhythm _____ Atrial rate/rhythm _____

PR interval _____ QRS duration _____ QT interval _____

Identification _____

76. Identify the rhythm (lead II).

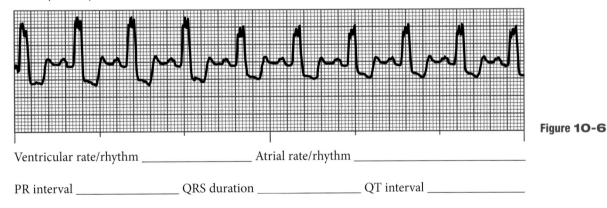

Figure 10-6

Ventricular rate/rhythm _____ Atrial rate/rhythm _____

PR interval _____ QRS duration _____ QT interval _____

Identification _____

77. Identify the rhythm (lead II).

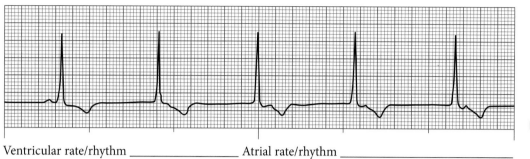

Figure 10-7

Ventricular rate/rhythm _____ Atrial rate/rhythm _____

PR interval _____ QRS duration _____ QT interval _____

Identification _____

78. Identify the rhythm.

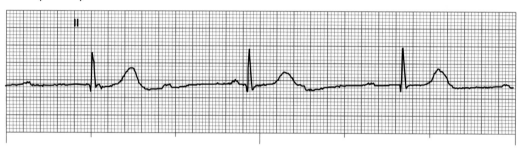

Figure 10-8

Ventricular rate/rhythm _____ Atrial rate/rhythm _____

PR interval _____ QRS duration _____ QT interval _____

Identification _____

79. Identify the rhythm (lead II).

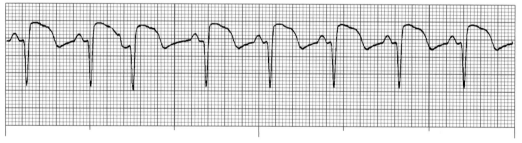

Figure 10-9

Ventricular rate/rhythm _____ Atrial rate/rhythm _____

PR interval _____ QRS duration _____ QT interval _____

Identification _____

80. This rhythm strip is from a 76-year-old woman complaining of back pain. Her medical history includes a myocardial infarction 2 years ago. Identify the rhythm (lead II).

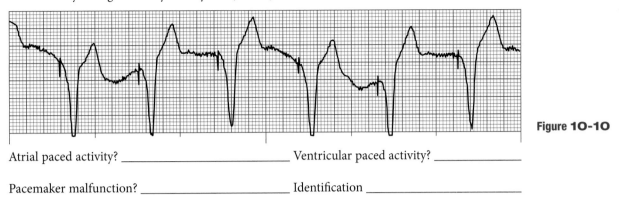

Figure 10-10

Atrial paced activity? _____ Ventricular paced activity? _____

Pacemaker malfunction? _____ Identification _____

81. Identify the rhythm (lead II).

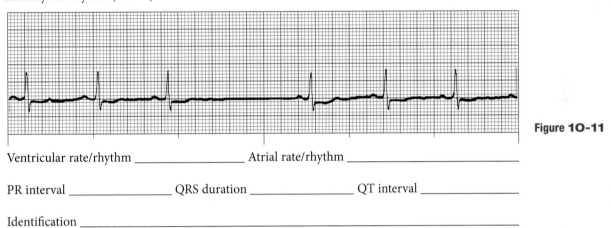

Figure 10-11

Ventricular rate/rhythm _____ Atrial rate/rhythm _____

PR interval _____ QRS duration _____ QT interval _____

Identification _____

82. This rhythm strip is from a 51-year-old man complaining of "dull chest pain" that began about 2 hours ago. He rates his discomfort as 6/10. His blood pressure is 70/48 mm Hg. His skin is cool, pale, and diaphoretic. Identify the rhythm.

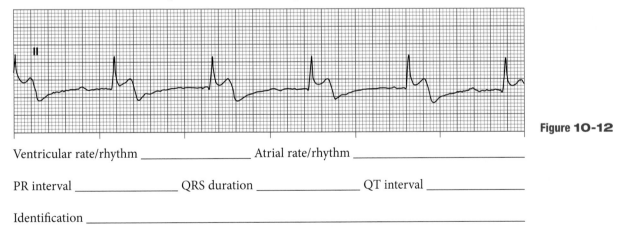

Figure 10-12

Ventricular rate/rhythm _____ Atrial rate/rhythm _____

PR interval _____ QRS duration _____ QT interval _____

Identification _____

83. This rhythm strip is from a 59-year-old man complaining of poor circulation in his legs. His blood pressure is 106/68 mm Hg. Identify the rhythm (lead II).

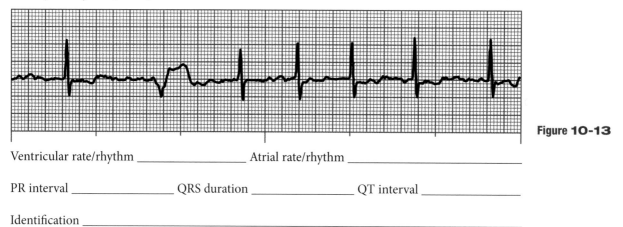

Figure 10-13

Ventricular rate/rhythm _____ Atrial rate/rhythm _____

PR interval _____ QRS duration _____ QT interval _____

Identification _____

84. Identify the rhythm (lead II).

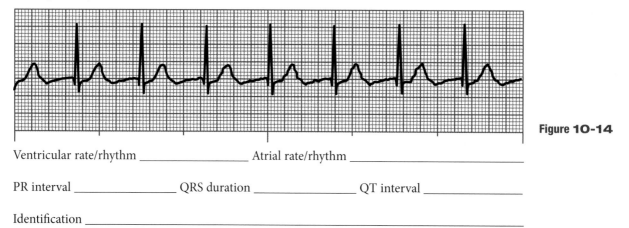

Figure 10-14

Ventricular rate/rhythm _____ Atrial rate/rhythm _____

PR interval _____ QRS duration _____ QT interval _____

Identification _____

85. Identify the rhythm (lead II).

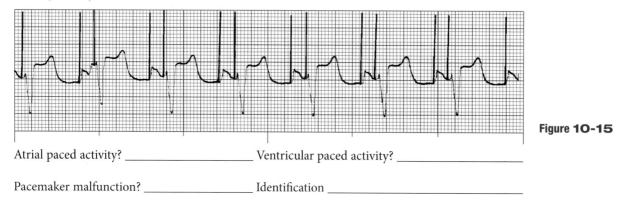

Figure 10-15

Atrial paced activity? _____ Ventricular paced activity? _____

Pacemaker malfunction? _____ Identification _____

86. These rhythm strips are from a 33-year-old man who is seeking medical attention because he wants "the voices in my head to stop." His blood pressure is 144/72 mm Hg, and his serum glucose is 99 mg/dL. Identify the rhythm.

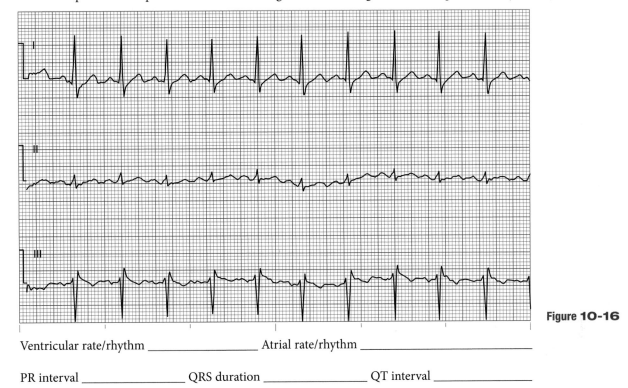

Figure 10-16

Ventricular rate/rhythm _____ Atrial rate/rhythm _____

PR interval _____ QRS duration _____ QT interval _____

Identification _____

87. Identify the rhythm (lead II).

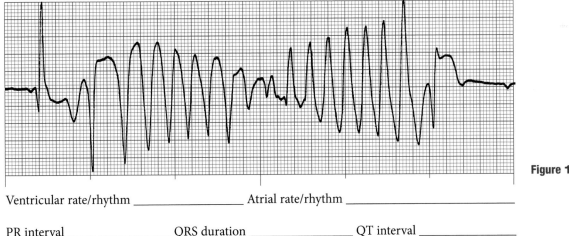

Figure 10-17

Ventricular rate/rhythm _____ Atrial rate/rhythm _____

PR interval _____ QRS duration _____ QT interval _____

Identification _____

88. Identify the rhythm (lead II).

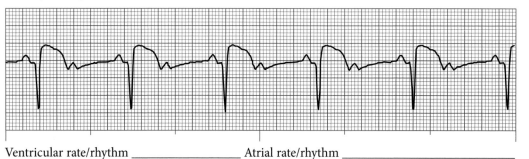

Figure **10-18**

Ventricular rate/rhythm _____ Atrial rate/rhythm _____

PR interval _____ QRS duration _____ QT interval _____

Identification _____

89. These rhythm strips are from a 58-year-old man who is complaining of palpitations. Identify the rhythm.

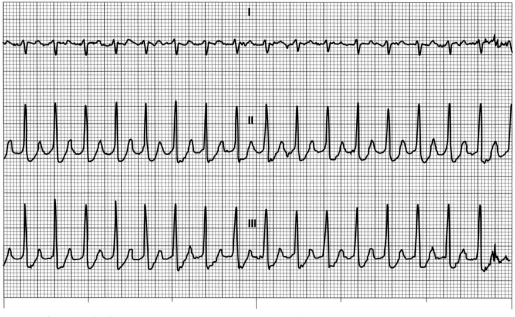

Figure **10-19**

Ventricular rate/rhythm _____ Atrial rate/rhythm _____

PR interval _____ QRS duration _____ QT interval _____

Identification _____

90. These rhythm strips are from an 82-year-old man complaining of back pain. Identify the rhythm.

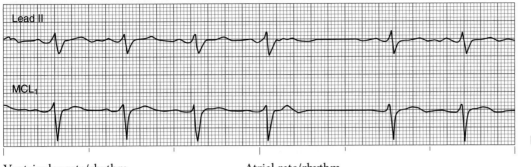

Figure 10-20

Ventricular rate/rhythm _____ Atrial rate/rhythm _____

PR interval _____ QRS duration _____ QT interval _____

Identification _____

91. Identify the rhythm (lead II).

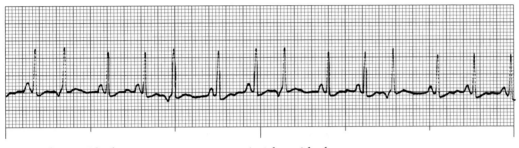

Figure 10-21

Ventricular rate/rhythm _____ Atrial rate/rhythm _____

PR interval _____ QRS duration _____ QT interval _____

Identification _____

92. Identify the rhythm (lead II).

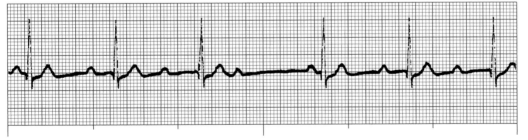

Figure 10-22

Ventricular rate/rhythm _____ Atrial rate/rhythm _____

PR interval _____ QRS duration _____ QT interval _____

Identification _____

93. Identify the rhythm (lead II).

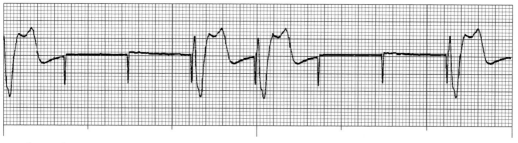

Figure 10-23

Atrial paced activity? _____ Ventricular paced activity? _____

Pacemaker malfunction? _____ Identification _____

94. Identify the rhythm (lead II).

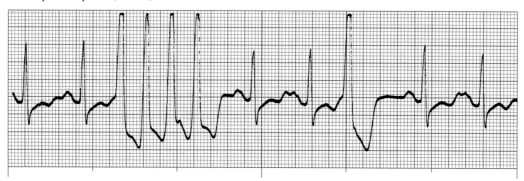

Figure 10-24

Ventricular rate/rhythm _____ Atrial rate/rhythm _____

PR interval _____ QRS duration _____ QT interval _____

Identification _____

95. These rhythm strips are from a 67-year-old woman complaining of dizziness and chest pain. She has a history of a three-vessel coronary artery bypass graft and hypertension. Identify the rhythm.

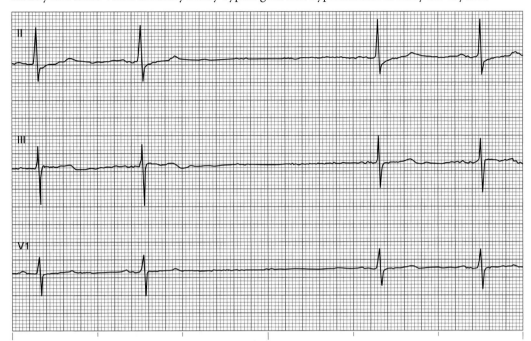

Figure 10-25

Ventricular rate/rhythm _____ Atrial rate/rhythm _____

PR interval _____ QRS duration _____ QT interval _____

Identification _____

96. Identify the rhythm (lead II).

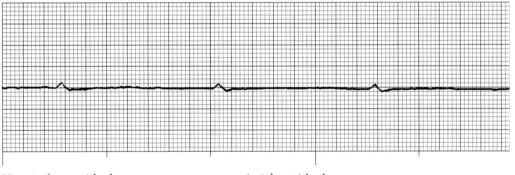

Figure 10-26

Ventricular rate/rhythm _____ Atrial rate/rhythm _____

PR interval _____ QRS duration _____ QT interval _____

Identification _____

97. Identify the rhythm (lead II).

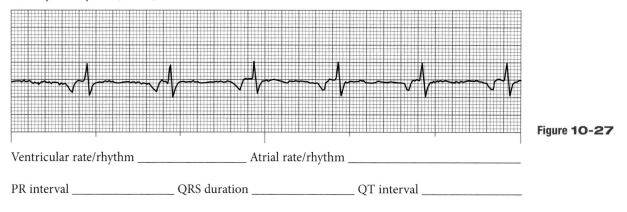

Figure **10-27**

Ventricular rate/rhythm _____ Atrial rate/rhythm _____

PR interval _____ QRS duration _____ QT interval _____

Identification _____

98. This rhythm strip is from a 90-year-old unresponsive woman. She has a history of heart failure. Her medications include furosemide and albuterol. Identify the rhythm (lead II).

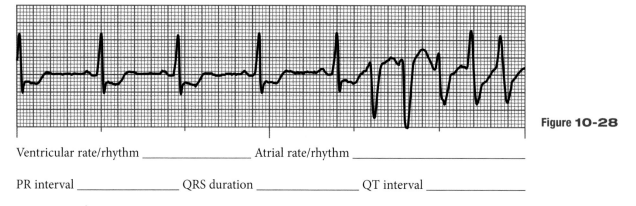

Figure **10-28**

Ventricular rate/rhythm _____ Atrial rate/rhythm _____

PR interval _____ QRS duration _____ QT interval _____

Identification _____

99. Identify the rhythm (lead II).

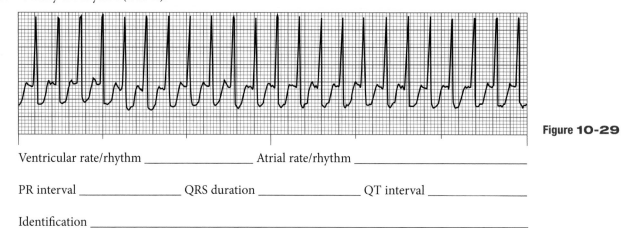

Figure **10-29**

Ventricular rate/rhythm _____ Atrial rate/rhythm _____

PR interval _____ QRS duration _____ QT interval _____

Identification _____

100. Identify the rhythm (lead II).

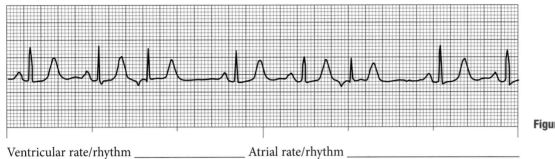

Figure 10-30

Ventricular rate/rhythm _____ Atrial rate/rhythm _____

PR interval _____ QRS duration _____ QT interval _____

Identification _____

101. This rhythm strip is from a 62-year-old woman who experienced a syncopal episode. Identify the rhythm (lead II).

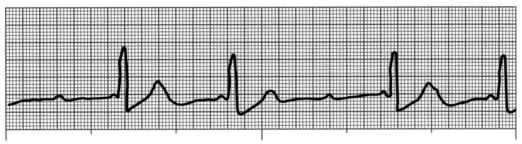

Figure 10-31

Ventricular rate/rhythm _____ Atrial rate/rhythm _____

PR interval _____ QRS duration _____ QT interval _____

Identification _____

102. Identify the rhythm (lead II).

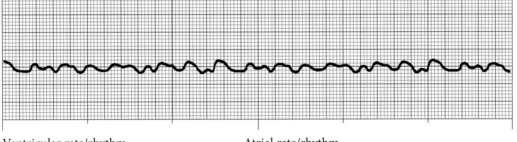

Figure 10-32

Ventricular rate/rhythm _____ Atrial rate/rhythm _____

PR interval _____ QRS duration _____ QT interval _____

Identification _____

103. Identify the rhythm (lead II).

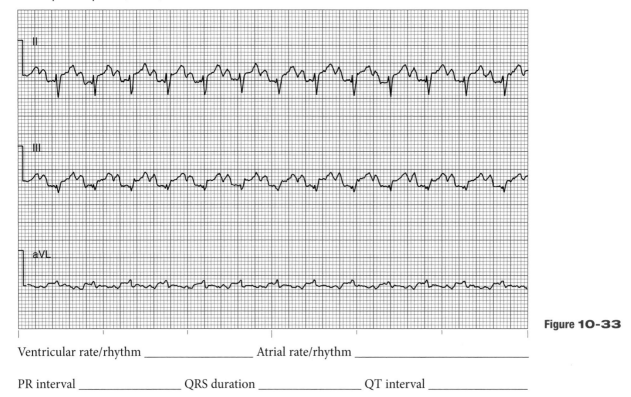

Figure 10-33

Ventricular rate/rhythm _____ Atrial rate/rhythm _____

PR interval _____ QRS duration _____ QT interval _____

Identification _____

104. Identify the rhythm (lead II).

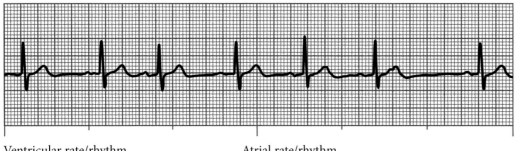

Figure 10-34

Ventricular rate/rhythm _____ Atrial rate/rhythm _____

PR interval _____ QRS duration _____ QT interval _____

Identification _____

105. These rhythm strips are from a 52-year-old man with syncope. Identify the rhythm.

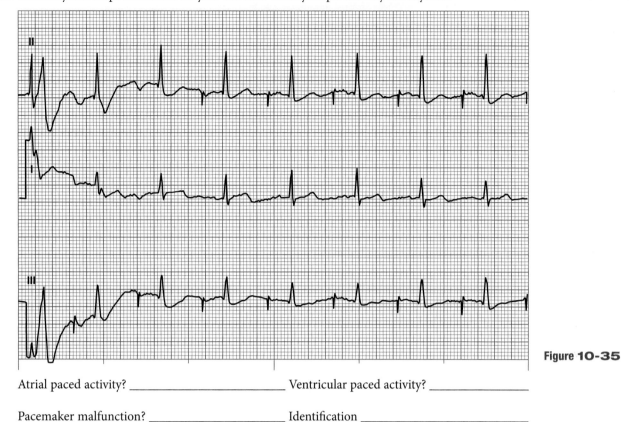

Figure 10-35

Atrial paced activity? _____ Ventricular paced activity? _____

Pacemaker malfunction? _____ Identification _____

106. This rhythm strip is from a 59-year-old man who was driving to work on the freeway when his internal defibrillator discharged. He was asymptomatic at the time this ECG was obtained a few minutes after the event. Identify the rhythm (lead II).

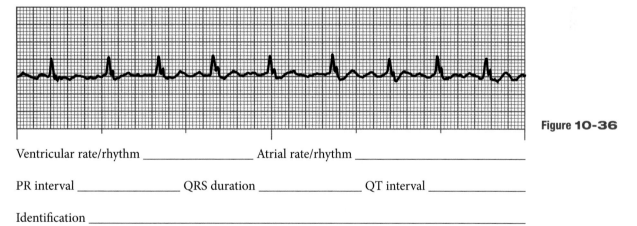

Figure 10-36

Ventricular rate/rhythm _____ Atrial rate/rhythm _____

PR interval _____ QRS duration _____ QT interval _____

Identification _____

107. Identify the rhythm.

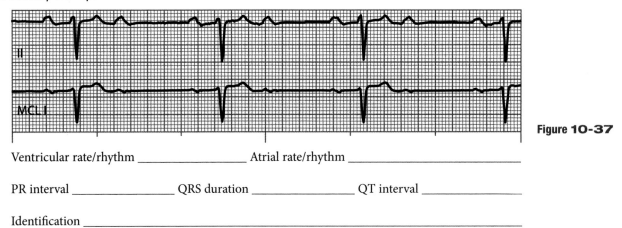

Figure 10-37

Ventricular rate/rhythm _____ Atrial rate/rhythm _____

PR interval _____ QRS duration _____ QT interval _____

Identification _____

108. Identify the rhythm (lead II).

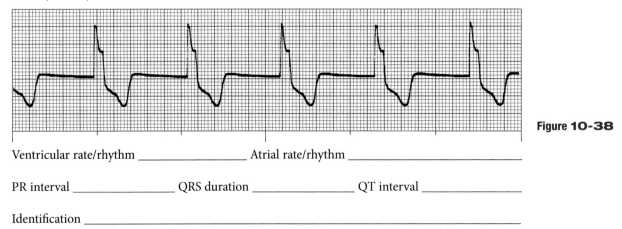

Figure 10-38

Ventricular rate/rhythm _____ Atrial rate/rhythm _____

PR interval _____ QRS duration _____ QT interval _____

Identification _____

109. This rhythm strip is from an 86-year-old woman complaining of weakness. Breath sounds are clear. Her skin is pale, cool, and dry, and her blood pressure is 180/84 mm Hg. Identify the rhythm.

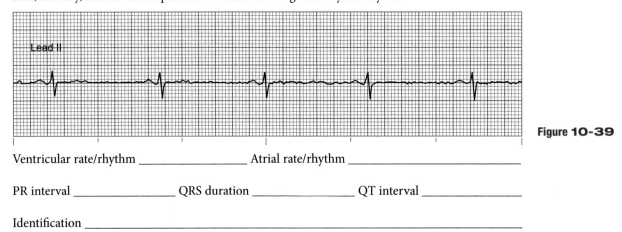

Figure 10-39

Ventricular rate/rhythm _____ Atrial rate/rhythm _____

PR interval _____ QRS duration _____ QT interval _____

Identification _____

110. This rhythm strip is from a 90-year-old woman with acute pulmonary edema. Identify the rhythm (lead II).

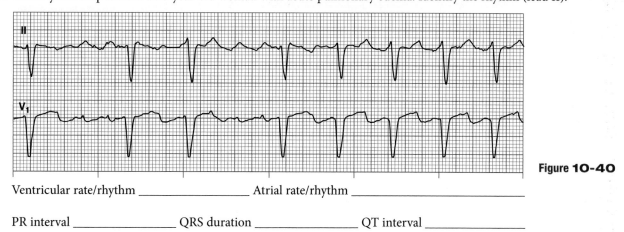

Figure 10-40

Ventricular rate/rhythm _____ Atrial rate/rhythm _____

PR interval _____ QRS duration _____ QT interval _____

Identification _____

111. This rhythm strip is from an 84-year-old man who is complaining of dizziness. He had a triple bypass four days ago. Identify the rhythm (lead II).

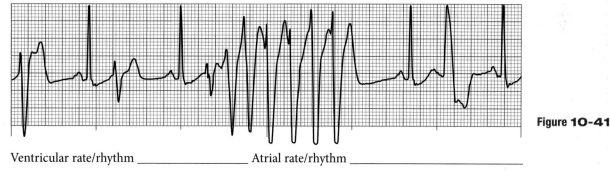

Figure 10-41

Ventricular rate/rhythm _____ Atrial rate/rhythm _____

PR interval _____ QRS duration _____ QT interval _____

Identification _____

112. Identify the rhythm.

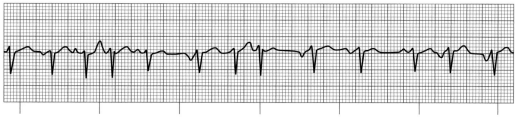

Figure 10-42

Ventricular rate/rhythm _____ Atrial rate/rhythm _____

PR interval _____ QRS duration _____ QT interval _____

Identification _____

113. This rhythm strip is from a 76-year-old woman who is complaining of back pain. Her medical history includes a myocardial infarction two years ago. Identify the rhythm (lead II).

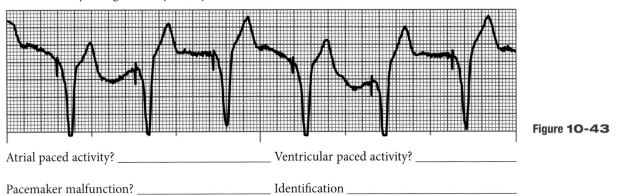

Figure 10-43

Atrial paced activity? _____ Ventricular paced activity? _____

Pacemaker malfunction? _____ Identification _____

114. Identify the rhythm (lead II).

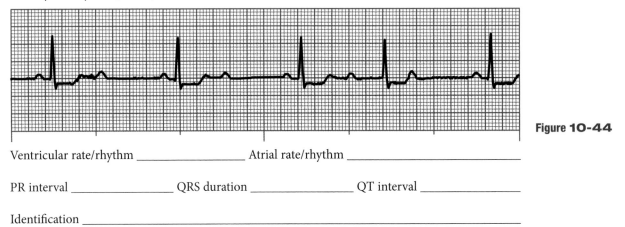

Figure 10-44

Ventricular rate/rhythm _____ Atrial rate/rhythm _____

PR interval _____ QRS duration _____ QT interval _____

Identification _____

115. Identify the rhythm (lead II).

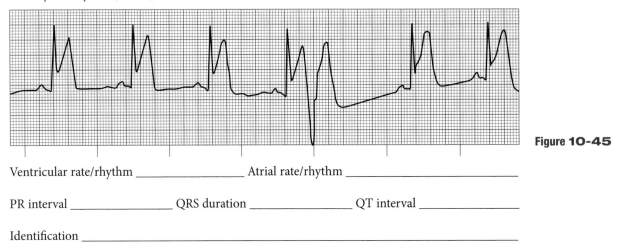

Figure 10-45

Ventricular rate/rhythm _____ Atrial rate/rhythm _____

PR interval _____ QRS duration _____ QT interval _____

Identification _____

116. Identify the rhythm (lead II).

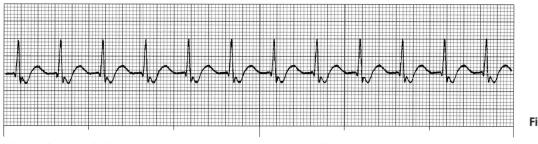

Figure 10-46

Ventricular rate/rhythm _____ Atrial rate/rhythm _____

PR interval _____ QRS duration _____ QT interval _____

Identification _____

117. Identify the rhythm (lead II).

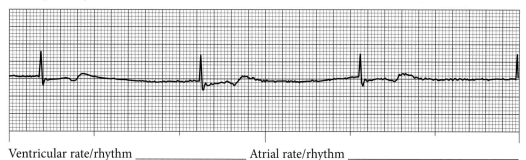

Figure 10-47

Ventricular rate/rhythm _____ Atrial rate/rhythm _____

PR interval _____ QRS duration _____ QT interval _____

Identification _____

118. Identify the rhythm (lead II).

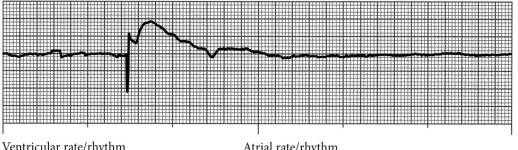

Figure 10-48

Ventricular rate/rhythm _____ Atrial rate/rhythm _____

PR interval _____ QRS duration _____ QT interval _____

Identification _____

119. These rhythm strips are from a 24-year-old woman who attempted suicide. Identify the rhythm.

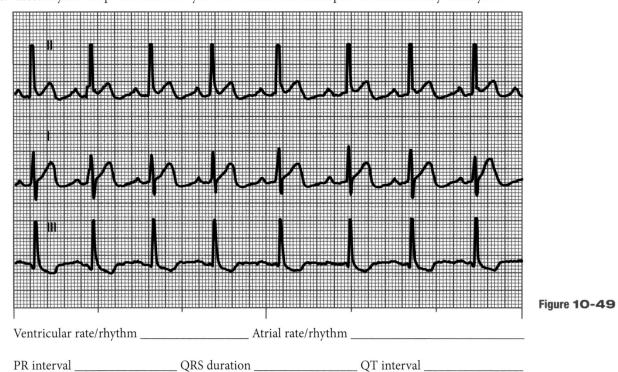

Figure 10-49

Ventricular rate/rhythm _____ Atrial rate/rhythm _____

PR interval _____ QRS duration _____ QT interval _____

Identification _____

120. Identify the rhythm (lead II).

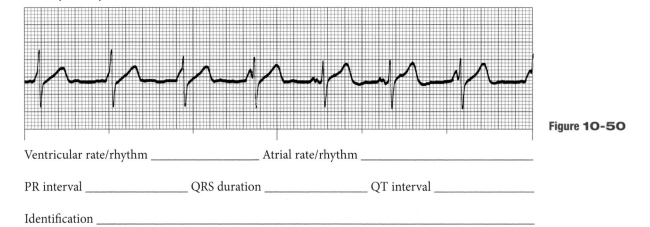

Figure 10-50

Ventricular rate/rhythm _____ Atrial rate/rhythm _____

PR interval _____ QRS duration _____ QT interval _____

Identification _____

121. Identify the rhythm (lead II).

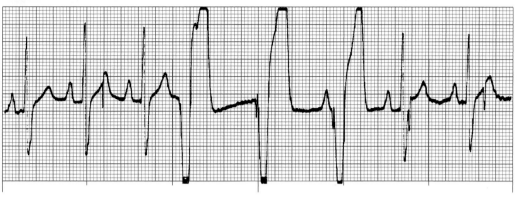

Figure 10-51

Atrial paced activity? _____ Ventricular paced activity? _____

Pacemaker malfunction? _____ Identification _____

122. Identify the rhythm (lead II).

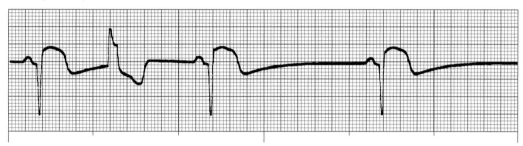

Figure 10-52

Ventricular rate/rhythm _____ Atrial rate/rhythm _____

PR interval _____ QRS duration _____ QT interval _____

Identification _____

123. Identify the rhythm (lead II).

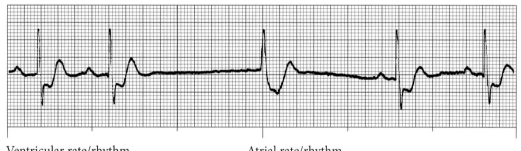

Figure 10-53

Ventricular rate/rhythm _____ Atrial rate/rhythm _____

PR interval _____ QRS duration _____ QT interval _____

Identification _____

124. This rhythm strip is from a 90-year-old woman with shortness of breath. Identify the rhythm (lead II).

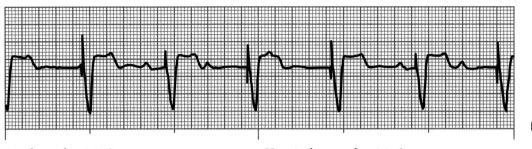

Figure 10-54

Atrial paced activity? _____ Ventricular paced activity? _____

Pacemaker malfunction? _____ Identification _____

125. Identify the rhythm (lead II).

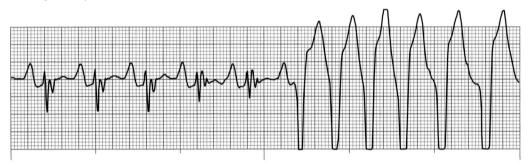

Figure 10-55

Ventricular rate/rhythm _____ Atrial rate/rhythm _____

PR interval _____ QRS duration _____ QT interval _____

Identification _____

126. Identify the rhythm (lead II).

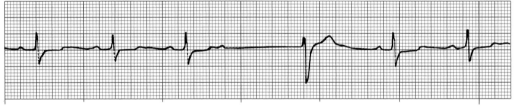

Figure 10-56

Ventricular rate/rhythm _____ Atrial rate/rhythm _____

PR interval _____ QRS duration _____ QT interval _____

Identification _____

127. This rhythm strip is from a 20-year-old woman who collapsed on the sidewalk of her residence. A family member states that she has a history of supraventricular tachycardia and takes atenolol. Identify the rhythm (lead II).

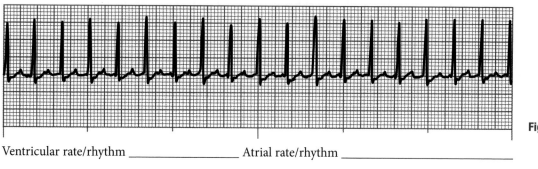

Figure 10-57

Ventricular rate/rhythm _____ Atrial rate/rhythm _____

PR interval _____ QRS duration _____ QT interval _____

Identification _____

128. This rhythm strip is from a 61-year-old woman complaining of shortness of breath. Identify the rhythm (lead II).

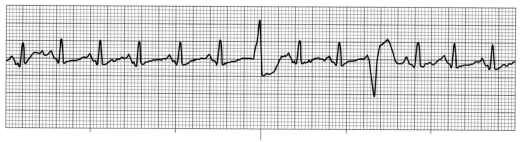

Figure 10-58

Ventricular rate/rhythm _____ Atrial rate/rhythm _____

PR interval _____ QRS duration _____ QT interval _____

Identification _____

129. Identify the rhythm.

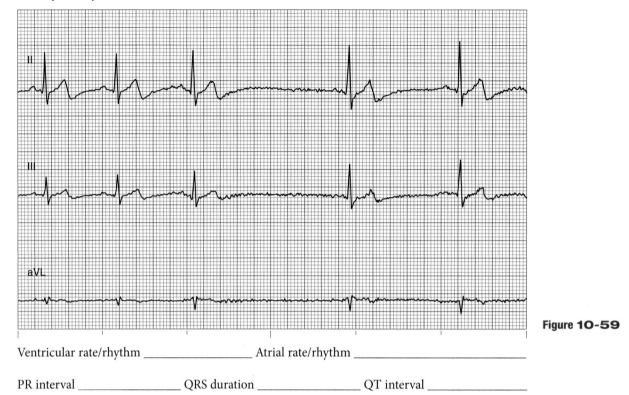

Figure 10-59

Ventricular rate/rhythm _____ Atrial rate/rhythm _____

PR interval _____ QRS duration _____ QT interval _____

Identification _____

130. Identify the rhythm.

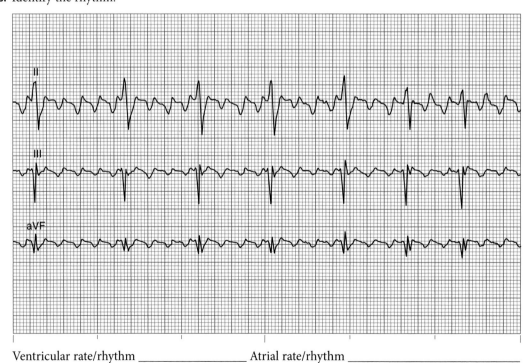

Figure 10-60

Ventricular rate/rhythm _____ Atrial rate/rhythm _____

PR interval _____ QRS duration _____ QT interval _____

Identification _____

131. This rhythm strip is from an asymptomatic 56-year-old man. Identify the rhythm (lead II).

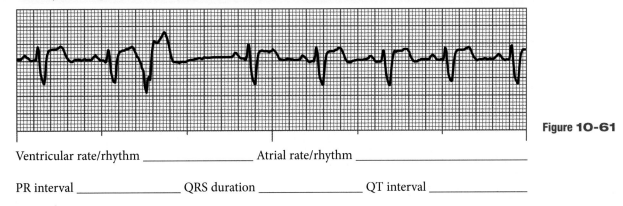

Figure 10-61

Ventricular rate/rhythm _____ Atrial rate/rhythm _____

PR interval _____ QRS duration _____ QT interval _____

Identification _____

132. Identify the rhythm (lead II).

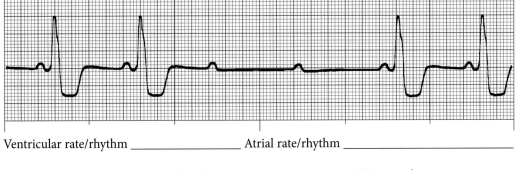

Figure 10-62

Ventricular rate/rhythm _____ Atrial rate/rhythm _____

PR interval _____ QRS duration _____ QT interval _____

Identification _____

133. These rhythm strips are from an 82-year-old man who is complaining of chest pain. Identify the rhythm.

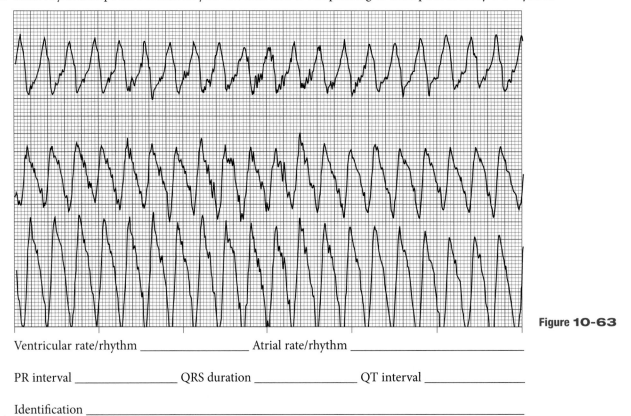

Figure 10-63

Ventricular rate/rhythm _____ Atrial rate/rhythm _____

PR interval _____ QRS duration _____ QT interval _____

Identification _____

134. These rhythm strips are from a 49-year-old woman complaining of chest pain with nausea and vomiting for 24 hours. She has a history of hypertension, stroke, and asthma. Identify the rhythm.

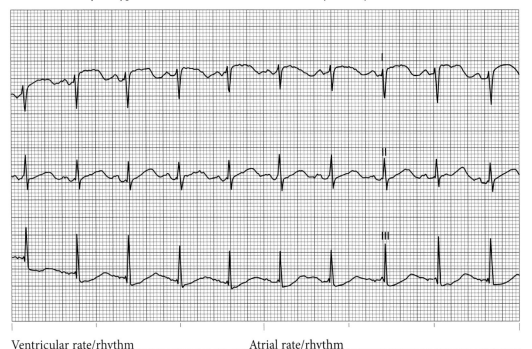

Figure 10-64

Ventricular rate/rhythm _____ Atrial rate/rhythm _____

PR interval _____ QRS duration _____ QT interval _____

Identification _____

135. Identify the rhythm (lead II).

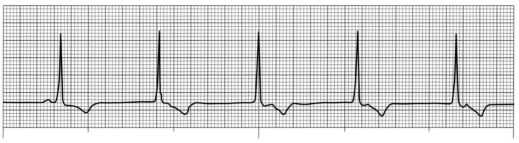

Figure 10-65

Ventricular rate/rhythm _____ Atrial rate/rhythm _____

PR interval _____ QRS duration _____ QT interval _____

Identification _____

136. Identify the rhythm (lead II).

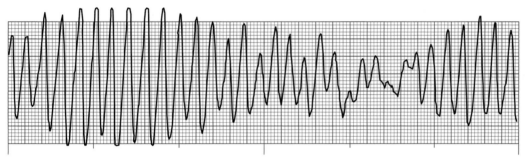

Figure 10-66

Ventricular rate/rhythm _____ Atrial rate/rhythm _____

PR interval _____ QRS duration _____ QT interval _____

Identification _____

137. These rhythm strips are from an 83-year-old woman with shortness of breath. Identify the rhythm.

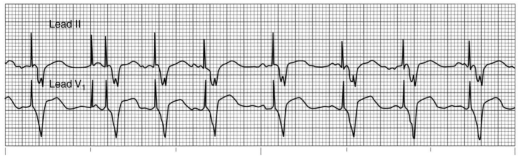

Figure 10-67

Atrial paced activity? _____ Ventricular paced activity? _____

Pacemaker malfunction? _____ Identification _____

138. This rhythm strip is from an 18-year-old male with a gunshot wound to his chest. Identify the rhythm (lead II).

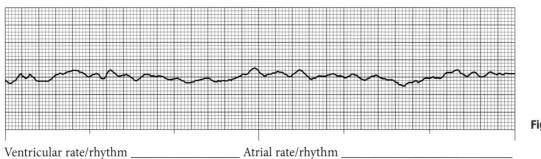

Figure **10-68**

Ventricular rate/rhythm _____ Atrial rate/rhythm _____

PR interval _____ QRS duration _____ QT interval _____

Identification _____

139. This rhythm strip is from a 44-year-old construction worker with a sudden onset of chest pressure. Identify the rhythm (lead II).

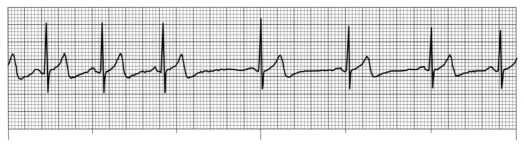

Figure **10-69**

Ventricular rate/rhythm _____ Atrial rate/rhythm _____

PR interval _____ QRS duration _____ QT interval _____

Identification _____

140. Identify the rhythm.

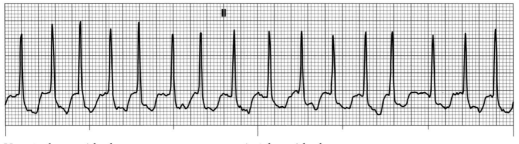

Figure **10-70**

Ventricular rate/rhythm _____ Atrial rate/rhythm _____

PR interval _____ QRS duration _____ QT interval _____

Identification _____

ANSWER SECTION

Multiple Choice

1. ANS: B
A branch of the right coronary artery supplies the right atrium and right ventricle with blood.
OBJ: Name the primary branches and areas of the heart supplied by the right and left coronary arteries.

2. ANS: D
Parasympathetic (inhibitory) nerve fibers supply the sinoatrial node, atrial muscle, and the atrioventricular (AV) bundle of the heart by the vagus nerves. Parasympathetic stimulation has the following actions:
- Slows the rate of discharge of the sinoatrial (SA) node
- Slows conduction through the AV node
- Decreases the strength of atrial contraction
- Can cause a small decrease in the force of ventricular contraction
OBJ: Compare and contrast the effects of sympathetic and parasympathetic stimulation of the heart.

3. ANS: B
The flow of blood from the superior and inferior venae cavae into the atria is normally continuous. About 70% of this blood flows directly through the atria and into the ventricles before the atria contract; this is called *passive filling*. When the atria contract, an additional 10% to 30% of the returning blood is added to filling of the ventricles. This additional contribution of blood resulting from atrial contraction is called *atrial kick*. Afterload is the pressure or resistance against which the ventricles must pump to eject blood. Cardiac output is the amount of blood pumped into the aorta each minute by the heart; it is defined as the stroke volume multiplied by the heart rate. Peripheral resistance is the resistance to the flow of blood determined by blood vessel diameter and the tone of the vascular musculature.
OBJ: Explain atrial kick.

4. ANS: A
The pulmonic and aortic valves are semilunar valves. The semilunar valves prevent backflow of blood from the aorta and pulmonary arteries into the ventricles. The tricuspid and mitral valves are atrioventricular valves, which separate the atria from the ventricles.
OBJ: Name and identify the location of the atrioventricular and semilunar valves.

5. ANS: D
The left main coronary artery supplies oxygenated blood to its two primary branches: the left anterior descending, which is also called the *anterior interventricular artery*, and the circumflex artery.
OBJ: Name the primary branches and areas of the heart supplied by the right and left coronary arteries.

6. ANS: B
In general, cardiac cells have either a mechanical (i.e., contractile) or an electrical (i.e., pacemaker) function. Pacemaker cells are specialized cells of the electrical conduction system. Pacemaker cells also may be referred to as *conducting cells* or *automatic cells*. They are responsible for the spontaneous generation and conduction of electrical impulses.
OBJ: Describe the two basic types of cardiac cells in the heart, where they are found, and their function.

7. ANS: B
During the absolute refractory period, the cell will not respond to further stimulation within itself. This means that the myocardial working cells cannot contract and that the cells of the electrical conduction system cannot conduct an electrical impulse, no matter how strong the internal electrical stimulus. On the ECG, the absolute refractory period begins with the onset of the QRS complex and terminates at approximately the apex of the T wave.
OBJ: Define the absolute, effective, relative refractory, and supranormal periods and their location in the cardiac cycle.

8. ANS: D
The QT interval, measured from the beginning of the QRS complex to the end of the T wave, represents the time from initial depolarization of the ventricles to the end of ventricular repolarization.
OBJ: Define and describe the significance of each of the following as they relate to cardiac electrical activity: the P wave, the QRS complex, the T wave, the U wave, the PR segment, the TP segment, the ST segment, the PR interval, the QRS duration, and the QT interval.

9. ANS: D
To evaluate the rhythmicity of the atrial rhythm, the interval between two consecutive P waves is measured and compared to succeeding P-P intervals.
OBJ: Describe a systematic approach to the analysis and interpretation of cardiac dysrhythmias.

10. ANS: A
A bipolar lead is an ECG lead that has a positive and negative electrode. Each lead records the difference in electrical potential (i.e., voltage) between two selected electrodes. Although all ECG leads are technically bipolar, leads I, II, and III use two distinct electrodes, one of which is connected to the positive input of the ECG machine and the other to the negative input.
OBJ: Describe correct anatomic placement of the standard limb leads, the augmented leads, and the chest leads.

11. ANS: A

In sinus arrhythmia, the heart rate increases gradually during inspiration (R-R intervals shorten) and decreases with expiration (R-R intervals lengthen). OBJ: Describe the ECG characteristics, possible causes, signs and symptoms, and emergency management of sinus arrhythmia.

12. ANS: D

The rate of a sinus bradycardia is less than 60 beats/min. R-R and P-P intervals are regular, P waves are positive in lead II and one precedes each QRS complex. The PR interval is within normal limits and the QRS duration is 0.11 second or less unless it is abnormally conducted. OBJ: Describe the ECG characteristics, possible causes, signs and symptoms, and emergency management of sinus bradycardia.

13. ANS: B

During sinoatrial (SA) block, which is also called *sinus exit block*, the pacemaker cells within the SA node initiate an impulse but it is blocked as it exits the SA node; thus, SA block is a disorder of impulse conduction. Sinus arrest, which is also called *sinus pause* or *sinoatrial arrest*, is a disorder of impulse formation. In sinus arrest, the pacemaker cells of the SA node fail to initiate an electrical impulse for one or more beats resulting in absent PQRST complexes on the ECG. OBJ: Describe the ECG characteristics, possible causes, signs and symptoms, and emergency management of sinoatrial block. Describe the ECG characteristics, possible causes, signs and symptoms, and emergency management of sinus arrest.

14. ANS: D

The heart's demand for oxygen increases as the heart rate increases. As the heart rate increases, there is less time for the ventricles to fill and less blood for the ventricles to pump out with each contraction, which can lead to decreased cardiac output. Because the coronary arteries fill when the ventricles are at rest, rapid heart rates decrease the time available for coronary artery filling. This decreases the heart's blood supply. Chest discomfort can result if the supplies of blood and oxygen to the heart are inadequate. OBJ: Describe the ECG characteristics, possible causes, signs and symptoms, and emergency management of sinus tachycardia.

15. ANS: B

OBJ: Describe the location, function, and (where appropriate), the intrinsic rate of the following structures: sinoatrial (SA) node, atrioventricular (AV) bundle, and Purkinje fibers.

16. ANS: C

Multiformed atrial rhythm is an updated term for the rhythm formerly known as wandering atrial pacemaker. With this rhythm, the size, shape, and direction of the P waves vary, sometimes from beat to beat. The difference in the look of the P waves is a result of the gradual shifting of the dominant pacemaker between the sinoatrial (SA) node, the atria, and the atrioventricular (AV) junction. Wandering atrial pacemaker is associated with a normal or slow rate and irregular P-P, R-R, and PR intervals because of the different sites of impulse formation. OBJ: Describe the ECG characteristics, possible causes, signs and symptoms, and initial emergency care for wandering atrial pacemaker (multiformed atrial rhythm).

17. ANS: D

Atrioventricular (AV) nodal reentrant tachycardia is the most common type of supraventricular tachycardia. OBJ: Describe the ECG characteristics, possible causes, signs and symptoms, and initial emergency care for atrioventricular nodal reentrant tachycardia.

18. ANS: D

Atrial flutter or atrial fibrillation (AFib) that has a ventricular rate of more than 100 beats/min is described as *uncontrolled*. The ventricular rate is considered rapid when it is 150 beats/min or more. New-onset atrial flutter or AFib is often associated with a rapid ventricular rate. Atrial flutter or AFib that has a ventricular rate of less than 100 beats/min, is described as *controlled*. A controlled ventricular rate may be the result of a healthy atrioventricular (AV) node protecting the ventricles from very fast atrial impulses or of drugs used to control (i.e., block) conduction through the AV node, thereby decreasing the number of impulses that reach the ventricles. OBJ: Describe the ECG characteristics, possible causes, signs and symptoms, and initial emergency care for atrial fibrillation.

19. ANS: C

The term *paroxysmal* is used to describe a rhythm that starts or ends suddenly. Atrial tachycardia that starts or ends suddenly is called *paroxysmal supraventricular tachycardia* (PSVT), once called *paroxysmal atrial tachycardia* (PAT). PSVT may last for minutes, hours, or days. If the onset or end of PSVT is not observed on the ECG, the dysrhythmia is simply called *supraventricular tachycardia*. OBJ: Explain the terms *paroxysmal atrial tachycardia* (PAT) and *paroxysmal supraventricular tachycardia* (PSVT).

20. ANS: A

AFib is the most common sustained dysrhythmia in adults and it occurs because of altered automaticity in one or several rapidly firing sites in the atria or reentry involving one or more circuits in the atria.

OBJ: Describe the ECG characteristics, possible causes, signs and symptoms, and initial emergency care for atrial fibrillation.

21. ANS: D

You can usually tell the difference between a premature atrial complex (PAC) and a premature junctional complex (PJC) by the P wave. A PAC typically has an upright P wave before the QRS complex in leads II, III, and aVF. A P wave may or may not be present with a PJC. If a P wave is present, it is inverted (retrograde) and may precede or follow the QRS. PJCs can be misdiagnosed when the P wave of a PAC is buried in the preceding T wave.

OBJ: Describe the ECG characteristics, possible causes, signs and symptoms, and initial emergency care for premature junctional complexes.

22. ANS: B

Characteristic ECG findings in Wolff-Parkinson-White syndrome include a short PR interval, QRS widening, and a delta wave. A delta wave is an initial slurred deflection at the beginning of the QRS complex that results from the initial activation of the QRS by conduction over the accessory pathway.

OBJ: Describe the ECG characteristics, possible causes, signs and symptoms, and initial emergency care for atrioventricular reentrant tachycardia.

23. ANS: D

In atrial flutter, atrial waveforms are produced that resemble the teeth of a saw, or a picket fence; these are called *flutter waves*, which are best observed in leads II, III, aVF, and V_1.

OBJ: Describe the ECG characteristics, possible causes, signs and symptoms, and initial emergency care for atrial flutter.

24. ANS: B

If the atrioventricular (AV) junction paces the heart, the electrical impulse must travel in a backward (retrograde) direction to activate the atria. If the atria depolarize before the ventricles, an inverted P wave will be seen *before* the QRS complex and the PR interval will usually measure 0.12 second or less. The PR interval is shorter than usual because an impulse that begins in the AV junction does not have to travel as far to stimulate the ventricles. If the atria and ventricles depolarize at the same time, a P wave will not be visible because it will be hidden in the QRS complex. When the atria are depolarized after the ventricles, the P wave typically distorts the end of the QRS complex and an inverted P wave will appear *after* the QRS.

OBJ: Describe the ECG characteristics, possible causes, signs and symptoms, and initial emergency care for a junctional escape rhythm.

25. ANS: C

Nonparoxysmal (i.e., gradual onset) junctional tachycardia usually starts as an accelerated junctional rhythm, but the heart rate gradually increases to more than 100 beats/min. The usual ventricular rate for nonparoxysmal junctional tachycardia is 101 to 140 beats/min. Paroxysmal junctional tachycardia, which is also known as focal or automatic junctional tachycardia, is an uncommon dysrhythmia that starts and ends suddenly and that is often precipitated by a premature junctional complex (PJC). The ventricular rate for paroxysmal junctional tachycardia is generally faster, at a rate of 140 beats/min or more.

OBJ: Describe the ECG characteristics, possible causes, signs and symptoms, and initial emergency care for junctional tachycardia.

26. ANS: B

Junctional (or ventricular) complexes may come early (before the next expected sinus beat) or late (after the next expected sinus beat). If the complex is *early* it is called a *premature junctional (or ventricular) complex*. If the complex is *late* it is called a *junctional (or ventricular) escape beat*. To determine if a complex is early or late, you need to see at least two sinus beats in a row to establish the regularity of the underlying rhythm.

OBJ: Explain the difference between premature junctional complexes and junctional escape beats.

27. ANS: B

The term *symptomatic bradycardia* is used to describe a patient who experiences signs and symptoms of hemodynamic compromise related to a slow heart rate. Treatment of a symptomatic bradycardia should include assessment of the patient's oxygen saturation level, and determining if signs of increased work of breathing are present (e.g., retractions, tachypnea, paradoxic abdominal breathing). Give supplemental oxygen if oxygenation is inadequate. Assist breathing if ventilation is inadequate, establish intravenous access, and obtain a 12-lead ECG. Atropine, administered intravenously, is the drug of choice for symptomatic bradycardia. Reassess the patient's response and continue monitoring the patient.

OBJ: Describe the ECG characteristics, possible causes, signs and symptoms, and initial emergency care for a junctional escape rhythm.

28. ANS: C

Three or more sequential PVCs are termed a *run* or *burst*, and three or more PVCs that occur in a row at a rate of more than 100 beats/min is considered a run of ventricular tachycardia.

OBJ: Explain the terms *bigeminy, trigeminy, quadrigeminy*, and *run* when used to describe premature complexes.

29. ANS: A

PVCs that look alike in the same lead and begin from the same anatomic site (i.e., focus) are called *uniform PVCs*.
OBJ: Describe the ECG characteristics, possible causes, signs and symptoms, and initial emergency care for premature ventricular complexes.

30. ANS: C

Polymorphic ventricular tachycardia is characterized by QRS complexes that vary in shape and amplitude from beat to beat and appear to twist from upright to negative or negative to upright and back, resembling a spindle. The ventricular rate is 150 to 300 beats/min and is typically 200 to 250 beats/min.
OBJ: Describe the ECG characteristics, possible causes, signs and symptoms, and initial emergency care for polymorphic ventricular tachycardia.

31. ANS: D

When a delay or interruption in impulse conduction from the atria to the ventricles occurs as a result of a transient or permanent anatomic or functional impairment, the resulting dysrhythmia is called an *atrioventricular block*. A bundle branch block is a disruption in impulse conduction from the bundle of His through either the right or left bundle branch to the Purkinje fibers. With sinoatrial (SA) block, which is also called *sinus exit block*, the pacemaker cells within the SA node initiate an impulse, but it is blocked as it exits the SA node. With sinus arrest, the pacemaker cells of the SA node fail to initiate an electrical impulse for one or more beats resulting in absent PQRST complexes on the ECG.
OBJ: Describe the ECG characteristics, possible causes, signs and symptoms, and emergency management for first-degree atrioventricular block.

32. ANS: B

The rSR' pattern is characteristic of right bundle branch block. The rSR' pattern is sometimes referred to as an "M" or "rabbit ear" pattern.
OBJ: Describe the appearance of right and left bundle branch block as seen in lead V₁.

33. ANS: B

A first-degree atrioventricular (AV) block is present when there is a 1:1 relationship between P waves and QRS complexes and the PR interval is prolonged (i.e., more than 0.20 second) and constant.
OBJ: Describe the ECG characteristics, possible causes, signs and symptoms, and emergency management for first-degree atrioventricular (AV) block.

34. ANS: D

Second-degree AV blocks are types of *incomplete* blocks because at least some of the impulses from the sinoatrial (SA) node are conducted to the ventricles. With third-degree AV block, there is a *complete* block in conduction of impulses between the atria and the ventricles.
OBJ: Describe the ECG characteristics, possible causes, signs and symptoms, and emergency management for third-degree atrioventricular (AV) block.

35. ANS: B

Second-degree 2:1 atrioventricular (AV) block is characterized by P waves that are normal in size and shape, but every other P wave is not followed by a QRS. The atrial rate is twice the ventricular rate. Because there are no two PQRST cycles in a row from which to compare PR intervals, 2:1 AV block cannot be conclusively classified as type I or type II. To determine the type of block with certainty, it is necessary to continue close ECG monitoring of the patient until the conduction ratio of P waves to QRS complexes changes to 3:2, 4:3, and so on, which would enable PR interval comparison. With second-degree AV block in the form of 2:1 AV block, the level of the block can be located within the AV node or within the His-Purkinje system.
OBJ: Describe 2:1 atrioventricular (AV) block and advanced second-degree AV block.

36. ANS: B

The terms *advanced* or *high-grade* second-degree atrioventricular (AV) block may be used to describe three or more consecutive P waves that are not conducted. For example, with 3:1 AV block, every third P wave is conducted (i.e., followed by a QRS complex); with 4:1 AV block, every fourth P wave is conducted.
OBJ: Describe 2:1 atrioventricular (AV) block and advanced second-degree AV block.

37. ANS: A

Once the presence of bundle branch block is suspected, an examination of V₁ can reveal whether the block affects the right or the left bundle branch.
OBJ: Describe the appearance of right and left bundle branch block as seen in lead V₁.

38. ANS: D

Capture refers to the successful conduction of an artificial pacemaker's impulse through the myocardium, resulting in depolarization. A pacemaker spike is a vertical line on the ECG that indicates the pacemaker has discharged. Sensitivity is the extent to which an artificial pacemaker recognizes intrinsic cardiac electrical activity. Inhibition is a pacemaker response in which the output pulse is suppressed when an intrinsic event is sensed.
OBJ: Discuss the terms *triggering*, *inhibition*, *pacing*, *capture*, *electrical capture*, *mechanical capture*, and *sensitivity*.

39. ANS: B

The 12-lead ECG provides a 2.5-second view of each lead because it is assumed that 2.5 seconds is long enough to capture at least one representative complex. However, a 2.5-second view is not long enough to properly assess rate and rhythm, so at least one continuous rhythm strip is usually included at the bottom of the tracing.
OBJ: Describe a systematic method for analyzing a 12-lead ECG.

40. ANS: C

Although a right ventricular infarction may occur by itself, it is more commonly associated with an inferior myocardial infarction (MI), and it should be suspected when ECG changes suggesting an inferior infarction are seen.

OBJ: Recognize the changes on the ECG that may reflect evidence of myocardial ischemia, injury, or infarction.

Completion

42. ANS: The right atrium receives deoxygenated blood from the <u>superior vena cava</u> (which carries blood from the head and upper extremities), the <u>inferior vena cava</u> (which carries blood from the lower body), and the <u>coronary sinus</u> (which receives blood from the intracardiac circulation).

OBJ: Identify and describe the chambers of the heart and the vessels that enter or leave each.

43. ANS: A beat originating from the AV junction that appears later than the next expected sinus beat is called a <u>junctional</u> <u>escape</u> <u>beat</u>.

OBJ: Describe the ECG characteristics and possible causes for junctional escape beats.

44. ANS: A rapid, wide-QRS rhythm associated with pulselessness, shock, or heart failure should be presumed to be <u>ventricular</u> <u>tachycardia</u>.

OBJ: Describe the ECG characteristics, possible causes, signs and symptoms, and initial emergency care for monomorphic ventricular tachycardia (VT).

45. ANS: PACs associated with a wide QRS complex are called <u>aberrantly</u> <u>conducted</u> PACs, indicating conduction through the ventricles is abnormal.

OBJ: Describe the ECG characteristics, possible causes, signs and symptoms, and initial emergency care for premature atrial complexes.

46. ANS: <u>Diastole</u> is the period of relaxation during which a heart chamber is filling.

OBJ: Identify and discuss each phase of the cardiac cycle.

47. ANS: The thick, muscular middle layer of the heart wall that contains the atrial and ventricular muscle fibers necessary for contraction is the <u>myocardium</u>.

OBJ: Identify the three cardiac muscle layers.

48. ANS: Delivery of an electrical current timed for delivery during the QRS complex is called <u>synchronized</u> <u>cardioversion</u>.

OBJ: Discuss the indications and procedure for synchronized cardioversion.

41. ANS: B

Poor R-wave progression is a phrase used to describe R waves that decrease in size from V_1 to V_4. This is often seen in an anteroseptal infarction but may be a normal variant in young persons, particularly in young women. Other causes of poor R-wave progression include left bundle branch block, left ventricular hypertrophy, and severe chronic obstructive pulmonary disease (particularly emphysema).

OBJ: Distinguish patterns of normal and abnormal R-wave progression.

49. ANS: Sometimes, when a premature atrial complex (PAC) occurs very prematurely and close to the T wave of the preceding beat, only a P wave may be seen with no QRS after it (appearing as a pause). This type of PAC is termed a "<u>nonconducted</u>" (or "blocked") PAC.

OBJ: Describe the ECG characteristics, possible causes, signs and symptoms, and initial emergency care for premature atrial complexes.

50. ANS: If the AV junction paces the heart, the electrical impulse must travel in a <u>backward</u> (retrograde) direction to activate the atria.

51. ANS: A demand pacemaker is also known as a <u>synchronous</u> or <u>noncompetitive</u> pacemaker.

OBJ: Explain the differences between single-chamber and dual-chamber pacemakers, and between fixed-rate and demand pacemakers.

52. ANS: The axes of leads I, II, and III form an equilateral triangle with the heart at the center (Einthoven's triangle). If the augmented limb leads are added to this configuration and the axes of the six leads moved in a way in which they bisect each other, the result is the <u>hexaxial</u> <u>reference</u> <u>system</u>.

OBJ: Explain the term *electrical axis* and its significance.

53. ANS:

Leads	Heart Surface Viewed
II, III, aVF	Inferior
V_1, V_2	Septal
V_3, V_4	Anterior
I, aVL, V_5, V_6	Lateral

OBJ: Relate the cardiac surfaces or areas represented by the ECG leads.

Short Answer

54. ANS:

The pathway of blood flow through the normal heart and lungs to the systemic circulation:

1. right atrium	9. left ventricle
8. mitral valve	5. pulmonary arteries
11. aorta	2. tricuspid valve
3. right ventricle	6. pulmonary veins
4. pulmonic valve	10. aortic valve
7. left atrium	12. systemic circulation

OBJ: Beginning with the right atrium, describe blood flow through the normal heart and lungs to the systemic circulation.

55. ANS:

1. Assess rhythmicity (atrial and ventricular)
2. Assess rate (atrial and ventricular)
3. Identify and examine waveforms
4. Assess intervals (PR, QRS, and QT) and examine ST segments
5. Interpret the rhythm (and assess its clinical significance)

OBJ: Describe a systematic approach to the analysis and interpretation of cardiac dysrhythmias.

56. ANS:

A dual-chamber pacemaker stimulates the right atrium and right ventricle sequentially (stimulating first the atrium, then the ventricle), mimicking normal cardiac physiology and thus preserving the atrial contribution to ventricular filling (atrial kick).

OBJ: Explain the differences between single-chamber and dual-chamber pacemakers, and between fixed-rate and demand pacemakers.

57. ANS:

ECG monitoring may be used to (1) monitor a patient's heart rate, (2) evaluate the effects of disease or injury on heart function, (3) evaluate pacemaker function, (4) evaluate the response to medications (e.g., antiarrhythmics), (5) obtain a baseline recording before, during, and after a medical procedure, and (6) evaluate for signs of myocardial ischemia, injury, and infarction.

OBJ: Explain the purpose of electrocardiographic monitoring.

58. ANS:

An abnormal (i.e., pathologic) Q wave is more than 0.04 second in duration or more than one third the height of the following R wave in that lead. Myocardial infarction is one possible cause of abnormal Q waves.

OBJ: Define and describe the significance of each of the following as they relate to cardiac electrical activity: the P wave, the QRS complex, the T wave, the U wave, the PR segment, the TP segment, the ST segment, the PR interval, the QRS duration, and the QT interval.

59. ANS:

A sinus rhythm has a rate of 60 to 100 beats/min. A sinus tachycardia has a rate of 101 to 180 beats/min.

OBJ: Describe the ECG characteristics, possible causes, signs and symptoms, and emergency management of sinus tachycardia.

60. ANS:

Artifact may be caused by loose electrodes, broken wires or ECG cables, muscle tremor, patient movement, external chest compressions, or 60-cycle interference.

OBJ: Define the term *artifact* and explain methods that may be used to minimize its occurrence.

61. ANS:

Coarse ventricular fibrillation (VF) is 3 mm or more in amplitude. Fine VF is less than 3 mm in amplitude.

OBJ: Describe the ECG characteristics, possible causes, signs and symptoms, and initial emergency care for ventricular fibrillation.

62. ANS:

The atrioventricular (AV) junction may assume responsibility for pacing the heart if:

• The sinoatrial (SA) node fails to discharge (such as sinus arrest).
• An impulse from the SA node is generated but blocked as it exits the SA node (such as SA block).
• The rate of discharge of the SA node is slower than that of the AV junction (such as a sinus bradycardia or the slower phase of a sinus arrhythmia).
• An impulse from the SA node is generated and is conducted through the atria but is not conducted to the ventricles (such as an AV block).

OBJ: Describe the location, function, and, where appropriate, the intrinsic rate of the following structures: the sinoatrial node, the atrioventricular bundle, and the Purkinje fibers.

63. ANS:

Because the atria do not contract effectively and expel all of the blood within them, blood may pool within them and form clots. A clot may dislodge on its own or because of conversion to a sinus rhythm. A stroke can result if a clot moves from the atria and lodges in an artery in the brain.

OBJ: Describe the ECG characteristics, possible causes, signs and symptoms, and initial emergency care for atrial fibrillation.

64. ANS:

On the ECG, the ST segment represents early ventricular repolarization and the T wave represents ventricular repolarization.

OBJ: Define and describe the significance of each of the following as they relate to cardiac electrical activity: the P wave, the QRS complex, the T wave, the U wave, the PR segment, the TP segment, the ST segment, the PR interval, the QRS duration, and the QT interval.

65. ANS:

ECG Finding	Atrioventricular Nodal Reentrant Tachycardia (AVNRT)	Atrial Flutter	Atrial Fibrillation
Rhythm	Ventricular rhythm is usually very regular	Atrial regular, ventricular regular or irregular	Ventricular rhythm usually irregularly irregular
Rate (beats/min)	150 to 250	Atrial rate 250 to 450, typically 300; ventricular rate variable—determined by atrioventricular (AV) blockade	Atrial rate 400 to 600; ventricular rate variable
P waves (lead II)	P waves often hidden in QRS complex	No identifiable P waves; saw-toothed "flutter" waves present	No identifiable P waves; fibrillatory waves present; erratic, wavy baseline
PR interval (PRI)	If P waves are seen, the PRI will usually measure 0.12 to 0.20 sec	Not measurable	Not measurable
QRS duration	0.11 sec or less unless abnormally conducted	0.11 sec or less unless abnormally conducted	0.11 sec or less unless abnormally conducted

OBJ: Describe the ECG characteristics, possible causes, signs and symptoms, and initial emergency care for atrioventricular nodal reentrant tachycardia. Describe the ECG characteristics, possible causes, signs and symptoms, and initial emergency care for atrial flutter. Describe the ECG characteristics, possible causes, signs and symptoms, and initial emergency care for atrial fibrillation.

66. ANS:

During pacing, the cardiac monitor is observed for electrical capture, usually evidenced by a wide QRS and broad T wave. In some patients, electrical capture is less obvious, indicated only as a change in the shape of the QRS. Mechanical capture is evaluated by assessing the patient's right upper extremity or right femoral pulses.
OBJ: Discuss the terms *triggering, inhibition, pacing, capture, electrical capture, mechanical capture,* and *sensitivity.*

69. ANS:

67. ANS:

The four primary characteristics of cardiac cells are: (1) automaticity, (2) excitability (i.e., irritability), (3) conductivity, and (4) contractility.
OBJ: Describe the primary characteristics of cardiac cells.

68. ANS:

The term *anatomically contiguous leads* refers to those leads that "see" the same area of the heart. Two leads are contiguous if they look at the same or adjacent areas of the heart or if they are numerically consecutive *chest* leads.
OBJ: Relate the cardiac surfaces or areas represented by the ECG leads.

	Second-Degree AV Block Type II	2:1 AV Block
Ventricular Rhythm	Irregular	Regular
PR Interval	Constant	Constant
QRS Width	Narrow or wide	Narrow or wide

OBJ: Describe 2:1 AV block and advanced second-degree AV block.

70. ANS:

ECG Finding	Idioventricular Rhythm	Accelerated Idioventricular Rhythm	Monomorphic Ventricular Tachycardia
Rhythm	Essentially regular	Essentially regular	Usually regular
Rate (beats/min)	20 to 40	41 to 100; some experts consider the rate 41 to 120	101 to 250; some experts consider the rate 121 to 250
P waves (lead II)	Usually absent	Usually absent	Usually absent
PR interval	None	None	None
QRS duration	0.12 sec or greater	0.12 sec or greater	0.12 sec or greater

OBJ: Describe the ECG characteristics, possible causes, signs and symptoms, and initial emergency care for an idioventricular rhythm. Describe the ECG characteristics, possible causes, signs and symptoms, and initial emergency care for an accelerated idioventricular rhythm. Describe the ECG characteristics, possible causes, signs and symptoms, and initial emergency care for monomorphic VT.

71. **Figure 10-1 answer**

Ventricular rate/rhythm	88 beats/min; regular
Atrial rate/rhythm	88 beats/min; regular
PR interval	0.24 sec
QRS duration	0.06 sec
QT interval	0.32 sec
Identification	Sinus rhythm with first-degree AV block at 88 beats/min, ST-segment depression

72. **Figure 10-2 answer**

Ventricular rate/rhythm	58 to 115 beats/min; irregular
Atrial rate/rhythm	58 to 115 beats/min; irregular
PR interval	0.18 sec (sinus beats)
QRS duration	0.06 sec (sinus beats)
QT interval	0.28 sec (sinus beats)
Identification	Sinus tachycardia 58 to 115 beats/min with uniform PVCs

73. **Figure 10-3 answer**

Ventricular rate/rhythm	55 beats/min; regular
Atrial rate/rhythm	Unable to determine
PR interval	Not measurable
QRS duration	0.08 sec
QT interval	Unable to determine
Identification	Atrial flutter at 55 beats/min

74. **Figure 10-4 answer**

Ventricular rate/rhythm	30 to 41 beats/min; irregular
Atrial rate/rhythm	None
PR interval	None
QRS duration	0.16 sec
QT interval	0.44 sec
Identification	Idioventricular rhythm at 30 to 41 beats/min

75. **Figure 10-5 answer**

Ventricular rate/rhythm	167 beats/min; regular
Atrial rate/rhythm	None
PR interval	None
QRS duration	0.16 sec
QT interval	Unable to determine
Identification	Monomorphic ventricular tachycardia at 167 beats/min

76. **Figure 10-6 answer**

Ventricular rate/rhythm	94 beats/min; regular
Atrial rate/rhythm	94 beats/min; regular
PR interval	0.18 sec
QRS duration	0.12 sec
QT interval	0.40 sec
Identification	Sinus rhythm at 94 beats/min with a wide QRS and ST-segment depression

77. **Figure 10-7 answer**

Ventricular rate/rhythm	52 beats/min; regular
Atrial rate/rhythm	None
PR interval	None
QRS duration	0.06 sec
QT interval	0.44 sec
Identification	Sinus beat to junctional rhythm at 52 beats/min; inverted T waves

78. **Figure 10-8 answer**

Ventricular rate/rhythm	32 beats/min; regular
Atrial rate/rhythm	79 beats/min; regular
PR interval	Varies
QRS duration	0.10 to 12 sec
QT interval	0.60 sec (prolonged)
Identification	Third-degree AV block at 32 beats/min

79. **Figure 10-9 answer**

Ventricular rate/rhythm	78 beats/min; regular except for the PAC
Atrial rate/rhythm	78 beats/min; regular except for the PAC
PR interval	0.16 sec
QRS duration	0.06 sec
QT interval	Unable to determine
Identification	Sinus rhythm at 78 beats/min with a PAC, ST-segment elevation

80. **Figure 10-10 answer**

Atrial paced activity?	No
Ventricular paced activity?	Yes
Pacemaker malfunction?	No
Identification	Ventricular paced rhythm with 100% capture at 65 pulses/min

81. Figure 10-11 answer

Ventricular rate/rhythm	36 to 71 beats/min; regular except for the event
Atrial rate/rhythm	36 to 71 beats/min; regular except for the event
PR interval	0.16 sec
QRS duration	0.06 sec
QT interval	0.32 sec
Identification	Sinus rhythm at 36 to 71 beats/min with an episode of sinoatrial block

82. Figure 10-12 answer

Ventricular rate/rhythm	48 beats/min; regular
Atrial rate/rhythm	71 beats/min; slightly irregular
PR interval	Varies
QRS duration	0.08 to 0.10 sec
QT interval	0.24 to 0.28 sec
Identification	Third-degree AV block at 48 beats/min with ST-segment elevation

83. Figure 10-13 answer

Ventricular rate/rhythm	68 to 88 beats/min; irregular
Atrial rate/rhythm	Unable to determine
PR interval	Unable to determine
QRS duration	0.08 sec (atrial beats)
QT interval	Unable to determine
Identification	Atrial fibrillation at 68 to 88 beats/min with a ventricular complex

84. Figure 10-14 answer

Ventricular rate/rhythm	79 beats/min; regular
Atrial rate/rhythm	None
PR interval	None
QRS duration	0.06 sec
QT interval	0.36 to 0.38 sec
Identification	Accelerated junctional rhythm at 79 beats/min

85. Figure 10-15 answer

Atrial paced activity?	Yes
Ventricular paced activity?	Yes
Pacemaker malfunction?	No
Identification	Dual-chamber paced rhythm with 100% capture at 71 pulses/min

86. Figure 10-16 answer

Ventricular rate/rhythm	115 beats/min; regular
Atrial rate/rhythm	115 beats/min; regular
PR interval	0.16 to 0.20 sec
QRS duration	0.08 sec
QT interval	0.32 to 0.36 sec
Identification	Sinus tachycardia at 115 beats/min

87. Figure 10-17 answer

Ventricular rate/rhythm	230 to 300 beats/min; irregular
Atrial rate/rhythm	Unable to determine
PR interval	Unable to determine
QRS duration	Varies
QT interval	Unable to determine
Identification	Supraventricular beat followed by polymorphic ventricular tachycardia at 230 to 300 beats/min

88. Figure 10-18 answer

Ventricular rate/rhythm	55 beats/min; regular
Atrial rate/rhythm	107 beats/min; regular
PR interval	0.16 sec
QRS duration	0.06 sec
QT interval	Unable to determine
Identification	2:1 AV block at 55 beats/min with ST-segment elevation

89. Figure 10-19 answer

Ventricular rate/rhythm	167 beats/min; regular
Atrial rate/rhythm	Unable to determine
PR interval	Unable to determine
QRS duration	0.06 sec
QT interval	0.24 sec
Identification	AV nodal reentrant tachycardia (AVNRT) at 167 beats/min with ST-segment depression

90. Figure 10-20 answer

Ventricular rate/rhythm	41 to 73 beats/min; irregular
Atrial rate/rhythm	56 to 125 beats/min; irregular
PR interval	0.20 sec
QRS duration	0.12 sec
QT interval	0.40 to 0.44 sec
Identification	Sinus rhythm at 41 to 73 beats/min with a nonconducted PAC

91. Figure 10-21 answer

Ventricular rate/rhythm	136 to 188 beats/min; irregular
Atrial rate/rhythm	136 to 188 beats/min; irregular
PR interval	0.10 sec
QRS duration	0.06 sec
QT interval	0.24 sec
Identification	Sinus tachycardia at 136 to 188 beats/min with frequent PJCs (the PJCs are beats 2, 5, 8, and 11 from the left)

92. Figure 10-22 answer

Ventricular rate/rhythm	43 to 60 beats/min; irregular
Atrial rate/rhythm	68 beats/min; regular
PR interval	Inconstant
QRS duration	0.06 sec
QT interval	0.32 to 0.36 sec
Identification	Second-degree AV block type I at 43 to 60 beats/min

93. Figure 10-23 answer

Atrial paced activity?	No
Ventricular paced activity?	Yes
Pacemaker malfunction?	Yes; failure to capture
Identification	Ventricular-paced rhythm with pacemaker malfunction (3 of 7 beats captured; 40% capture)

94. Figure 10-24 answer

Ventricular rate/rhythm	88 (sinus beats), regular except for the events
Atrial rate/rhythm	88 (sinus beats), regular except for the events
PR interval	0.20 sec (sinus beats)
QRS duration	0.08 sec (sinus beats)
QT interval	0.36 sec (sinus beats)
Identification	Sinus rhythm at 88 beats/min with a run of VT and a PVC, ST-segment depression, inverted T waves

95. Figure 10-25 answer

Ventricular rate/rhythm	49 beats/min; regular except for the event
Atrial rate/rhythm	49 beats/min; regular except for the event
PR interval	0.20 sec
QRS duration	0.08 sec
QT interval	0.44 to 0.48 sec
Identification	Sinus bradycardia at 49 beats/min with an episode of sinus arrest

96. Figure 10-26 answer

Ventricular rate/rhythm	None
Atrial rate/rhythm	40 beats/min; regular
PR interval	None
QRS duration	None
QT interval	None
Identification	P-wave asystole at 40 beats/min

97. Figure 10-27 answer

Ventricular rate/rhythm	62 beats/min; regular
Atrial rate/rhythm	62 beats/min; regular
PR interval	0.14 sec
QRS duration	0.08 sec
QT interval	Unable to determine
Identification	Accelerated junctional rhythm at 62 beats/min

98. Figure 10-28 answer

Ventricular rate/rhythm	65 beats/min (sinus beats) to approximately 167 beats/min (ventricular beats); regular to irregular
Atrial rate/rhythm	65 beats/min (sinus beats); regular (sinus beats)
PR interval	0.16 sec (sinus beats)
QRS duration	0.10 to 0.12 sec (sinus beats)
QT interval	0.32 sec (sinus beats)
Identification	Sinus rhythm at 65 beats/min with ST-segment depression to polymorphic VT at 167 beats/min

99. Figure 10-29 answer

Ventricular rate/rhythm	231 beats/min; regular
Atrial rate/rhythm	Unable to determine
PR interval	Unable to determine
QRS duration	0.06 sec
QT interval	Unable to determine
Identification	AVNRT at 231 beats/min with ST-segment depression

100. Figure 10-30 answer

Ventricular rate/rhythm	60 to 88 beats/min; irregular
Atrial rate/rhythm	60 to 88 beats/min; irregular
PR interval	0.16 sec (sinus beats)
QRS duration	0.04 to 0.06 sec (sinus beats)
QT interval	0.40 sec (sinus beats)
Identification	Sinus rhythm at 60 to 88 beats/min with PJCs

101. Figure 10-31 answer

Ventricular rate/rhythm	33 to 47 beats/min; irregular
Atrial rate/rhythm	100 beats/min; regular
PR interval	0.14 sec
QRS duration	0.10 to 0.12 sec
QT interval	0.48 to 0.52 sec
Identification	Second-degree AV block type II at 33 to 47 beats/min

102. Figure 10-32 answer

Ventricular rate/rhythm	Unable to determine
Atrial rate/rhythm	None
PR interval	None
QRS duration	Unable to determine
QT interval	None
Identification	Ventricular fibrillation

103. Figure 10-33 answer

Ventricular rate/rhythm	136 beats/min; regular
Atrial rate/rhythm	136 beats/min; regular
PR interval	0.16 sec
QRS duration	0.08 sec
QT interval	0.24 sec
Identification	Sinus tachycardia at 136 beats/min; ST-segment elevation

104. Figure 10-34 answer

Ventricular rate/rhythm	67 to 73 beats/min (sinus beats); irregular
Atrial rate/rhythm	67 to 73 beats/min (sinus beats); irregular
PR interval	0.16 sec (sinus beats)
QRS duration	0.08 sec (sinus beats)
QT interval	0.32 sec (sinus beats)
Identification	Sinus rhythm at 67 to 73 beats/min with a PAC and a nonconducted PAC

105. Figure 10-35 answer

Atrial paced activity?	Yes
Ventricular paced activity?	No
Pacemaker malfunction?	No
Identification	Atrial-paced rhythm with 100% capture at 79 pulses/min

106. Figure 10-36 answer

Ventricular rate/rhythm	83 to 115 beats/min; irregular
Atrial rate/rhythm	Unable to determine
PR interval	Unable to determine
QRS duration	0.08 to 0.10 sec
QT interval	Unable to determine
Identification	Atrial fibrillation at 83 to 115 beats/min

107. Figure 10-37 answer

Ventricular rate/rhythm	36 beats/min; regular
Atrial rate/rhythm	75 beats/min; regular
PR interval	0.32 sec
QRS duration	0.10 sec
QT interval	0.36 sec
Identification	2:1 AV block at 36 beats/min

108. Figure 10-38 answer

Ventricular rate/rhythm	56 beats/min; regular
Atrial rate/rhythm	None
PR interval	None
QRS duration	0.12 sec
QT interval	0.40 sec
Identification	Accelerated idioventricular rhythm (AIVR) at 56 beats/min; ST-segment depression

109. Figure 10-39 answer

Ventricular rate/rhythm	51 beats/min; essentially regular
Atrial rate/rhythm	51 beats/min; essentially regular
PR interval	0.16 sec
QRS duration	0.08 sec
QT interval	Unable to determine
Identification	Sinus bradycardia at 51 beats/min

110. Figure 10-40 answer

Ventricular rate/rhythm	54 to 94 beats/min; irregular
Atrial rate/rhythm	Unable to determine
PR interval	Not measurable
QRS duration	0.10 to 0.12 sec
QT interval	Unable to determine
Identification	Atrial flutter at 54 to 94 beats/min

111. Figure 10-41 answer

Ventricular rate/rhythm	56 beats/min (sinus beats); irregular
Atrial rate/rhythm	56 beats/min (sinus beats); irregular
PR interval	0.16 sec (sinus beats)
QRS duration	0.06 sec (sinus beats)
QT interval	Unable to determine
Identification	Sinus bradycardia at 56 beats/min with multiform ventricular bigeminy, a run of VT, and ST-segment depression

112. Figure 10-42 answer

Ventricular rate/rhythm	88 to 200 beats/min; irregular
Atrial rate/rhythm	88 to 200 beats/min; irregular
PR interval	Varies
QRS duration	0.08 sec
QT interval	Varies
Identification	Multifocal atrial tachycardia at 88 to 200 beats/min

113. Figure 10-43 answer

Atrial paced activity?	No
Ventricular paced activity?	Yes
Pacemaker malfunction?	No
Identification	Ventricular-paced rhythm with 100% capture at 65 pulses/min

114. Figure 10-44 answer

Ventricular rate/rhythm	41 to 63 beats/min; irregular
Atrial rate/rhythm	88 beats/min; regular
PR interval	Inconstant
QRS duration	0.08 to 0.10 sec
QT interval	0.40 to 0.44 sec
Identification	Second-degree AV block type I at 41 to 63 beats/min with ST-segment depression; note the presence of 2:1 AV block at the start of the rhythm strip

115. Figure 10-45 answer

Ventricular rate/rhythm	63 beats/min (sinus beats); regular except for the event
Atrial rate/rhythm	63 beats/min (sinus beats); regular except for the event
PR interval	0.16 to 0.18 sec (sinus beats)
QRS duration	0.08 to 0.10 sec (sinus beats)
QT interval	0.28 sec (sinus beats)
Identification	Sinus rhythm at 63 beats/min with an R-on-T PVC and ST-segment elevation

116. Figure 10-46 answer

Ventricular rate/rhythm	120 beats/min; regular
Atrial rate/rhythm	120 beats/min; regular
PR interval	None
QRS duration	0.10 sec
QT interval	0.36 sec
Identification	Junctional tachycardia at 120 beats/min

117. Figure 10-47 answer

Ventricular rate/rhythm	32 beats/min; regular
Atrial rate/rhythm	32 beats/min; regular
PR interval	None
QRS duration	0.06 to 0.08 sec
QT interval	0.44 to 0.48 sec
Identification	Junctional bradycardia at 32 beats/min with ST-segment depression and inverted T waves

118. Figure 10-48 answer

Ventricular rate/rhythm	None
Atrial rate/rhythm	None
PR interval	None
QRS duration	None
QT interval	None
Identification	Asystole

119. Figure 10-49 answer

Ventricular rate/rhythm	79 to 88 beats/min; irregular
Atrial rate/rhythm	79 to 88 beats/min; irregular
PR interval	0.18 sec
QRS duration	0.08 sec
QT interval	0.28 sec
Identification	Sinus arrhythmia at 79 to 88 beats/min

120. Figure 10-50 answer

Ventricular rate/rhythm	70 beats/min; regular
Atrial rate/rhythm	70 beats/min (sinus beats); unable to determine
PR interval	Varies
QRS duration	Varies
QT interval	0.44 sec
Identification	Underlying rhythm is sinus but pacemaker site varies; ventricular rate about 70 beats/min; patient with known Wolff-Parkinson-White syndrome; note the delta waves

121. Figure 10-51 answer

Atrial paced activity?	No
Ventricular paced activity?	Yes
Pacemaker malfunction?	Yes; failure to sense
Identification	Pacemaker malfunction (undersensing); underlying rhythm is a sinus rhythm at 88 beats/min; note the pacer spikes in the T waves of the second and eighth beats from the left

122. Figure 10-52 answer

Ventricular rate/rhythm	30 beats/min (sinus beats); regular
Atrial rate/rhythm	30 beats/min (sinus beats); regular
PR interval	0.16 sec
QRS duration	0.06 sec
QT interval	0.36 sec
Identification	Sinus bradycardia at 30 beats/min with an interpolated PVC and ST-segment elevation

123. Figure 10-53 answer

Ventricular rate/rhythm	71 beats/min (sinus beats); regular except for the event
Atrial rate/rhythm	71 beats/min (sinus beats); regular except for the event
PR interval	0.24 sec
QRS duration	0.08 sec
QT interval	0.28 sec
Identification	Sinus rhythm at 71 beats/min with a first-degree AV block, an episode of sinus arrest and a junctional escape beat; ST-segment depression

124. Figure 10-54 answer

Atrial paced activity?	No
Ventricular paced activity?	Yes
Pacemaker malfunction?	No
Identification	Ventricular-paced rhythm at 60 pulses/min with 100% capture; underlying rhythm appears to be a third-degree AV block

125. Figure 10-55 answer

Ventricular rate/rhythm	100 beats/min (sinus beats); regular; 150 beats/min (VT); regular
Atrial rate/rhythm	100 beats/min (sinus beats); regular
PR interval	0.24 sec (sinus beats)
QRS duration	0.08 sec (sinus beats)
QT interval	0.28 to 0.30 sec (sinus beats)
Identification	Sinus rhythm at 100 beats/min with first-degree AV block to monomorphic VT at 150 beats/min

126. Figure 10-56 answer

Ventricular rate/rhythm	63 beats/min (sinus beats); regular (sinus beats)
Atrial rate/rhythm	63 to 88 beats/min; irregular
PR interval	0.22 to 0.24 sec
QRS duration	0.08 sec (sinus beats)
QT interval	0.36 to 0.40 sec
Identification	Sinus rhythm at 63 beats/min with a first-degree AV block, nonconducted PAC, and a ventricular escape beat

127. Figure 10-57 answer

Ventricular rate/rhythm	188 beats/min; regular
Atrial rate/rhythm	Unable to determine
PR interval	Unable to determine
QRS duration	0.06 sec
QT interval	0.20 to 0.24 sec
Identification	AVNRT at 188 beats/min

128. Figure 10-58 answer

Ventricular rate/rhythm	125 beats/min; essentially regular except for events
Atrial rate/rhythm	125 beats/min; essentially regular except for events
PR interval	0.12 sec (sinus beats)
QRS duration	0.06 sec (sinus beats)
QT interval	Unable to determine
Identification	Sinus tachycardia at 125 beats/min with multiform PVCs

129. Figure 10-59 answer

Ventricular rate/rhythm	65 beats/min; regular except for the event
Atrial rate/rhythm	65 beats/min; regular except for the event
PR interval	0.16 sec
QRS duration	0.08 sec
QT interval	0.32 to 0.36 sec
Identification	Sinus rhythm at 65 beats/min with an episode of sinoatrial block

130. Figure 10-60 answer

Ventricular rate/rhythm	58 to 68 beats/min; irregular
Atrial rate/rhythm	Unable to determine
PR interval	Not measurable
QRS duration	0.12 sec
QT interval	Unable to determine
Identification	Atrial flutter at 58 to 68 beats/min

131. Figure 10-61 answer

Ventricular rate/rhythm	79 beats/min (sinus beats); regular except for the event
Atrial rate/rhythm	79 beats/min (sinus beats); regular except for the event
PR interval	0.16 to 0.18 sec (sinus beats)
QRS duration	0.12 sec (sinus beats)
QT interval	0.32 sec (sinus beats)
Identification	Sinus rhythm at 79 beats/min with a wide-QRS and an R-on-T PVC

132. Figure 10-62 answer

Ventricular rate/rhythm	Less than 20 to 60 beats/min; irregular
Atrial rate/rhythm	60 beats/min; regular
PR interval	0.16 sec
QRS duration	0.12 sec
QT interval	Unable to determine
Identification	Advanced second-degree AV block at less than 20 to 60 beats/min; ST-segment depression

133. Figure 10-63 answer

Ventricular rate/rhythm	245 beats/min; regular
Atrial rate/rhythm	None
PR interval	None
QRS duration	0.28 sec
QT interval	Unable to determine
Identification	Monomorphic ventricular tachycardia at 245 beats/min

134. Figure 10-64 answer

Ventricular rate/rhythm	96 beats/min; regular
Atrial rate/rhythm	96 beats/min; regular
PR interval	0.16 sec
QRS duration	0.08 to 0.10 sec
QT interval	0.36 sec
Identification	Sinus rhythm at 96 beats/min with ST-segment elevation in leads I and II

135. Figure 10-65 answer

Ventricular rate/rhythm	52 beats/min; regular
Atrial rate/rhythm	None
PR interval	None
QRS duration	0.06 sec
QT interval	0.40 sec
Identification	Sinus beat to a junction escape rhythm at 52 beats/min; inverted T waves

136. Figure 10-66 answer

Ventricular rate/rhythm	300 to 375 beats/min; irregular
Atrial rate/rhythm	None
PR interval	None
QRS duration	Varies
QT interval	Unable to determine
Identification	Polymorphic ventricular tachycardia at 300 to 375 beats/min

137. Figure 10-67 answer

Atrial paced activity?	Yes
Ventricular paced activity?	Yes
Pacemaker malfunction?	No
Identification	Dual-chamber paced rhythm with an atrial paced interval of 79 pulses/min and a ventricular paced interval of 85 pulses/min

138. Figure 10-68 answer

Ventricular rate/rhythm	None
Atrial rate/rhythm	None
PR interval	None
QRS duration	None
QT interval	None
Identification	Ventricular fibrillation

139. Figure 10-69 answer

Ventricular rate/rhythm	52 to 94 beats/min; irregular
Atrial rate/rhythm	52 to 94 beats/min; irregular
PR interval	0.12 sec
QRS duration	0.08 sec
QT interval	0.24 to 0.28 sec
Identification	Sinus arrhythmia at 52 to 94 beats/min

140. Figure 10-70 answer

Ventricular rate/rhythm	125 to 158 beats/min; irregular
Atrial rate/rhythm	Unable to determine
PR interval	None
QRS duration	0.06 sec
QT interval	Unable to determine
Identification	Atrial fibrillation (uncontrolled) at 125 to 158 beats/min with ST-segment depression

Glossary

Absolute refractory period Corresponds with the onset of the QRS complex to approximately the peak of the T wave; cardiac cells cannot be stimulated to conduct an electrical impulse, no matter how strong the stimulus

Accelerated idioventricular rhythm (AIVR) Dysrhythmia originating in the ventricles with a rate between 41 and 100 beats/min

Action potential A five-phase cycle that reflects the difference in the concentration of charged particles across the cell membrane at any given time

Acute coronary syndrome (ACS) A term used to refer to distinct conditions caused by a similar sequence of pathologic events—a temporary or permanent blockage of a coronary artery; these conditions are characterized by an excessive demand or inadequate supply of oxygen and nutrients to the heart muscle associated with plaque disruption, thrombus formation, and vasoconstriction. ACSs consist of three major syndromes: unstable angina (UA), non–ST-segment elevation myocardial infarction (NSTEMI), and ST-segment elevation myocardial infarction (STEMI).

Adrenergic Having the characteristics of the sympathetic division of the autonomic nervous system

Afterload The pressure or resistance against which the ventricles must pump to eject blood

Agonal rhythm Dysrhythmia similar in appearance to an idioventricular rhythm but occurring at a rate of less than 20 beats/min; dying heart

Altered automaticity A disorder of impulse formation in which cardiac cells fire and initiate impulses before a normal sinoatrial node impulse

Amplitude Height (voltage) of a waveform on the ECG

Angina pectoris Chest discomfort or other related symptoms of sudden onset that may occur because the increased oxygen demand of the heart temporarily exceeds the blood supply

Aortic valve Semilunar valve on the left side of the heart; separates the left ventricle from the aorta

Apex of the heart Lower portion of the heart that is formed by the tip of the left ventricle

Arrhythmia Abnormal heart rhythm

Arteriosclerosis A chronic disease of the arterial system characterized by abnormal thickening and hardening of the vessel walls

Artifact Distortion of an ECG tracing by electrical activity that is noncardiac in origin (e.g., electrical interference, poor electrical conduction, patient movement)

Asystole A total absence of ventricular electrical activity

Atherosclerosis A form of arteriosclerosis in which the thickening and hardening of the vessel walls are caused by a buildup of fatty deposits in the inner lining of large and middle-sized muscular arteries (from *athero*, meaning "gruel" or "paste," and *sclerosis*, meaning "hardness")

Atria Two upper chambers of the heart (singular, atrium)

Atrial kick Blood pushed into the ventricles because of atrial contraction

Atrioventricular (AV) block A delay or interruption in impulse conduction from the atria to the ventricles that occurs as a result of a transient or permanent anatomic or functional impairment

Atrioventricular bundle The bundle of His

Atrioventricular node A group of cells that conduct an electrical impulse through the heart; located in the floor of the right atrium immediately behind the tricuspid valve and near the opening of the coronary sinus

Atrioventricular valve Valve located between each atrium and ventricle; the tricuspid separates the right atrium from the right ventricle, and the mitral (bicuspid) separates the left atrium from the left ventricle

Atypical presentation Uncharacteristic signs and symptoms perceived by some patients experiencing a medical condition, such as an acute coronary syndrome

Augmented limb lead Leads aVR, aVL, and aVF; these leads record the difference in electrical potential at one location relative to zero potential rather than relative to the electrical potential of another extremity

Automated external defibrillator (AED) A machine with a sophisticated computer system that analyzes a patient's heart rhythm using an algorithm to distinguish shockable rhythms from nonshockable rhythms and provides visual and auditory instructions to the rescuer to deliver an electrical shock, if indicated

Automaticity Ability of cardiac pacemaker cells to spontaneously initiate an electrical impulse without being stimulated from another source (such as a nerve)

AV bundle The bundle of His

AV dissociation Any dysrhythmia in which the atria and ventricles beat independently (e.g., ventricular tachycardia, third-degree AV block)

AV interval In dual-chamber pacing, the length of time between an atrial sensed or atrial paced event and the delivery of a ventricular pacing stimulus; analogous to the PR interval of intrinsic waveforms; also called the artificial or electronic PR interval

AV node Specialized cells located in the lower portion of the right atrium; delays the electrical impulse to allow the atria to contract and complete filling of the ventricles

Axis Imaginary line joining the positive and negative electrodes of a lead

Base of the heart Posterior surface of the heart

Base rate Rate at which the pacemaker's pulse generator initiates impulses when no intrinsic activity is detected; expressed in pulses/minute (ppm)

Baseline Straight line recorded on ECG graph paper when no electrical activity is detected

Biphasic Waveform that is partly positive and partly negative

Bipolar limb lead ECG lead consisting of a positive and negative electrode

Blood pressure Force exerted by the blood against the walls of the arteries as the ventricles of the heart contract and relax

Bundle branch block (BBB) A disruption in impulse conduction from the bundle of His through the right or left bundle branch to the Purkinje fibers; a BBB may be intermittent or permanent

Bundle of His Fibers located in the upper portion of the interventricular septum that receive an electrical impulse from the AV node and conduct the impulse to the right and left bundle branches

Burst Three or more sequential ectopic beats; also referred to as a *salvo* or *run*

Capture The successful conduction of an artificial pacemaker's impulse through the myocardium, resulting in depolarization

Cardiac output The amount of blood pumped into the aorta each minute by the heart; defined as the stroke volume multiplied by the heart rate

Catecholamines Natural chemicals produced by the body that have sympathetic actions; epinephrine, norepinephrine, dopamine

Cholinergic Having the characteristics of the parasympathetic division of the autonomic nervous system

Chordae tendineae (tendinous cords) Thin strands of fibrous connective tissue that extend from the AV valves to the papillary muscles that prevent the AV valves from bulging back into the atria during ventricular systole (contraction)

Chronotropy A change in (heart) rate

Circumflex artery Division of the left coronary artery

Coarse ventricular fibrillation Ventricular fibrillation with fibrillatory waves greater than 3 mm in height

Complex Several waveforms

Conduction system A system of pathways in the heart composed of specialized electrical (pacemaker) cells

Conductivity Ability of a cardiac cell to receive an electrical stimulus and conduct that impulse to an adjacent cardiac cell

Contractility Ability of cardiac cells to shorten, causing cardiac muscle contraction in response to an electrical stimulus

Coronary sinus Outlet that drains five coronary veins into the right atrium

Couplet Two consecutive complexes

Current The flow of an electrical charge from one point to another

Defibrillation Delivery of an electrical current across the heart muscle over a very brief period to terminate an abnormal heart rhythm; also called *unsynchronized countershock* or *asynchronous countershock* because the delivery of current has no relationship to the cardiac cycle

Delta wave Slurring of the beginning portion of the QRS complex, caused by preexcitation

Demand pacemaker Pacemaker that discharges only when the patient's heart rate drops below the preset rate for the pacemaker; also known as a *synchronous* or *noncompetitive pacemaker*

Depolarization Movement of ions across a cell membrane, causing the inside of the cell to become more positive; an electrical event expected to result in contraction

Diastole Phase of the cardiac cycle in which the atria and ventricles relax between contractions and blood enters these chambers; when the term is used without reference to a specific chamber of the heart, the term implies ventricular diastole

Dromotropy Refers to the speed of conduction through the AV junction

Dual-chamber pacemaker Pacemaker that stimulates the atrium and ventricle; dual-chamber pacing is also called *physiologic pacing*

Dysrhythmia Any disturbance or abnormality in a normal rhythmic pattern; any cardiac rhythm other than a sinus rhythm

Ectopic Impulse(s) originating from a source other than the sinoatrial node

Effective refractory period Period of the cardiac action potential that includes the absolute refractory period and the first half of the relative refractory period

Ejection fraction The percentage of blood pumped out of a heart chamber with each contraction

Electrode An adhesive pad that contains a conductive gel and is applied at specific locations on the patient's chest wall and extremities and connected by cables to an ECG machine

Electrolytes Elements or compounds that break into charged particles (ions) when melted or dissolved in water or another solvent

Endocardium Innermost layer of the heart that lines the inside of the myocardium and covers the heart valves

Enhanced automaticity Abnormal condition in which cardiac cells not normally associated with the property of automaticity begin to depolarize spontaneously or when escape pacemaker sites increase their firing rate beyond that considered normal

Epicardium Also known as the *visceral pericardium*; the external layer of the heart wall that covers the heart muscle

Escape interval Time measured between a sensed cardiac event and the next pacemaker output

Excitability The ability of cardiac muscle cells to respond to an outside stimulus

f waves Fibrillation waves; irregularly shaped atrial waves associated with atrial fibrillation, occurring at a rate of 400 to 600 beats/min

F waves Flutter waves; atrial waves associated with atrial flutter; usually shaped like the teeth of a saw or a picket fence

Failure to capture A pacemaker malfunction that occurs when the artificial pacemaker stimulus is unable to depolarize the myocardium

Failure to pace A pacemaker malfunction that occurs when the pacemaker fails to deliver an electrical stimulus at its programmed time; also referred to as *failure to fire* or *failure of pulse generation*

Fine ventricular fibrillation VF with fibrillatory waves less than 3 mm in height

Fixed-rate pacemaker Pacemaker that continuously discharges at a preset rate regardless of the patient's intrinsic activity; also known as an *asynchronous pacemaker*

Focal atrial tachycardia AT that begins in a small area (focus) within the heart

Fusion beat Beat that occurs because of simultaneous activation of one cardiac chamber by two sites (foci); in pacing, the ECG waveform that results when an intrinsic depolarization and a pacing stimulus occur simultaneously and both contribute to depolarization of that cardiac chamber

Great vessels Large vessels that carry blood to and from the heart superior and inferior venae cavae, pulmonary veins, aorta, and pulmonary trunk

Ground electrode Third ECG electrode (the first and second are the positive and negative electrodes), which minimizes electrical activity from other sources

Heart failure A condition in which the heart is unable to pump enough blood to meet the metabolic needs of the body; it may result from any condition that impairs preload, afterload, cardiac contractility, or heart rate

His-Purkinje system Portion of the conduction system consisting of the bundle of His, bundle branches, and Purkinje fibers

Hypovolemia Inadequate tissue perfusion caused by inadequate vascular volume

Indicative changes ECG changes observed in leads that look directly at the affected area of the heart; indicative changes are significant when they are seen in two anatomically contiguous leads.

Infarction Death of tissue because of an inadequate blood supply

Inherent Natural, intrinsic

Inhibition Pacemaker response in which the output pulse is suppressed when an intrinsic event is sensed

Inotropy Refers to a change in myocardial contractility

Interpolated PVC PVC that occurs between two normally conducted QRS complexes and that does not disturb the next ventricular depolarization or sinoatrial node activity

Interval Waveform and a segment; in pacing, the period, measured in milliseconds, between any two designated cardiac events

Intrinsic rate Rate at which a pacemaker of the heart normally generates impulses

Ion Electrically charged particle

Ischemia Decreased supply of oxygenated blood to a body part or organ

Isoelectric line Absence of electrical activity; observed on the ECG as a straight line

J-point Point where the QRS complex and ST segment meet

Junctional bradycardia A rhythm that begins in the AV bundle with a rate of less than 40 beats/min

Junctional escape rhythm A rhythm that begins in the AV bundle; characterized by a very regular ventricular rate of 40 to 60 beats/min

Junctional tachycardia A rhythm that begins in the AV bundle with a ventricular rate of more than 100 beats/min

Lead Electrical connection attached to the body to record electrical activity

Left anterior descending artery Division of the left coronary artery

Mediastinum Middle area of the thoracic cavity; contains the heart, great vessels, trachea, and esophagus, among other structures; extends from the sternum to the vertebral column

Membrane potential Difference in electrical charge across the cell membrane

Millivolt (mV) Difference in electrical charge between two points in a circuit

Mitochondria The energy-producing parts of a cell

Monomorphic Having the same shape

Multiformed atrial rhythm Dysrhythmia that occurs because of impulses originating from various sites, including the SA node, the atria, and/or the AV junction; requires at least three different P waves, seen in the same lead, for proper diagnosis

Myocardial cells Working cells of the myocardium that contain contractile filaments and form the muscular layer of the atrial walls and the thicker muscular layer of the ventricular walls

Myocardium Middle and thickest layer of the heart; contains the cardiac muscle fibers that cause contraction of the heart and contains the conduction system and blood supply

Myofibril Slender, striated strand of muscle tissue

Neurotransmitter A chemical released from one nerve that crosses the synaptic cleft to reach a receptor

Nonconducted PAC (blocked PAC) Premature atrial complex that is not followed by a QRS complex

Noncompensatory pause A pause that often follows a premature atrial complex that represents the delay during which the SA node resets its rhythm for the next beat; the pause is noncompensatory if the normal beat following the premature complex occurs before it was expected (i.e., the period between the complex before and after the premature beat is less than two normal R-R intervals)

Oversensing A pacemaker malfunction that results from inappropriate sensing of extraneous electrical signals

P wave First wave in the cardiac cycle; represents atrial depolarization and the spread of the electrical impulse throughout the right and left atria

Paced interval Period between two consecutive paced events in the same cardiac chamber; also known as the *automatic interval*

Pacemaker A battery-powered device that delivers an electrical current to the heart to stimulate depolarization

Pacemaker cells Specialized cells of the heart's electrical conduction system, capable of spontaneously generating and conducting electrical impulses

Paired beats Two consecutive complexes

Palpitations An unpleasant awareness of one's heartbeat

Paroxysmal atrial tachycardia (PAT) AT that starts or ends suddenly

Paroxysmal supraventricular tachycardia (PSVT) A regular, narrow-QRS tachycardia that starts or ends suddenly; also called *paroxysmal atrial tachycardia (PAT)*

Pericardium A double-walled sac that encloses the heart and helps protect it from trauma and infection

Peripheral resistance Resistance to the flow of blood determined by blood vessel diameter and the tone of the vascular musculature

Permeability Ability of a membrane channel to allow passage of electrolytes once it is open

Polarized state Period after repolarization of a myocardial cell (also called the *resting state*) when the outside of the cell is positive and the interior of the cell is negative

Polymorphic Varying in shape

Preexcitation Term used to describe rhythms that originate from above the ventricles but in which the impulse travels by a pathway other than the AV node and bundle of His; thus the supraventricular impulse excites the ventricles earlier than normal

Preload Force exerted by the blood on the walls of the ventricles at the end of diastole

Premature complex Early beat occurring before the next expected beat; can be atrial, junctional, or ventricular

PR interval P wave plus the PR segment; reflects depolarization of the right and left atria (P wave) and the spread of the impulse through the AV node, AV bundle, right and left bundle branches, and the Purkinje fibers (PR segment)

Prophylaxis Preventive treatment

Proximal Location nearer to the midline of the body or the point of attachment than something else is

Pulmonary circulation Flow of unoxygenated (venous) blood from the right ventricle to the lungs and oxygenated blood from the lungs to the left atrium

Purkinje fibers Fibers found in both ventricles that conduct an electrical impulse through the heart

QRS complex Several waveforms (i.e., the Q wave, the R wave, and the S wave) that represent the spread of an electrical impulse through the ventricles (i.e., ventricular depolarization)

Quadrigeminy Dysrhythmia in which every fourth beat is a premature ectopic beat

R wave On an EGG, the first positive deflection in the QRS complex, representing ventricular depolarization; in pacing, R wave refers to the entire QRS complex, denoting an intrinsic ventricular event

Reciprocal change ECG changes observed in leads opposite the affected area of the heart; also called *mirror image* changes

Reentry Spread of an impulse through tissue already stimulated by that same impulse.

Refractoriness Period of recovery that cells need after being discharged before they are able to respond to a stimulus

Relative refractory period Corresponds with the downslope of the T wave; cardiac cells can be stimulated to depolarize if the stimulus is strong enough.

Repolarization Movement of ions across a cell membrane in which the inside of the cell is restored to its negative charge

Retrograde Moving backward; moving in the opposite direction to that which is considered normal

Run Three or more sequential ectopic beats; also referred to as a *salvo* or *burst*

Salvo Three or more sequential ectopic beats; also referred to as a *run* or *burst*

Sarcolemma Membrane that covers smooth, striated, and cardiac muscle fibers

Sarcomere Smallest functional unit of a myofibril

Sarcoplasm Semifluid cytoplasm of muscle cells

Sarcoplasmic reticulum Network of tubules and sacs that plays an important role in muscle contraction and relaxation by releasing and storing calcium ions

Segment Line between waveforms; named by the waveform that precedes and follows it

Semilunar valves Valves shaped like half-moons that separate the ventricles from the aorta and pulmonary artery

Sensitivity The extent to which an artificial pacemaker recognizes intrinsic cardiac electrical activity

Septum An internal wall of connective tissue

Shock Inadequate tissue perfusion that results from the failure of the cardiovascular system to deliver sufficient oxygen and nutrients to sustain vital organ function

Sinoatrial (SA) node Normal pacemaker of the heart that normally discharges at a rhythmic rate of 60 to 100 beats/min

Sinus arrhythmia Dysrhythmia originating in the SA node that occurs when the SA node discharges irregularly; sinus arrhythmia is a normal phenomenon associated with the phases of breathing and changes in intrathoracic pressure

Sinus bradycardia Dysrhythmia originating in the SA node with a ventricular response of less than 60 beats/min

Sinus rhythm A normal heart rhythm; sometimes called a *regular sinus rhythm (RSR)* or *normal sinus rhythm (NSR)*

Sinus tachycardia Dysrhythmia originating in the SA node with a ventricular response between 101 and 180 beats/min

Stroke volume The amount of blood ejected from a ventricle with each heartbeat

ST segment Portion of the ECG representing the end of ventricular depolarization (end of the R wave) and the beginning of ventricular repolarization (T wave)

Sulcus Groove

Supranormal period Period during the cardiac cycle when a weaker-than-normal stimulus can cause cardiac cells to depolarize; extends from the end of phase 3 to the beginning of phase 4 of the cardiac action potential

Supraventricular Originating from a site above the bifurcation of the bundle of His, such as the SA node, atria, or AV junction

Syncytium Unit of combined cells

Systole Contraction of the heart (usually referring to ventricular contraction) during which blood is propelled into the pulmonary artery and aorta; when the term is used without reference to a specific chamber of the heart, the term implies ventricular systole

T wave Waveform that follows the QRS complex and represents ventricular repolarization

Tone A term that may be used when referring to the normal state of balanced tension in body tissues

Torsades de pointes (TdP) Type of polymorphic VT associated with a prolonged QT interval; the QRS changes in shape, amplitude, and width and appears to "twist" around the isoelectric line, resembling a spindle

TP segment Interval between two successive PQRST complexes during which electrical activity of the heart is absent; begins with the end of the T wave through the onset of the following P wave and represents the period from the end of ventricular repolarization to the onset of atrial depolarization

Trigeminy Dysrhythmia in which every third beat is a premature ectopic beat

Triggered activity A disorder of impulse formation that occurs when escape pacemaker and myocardial working cells fire more than once after stimulation by a single impulse, resulting in atrial or ventricular beats that occur alone, in pairs, in runs, or as a sustained ectopic rhythm

Undersensing A pacemaker malfunction that occurs when the artificial pacemaker fails to recognize spontaneous myocardial depolarization

Unipolar lead Lead that consists of a single positive electrode and a reference point

Vagal maneuver Methods used to stimulate the vagus nerve in an attempt to slow conduction through the AV node, resulting in slowing of the heart rate

Venous return Amount of blood flowing into the right atrium each minute from the systemic circulation

Ventricle Either of the two lower chambers of the heart

Ventricular tachycardia (VT) Dysrhythmia originating in the ventricles with a ventricular response greater than 100 beats/min

Voltage Difference in electrical charge between two points

Wandering atrial pacemaker (multiformed atrial rhythm) Cardiac dysrhythmia that occurs because of impulses originating from various sites, including the SA node, the atria, and/or the AV junction; requires at least three different P waves, seen in the same lead, for proper diagnosis

Waveform Movement away from the baseline in either a positive or negative direction

Wolff-Parkinson-White syndrome Type of preexcitation syndrome, characterized by a slurred upstroke of the QRS complex (delta wave) and wide QRS

Illustration Credits

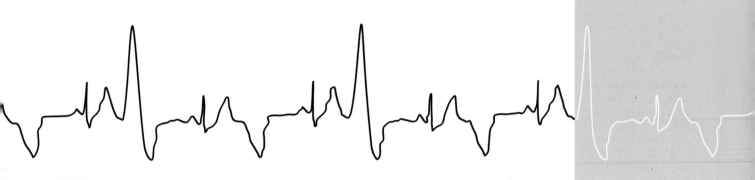

CHAPTER 1

Figures 1-1, 1-3, 1-4, 1-13, 1-14, 1-16, 1-22 Drake R, Vogl AW, Mitchell AWM: *Gray's anatomy for students*, ed 2, New York, 2010, Churchill Livingstone.

Figure 1-2 Courtesy Patricia Kane, Indiana University Medical School.

Figures 1-5 to 1-7, 1-11 Gosling JA: *Human anatomy: color atlas and text*, ed 4, London, 2002, Mosby Ltd.

Figures 1-8, 1-10, 1-12, 1-17, 1-23, 1-25, 1-26 Patton KT, Thibodeau GA: *Anatomy & physiology*, ed 8, St Louis, 2013, Mosby.

Figure 1-9 Patton KT, Thibodeau GA: *Anatomy & physiology*, ed 4, St Louis, 1999, Mosby.

Figures 1-15, 1-19 Keoppen BM, Stanton BA: *Berne & Levy physiology*, ed 6, St Louis, 2008, Mosby.

Figures 1-20, 1-21 Weiderhold R: *Electrocardiography: the monitoring and diagnostic leads*, ed 2, Philadelphia, 1999, Saunders.

Figure 1-24 Herlihy B, Maebius NK: *The human body in health and illness*, ed 3, St Louis, 2007, Mosby.

CHAPTER 2

Figures 2-1, 2-2, 2-10, 2-15, 2-25 Boron WF: *Medical physiology*, ed 2 updated edition, Philadelphia, 2011, Saunders.

Figures 2-3 to 2-5 Herlihy B, Maebius NK: *The human body in health and illness*, ed 3, St Louis, 2007, Mosby.

Figure 2-6 Keoppen BM, Stanton BA: *Berne & Levy physiology*, ed 6, St Louis, 2008, Mosby.

Figures 2-7 to 2-9 Costanzo LS: *Physiology*, ed 4, Philadelphia, 2009, Saunders.

Figures 2-11, 2-16 Hall JE: *Guyton and Hall textbook of medical physiology*, ed 12, Philadelphia, 2010, Saunders.

Figures 2-12, 2-43 Crawford MV, Spence MI: *Commonsense approach to coronary care*, rev ed 6, St Louis, 1994, Mosby.

Figures 2-13, 2-17 to 2-19, 2-23, 2-24 Copstead-Kirkhorn LE, Banasik JL: *Pathophysiology*, ed 4, Philadelphia, 2009, Saunders.

Figure 2-14AB Courtesy Philips Medical Systems, Andover, MA.

Figure 2-20 Drew BJ, Ide B: Right ventricular infarction, *Prog Cardiovascular Nurs* 10:46, 1195.

Figure 2-21 AACN: *AACN procedure manual for critical care*, ed 6, Philadelphia, 2010, St Louis.

Figures 2-22, 2-28 Phalen T, Aehlert BJ: *The 12-lead ECG in acute coronary syndromes*, ed 3, St. Louis, 2012, Mosby.

Figures 2-27, 2-31, 2-33, 2-34, 2-42 Urden LD, Stacy KM, Lough ME: *Critical care nursing: diagnosis and management*, ed 6, St Louis, 2009, Mosby.

Figure 2-29 Irwin S, Tecklin JS: *Cardiopulmonary physical therapy: a guide to practice*, ed 4, St Louis, 2004, Mosby.

Figures 2-35, 2-37 Grauer K: *A practical guide to ECG interpretation*, ed 2, St Louis, 1998, Mosby.

Figure 2-36 Goldberger A: *Clinical electrocardiography: a simplified approach*, ed 6, St Louis, 1999, Mosby.

Figures 2-38 to 2-40 Sanders M: *Mosby's paramedic textbook*, ed 4, Burlington, 2012, Jones & Bartlett Learning.

Figure 2-41 Sole, ML, Goldenberg Klein D, Moseley MJ: *Introduction to critical care nursing*, ed 5, Philadelphia, 2008, Saunders.

Skill 2-1, 2-2, 2-3, 2-4 B-E Aehlert B: *Paramedic practice today*, RR Burlington, 2011, Jones and Bartlett Learning.

CHAPTER 3

Figure 3-1 Boron WF, Boulpaep EL: *Medical physiology*, ed 2 updated ed, Philadelphia, 2011, Saunders.

Figures 3-9 to 3-11, 3-13, 3-17, 3-19, 3-21, 3-23, 3-25 to 3-30 Aehlert B: *ECG study cards*, St. Louis, 2004, Mosby.

CHAPTER 4

Figure 4-1 Crawford: *Common sense approach to coronary care*, ed 6, St. Louis, 1994, Mosby.

Figures 4-4, 4-7 Paul S, Hebra JD: *The nurse's guide to cardiac rhythm interpretation: Implications for patient care*, Philadelphia, 1998, Saunders.

Figures 4-5, 4-11 Kinney MP, Packa DR: *Andreoli's comprehensive cardiac care*, ed 8, St. Louis, 1996, Mosby.

Figure 4-8 Braunwald E, Libby P, Zipes DP, et al: *Heart disease: a textbook of cardiovascular medicine*, ed 6, St. Louis, 2001, Mosby.

Figure 4-9 Conover MB: *Understanding electrocardiography*, ed 7, St. Louis, 1995, Mosby.

Figures 4-10, 4-12, 4-22, 4-30 Goldberger AL: *Clinical electrocardiography: a simplified approach*, St. Louis, 2006, Mosby.

Figure 4-13 Andreoli TE, Benjamin I, Griggs R, et al: *Andreoli and Carpenter's Cecil essentials of medicine*, Philadelphia, 2011, Saunders.

Figures 4-14 to 4-19 Aehlert B: *Paramedic practice today: above and beyond*, Burlington, 2011, Jones and Bartlett Learning.

Figure 4-20 Braunwald E, Goldman L, Menz C: *Primary cardiology*, ed 2, Philadelphia, 2003, Saunders.

Figure 4-23 Chou: *Electrocardiography in clinical practice: adult and pediatric*, Philadelphia, 1994, Saunders.

Figures 4-24, 4-27 Grauer K: *A practical guide to ECG interpretation*, ed 2, St. Louis, 1998, Mosby.

Figure 4-25 Zipes DP, Jalife J: *Cardiac electrophysiology: from cell to bedside*, ed 3, Philadelphia, 2000, Saunders.

Figures 4-29, 4-33, 4-35 to 4-40, 4-42, 4-45, 4-48, 4-49, 4-52, 4-54 to 4-60 Aehlert B: *ECG study cards*, St. Louis, 2004, Mosby.

CHAPTER 5

Figure 5-1 Ignatavicius DD: *Medical-surgical nursing: patient-centered collaborative care*, ed 6, Philadelphia, 2009, Saunders.

Figures 5-3, 5-4 Grauer K: *A practical guide to ECG interpretation*, ed 2, St. Louis, 1998, Mosby.

Figures 5-13, 5-15, 5-16, 5-17, 5-18, 5-19, 5-20, 5-26, 5-27, 5-29, 5-30 Aehlert B: *ECG study cards*, St. Louis, 2004, Mosby.

CHAPTER 6

Figure 6-1 Ignatavicius DD: *Medical-surgical nursing: patient-centered collaborative care*, ed 6, Philadelphia, 2009, Saunders.

Figures 6-2, 6-5 Urden LD: *Critical care nursing: diagnosis and management*, ed 6, St. Louis, 2009, Mosby.

Figures 6-3, 6-22 Grauer K: *A practical guide to ECG interpretation*, ed 2, St. Louis, 1998, Mosby.

Figures 6-4, 6-15 Crawford MV, Spence M: *Common sense approach to coronary care*, ed 6, St. Louis, 1994, Mosby.

Figure 6-7, 6-31 to 6-33, 6-35 to 6-40, 6-42 to 6-44, 6-47, 6-49, 6-50 Aehlert B: *ECG study cards*, St. Louis, 2004, Mosby.

Figure 6-12 Chou: *Electrocardiography in clinical practice: adult and pediatric*, Philadelphia, 1994, Saunders.

Figure 6-19 Goldman L, Ausiello DA, Arend W, et al: *Cecil medicine*, ed 23, Philadelphia, 2007, Saunders.

Figures 6-23 to 6-26 Aehlert B: *Paramedic practice today: above and beyond*, Burlington, 2011, Jones & Bartlett Learning.

CHAPTER 7

Figure 7-1 Ignatavicius DD: *Medical-surgical nursing: patient-centered collaborative care*, ed 6, Philadelphia, 2009, Saunders.

Figures 7-7, 7-10, 7-13, 7-23 to 7-27, 7-33, 7-34, 7-36, 7-38 to 7-42 Aehlert B: *ECG study cards*, St. Louis, 2004, Mosby.

Figure 7-12 Monahan FD, Sands JK, Neighbors M, et al: *Phipps' medical-surgical nursing: health and illness perspectives*, 8 ed, St. Louis, 2006, Mosby.

Figure 7-15 Andreoli, TE, Benjamin I, Griggs R, et al: *Andreoli and Carpenter's Cecil essentials of medicine*, Philadelphia, 2011, Saunders.

Figures 7-16 to 7-19 Urden, LD, Stacey KM, Lough ME: *Critical care nursing: diagnosis and management*, 6 ed, St. Louis, 2009, Mosby.

Figures 7-20 to 7-22 Phalen T, Aehlert BJ: *The 12-lead ECG in acute coronary syndromes*, ed 3, St. Louis, 2012, Mosby.

CHAPTER 8

Figures 8-1, 8-4 to 8-7 Courtesy Medtronic, Inc. Minneapolis, MN.

Figure 8-2 Forbes C, Jackson W: *Color atlas and text of clinical medicine*, St. Louis, 2003, Mosby.

Figures 8-3, 8-8 Urden, LD, Stacey KM, Lough ME: *Critical care nursing: diagnosis and management*, 6 ed, St. Louis, 2009, Mosby.

Figure 8-11, Skill 8-1 Aehlert B: *Paramedic practice today: above and beyond*, Burlington, 2011, Jones & Bartlett Learning.

Figures 8-13, 8-14 Goldberger AL: *Clinical electrocardiography: a simplified approach*, St. Louis, 2006, Mosby.

Figures 8-15, 8-16, 8-19 AACN, Wiegand DL: *AACN procedure manual for critical care*, ed 6, Philadelphia, 2010, Saunders.

Figure 8-20, 8-22, 8-23, 8-25 to 8-27 Aehlert B: *ECG study cards*, St. Louis, 2004, Mosby.

Figure 8-21 Phalen T, Aehlert BJ: *The 12-lead ECG in acute coronary syndromes*, ed 3, St. Louis, 2012, Mosby.

Figures 8-24, 8-28 Sole ML, Klein DG, Moseley MJ: *Introduction to critical care nursing*, ed 5, Philadelphia, 2008, Saunders.

CHAPTER 9

Figure 9-1, 9-8 to 9-14, 9-16, 9-25, 9-27 to 9-38 Phalen T, Aehlert BJ: *The 12-lead ECG in acute coronary syndromes*, ed 3, St. Louis, 2012, Mosby.

Figure 9-2 Chou: *Electrocardiography in clinical practice: adult and pediatric*, Philadelphia, 1994, Saunders.

Figure 9-3 Goldman L, Ausiello DA, Arend W, et al: *Cecil medicine*, ed 23, Philadelphia, 2007, Saunders.

Figure 9-4 Urden, LD, Stacey KM, Lough ME: *Critical care nursing: diagnosis and management*, 6 ed, St. Louis, 2009, Mosby.

Figure 9-5 Butler HA, Caplin M, McCully E, et al: *Managing major diseases: cardiac disorders*, vol 2, St. Louis, 1999, Mosby.

Figure 9-6 Thelan LA: *Critical care nursing: diagnosis and management*, ed 2, St. Louis, 1994, Mosby.

Figure 9-7A Sanders M: *Mosby's paramedic textbook*, ed 4, Burlington, 2001, Jones & Bartlett Learning.

Figure 9-7B, 9-17 Grauer K: *A practical guide to ECG interpretation*, ed 2, St. Louis, 1998, Mosby.

Figure 9-15 Surawicz B, Knilans TK: Chou's electrocardiography in clinical practice: adult and pediatric, ed 5, Philadelphia, 2001, Saunders.

Figure 9-18, 9-24 Andreoli TE, Benjamin I, Griggs RC, et al: *Andreoli and Carpenter's Cecil essentials of medicine*, Philadelphia, 2010, Saunders.

Figure 9-21 Conover MB: *Understanding electrocardiography*, ed 7, St. Louis, 1995, Mosby.

Figure 9-26 Johnson R, Swartz MH: *A simplified approach to electrocardiography*, Philadelphia, 1986, Saunders.

CHAPTER 10

Figures 10-1, 10-2, 10-3, 10-4, 10-5, 10-6, 10-13, 10-14, 10-27, 10-28, 10-30, 10-31, 10-34, 10-36, 10-37, 10-41, 10-43, 10-44, 10-48, 10-49, 10-54, 10-57, 10-61 Aehlert B: *ECG study cards*, St. Louis, 2004, Mosby.

Figure 10-42 Sole ML, Klein DG, Moseley MJ: *Introduction to critical care nursing*, ed 5, Philadelphia, 2008, Saunders.

Figure 10-45 Modified from Sole ML, Klein DG, Moseley MJ: *Introduction to critical care nursing*, ed 5, Philadelphia, 2008, Saunders.

Index

345